DRUG TOXICITY

DRUG TOXICITY

Edited by

J.W. GORROD

Chelsea College
University of London

TAYLOR & FRANCIS LTD
10-14 Macklin Street, London WC2B 5NF
1979

First published 1979 by Taylor & Francis Ltd,
10-14 Macklin Street, London WC2B 5NF.

©1979 Taylor & Francis Ltd

Typeset by Red Lion Setters, Holborn, London
Printed and bound in Great Britain by
Taylor & Francis (Printers) Ltd.
Rankine Road, Basingstoke, Hampshire RG24 0PR

British Library Cataloging in Publication Data

Aspects of Drug Toxicity (*Conference*), *London, 1978*
    Drug Toxicity.
    1. Drugs — Toxicology — Congresses
    I. Title   II. Gorrod, John W
    615.9   RA1238

ISBN 0-85066-179-X

Contents

Preface

The material contained in this volume was originally presented at the Pharmaceutical Society's Easter School in April 1978 on Aspects of Drug Toxicity. The lecturers at this school were all experts in their topics, which were chosen to present as wide a view as possible of the contemporary situation of drug toxicity. In a volume of this size, it is not possible to cover every aspect of the subject, but it is hoped that the data presented will enable practising pharmacists and others to assess the likelihood of an adverse reaction having occurred, to propose mechanisms for its initiation, and to suggest means for preventing toxic reactions.

This volume is a sister volume to *Drug Metabolism in Man* and basic data presented in the earlier book have generally been omitted from this one. The first chapter deals with metabolic processes which are available, and for which evidence exists as toxication reactions (Gorrod). This is followed by chapters indicating how these reactions can be modified due to physiological or pharmacological factors. Amongst the topics considered are age (Jondorf), diet (Greaves & McClean), genetics (Boobis). Then follows a chapter on the influence of drug formulation or drug toxicity (Groves). Parke then considers the toxicological consequences produced via enzyme induction or inhibition and Connors deals with the possibility of neoplasia being produced during drug therapy.

Other authors then deal with the effect of drugs and foreign compounds on specific organs or systems. The organs covered are the liver (Slater), the lung (Orme), blood and blood-forming systems (Girdwood), the nervous system (Marsden & Jenner), the foetus (Beck), the optical system (Bron) and the skin (Felix).

Levene presents data which show how chemicals toxic to connective tissue have the potential to be developed into useful drugs. The last chapter deals with untoward effects which may be found during treatment with radiopharmaceuticals (Keeling).

As we live in a world where we are increasingly exposed to small amounts of chemicals in our environment and in our food and drink, the implications of much of this material go far beyond drugs. During the last decade, increasing demands have been made on manufacturers to provide materials which are 'safe'. It is hoped that this volume will help newcomers to the field of toxicology, in that it provides a broad-based basic text, that nevertheless points to the direction in which toxicology is now rapidly moving.

It is a pleasure to record the encouragement I have received from Professor A. H. Beckett, Head of the School of Pharmacy, Chelsea College, the representatives of the Pharmaceutical Society and the contributors.

It was again a pleasure working with Dr. J. Cheney of Taylor & Francis whose expertise made my lot that much easier.

The contributors to this volume

F. Beck, Department of Anatomy, School of Medicine, University of Leicester

A. R. Boobis, Department of Clinical Pharmacology, Royal Postgraduate Medical School, London

A. J. Bron, Department of Ophthalmology, University of Oxford

T. A. Connors, Medical Research Council Toxicology Unit, Carshalton, Surrey

R.H. Felix, Frimley Park Hospital, Camberley, Surrey

R. H. Girdwood, Department of Therapeutics, School of Medicine, University of Edinburgh

J. W. Gorrod, Department of Pharmacy, Chelsea College, London

M. Angeli-Greaves, University College Hospital Medical School, London

M. Groves, Department of Pharmacy, Chelsea College, London

P. Jenner, Institute of Psychiatry, University of London

W. R. Jondorf, Racecourse Security Services Laboratories, Newmarket, Suffolk

D. H. Keeling, Plymouth General Hospital, Plymouth, Devon

C. I. Levene, Department of Pathology, University of Cambridge

C. D. Marsden, School of Medicine, King's College, University of London

A. E. M. McLean, University College Hospital Medical School, London

M. Orme, Department of Pharmacology and Therapeutics, University of Liverpool

D. V. Parke, Department of Biochemistry, University of Surrey, Guildford, Surrey

T. F. Slater, Department of Biochemistry, Brunel University, Uxbridge, Middlesex

This volume is dedicated to

E. Boyland, D.Sc.
Professor Emeritus of the University of London

whose recognition of epoxides as active metabolites
paved the way for recent developments
in molecular toxicology

1. Toxic products produced during metabolism of drugs and foreign compounds

J. W. Gorrod

Introduction

In order for a compound to produce a deleterious effect upon a biological system, a reaction between the compound, or a substance derived from it, and a component of the biological system must occur. These reactions may be proximate, i.e. acting at a site directly involved in the advent of the toxic response or they may occur by reacting with a component involved in a sequence of biochemical processes, the disturbance of which precipitates the toxic crisis (Table 1.1). Even within these groups, the nature of the chemical

Table 1.1. Examples of toxicants acting via a direct or indirect reaction within cell.

Toxicant	Reaction	Consequences
Direct reaction		
Cyanide	Complexes with Cytochrome	Block Oxidative Phosphorylation & Respiration
Phenylhydroxylamine	Oxidizes Haemoglobin	Prevents Oxygen Transport
Fluorocitrate	Inhibits Aconitase	Blocks T.C.A Cycle
6-Aminonicotinamide	Forms analogues of coenzymes	Blocks Pentose Pathway
Indirect reaction		
Silica	Absorbed into lyosomes	Releases hydrolytic enzymes
Free Radicals	React with lipids	Initiate lipid peroxidation
Mercurials	React with thiols	Removes protection and upsets cell oxidn/redn. potential

reaction is often poorly defined and whilst in many cases evidence has been obtained for the formation of covalent bonds between toxicants and cellular constituents, this is by no means a prerequisite for a toxic response. In other cases, reaction via an ionic band or a charge-transfer complex may play a role in initiating an adverse response to a drug. Thus the ability of a compound to react with an enzyme or a membrane or a discrete molecule may arise by several mechanisms.

The nature of the bond formed is important in determining the duration of the compounds within the body; in certain cases the bond may be easily destroyed, as in the dissociation of certain inhibitors from enzymes or by hydrolysis, as in the breakdown of Schiff bases. The alternative situation may occur where the covalent bond formed between a toxicant and a macromolecule is extremely stable and only excision of the affected portion of molecule allows the release of the toxicant.

While the majority of compounds which are able to produce toxic effects require metabolism in order to produce a more reactive molecule, this is not always the case, and many molecules which are used in human therapy possess an inherent reactivity which allows reaction with cellular components. Examples of this type include various alkylating agents, including those based on strained rings, cyclic lactones and lactams. Some structures of this type of reactive compound are shown in Figure 1.1. This reactivity may enable drugs to produce antigenic material by reaction with protein and thereby produce an unwanted immunological response (Erlanger, 1973).

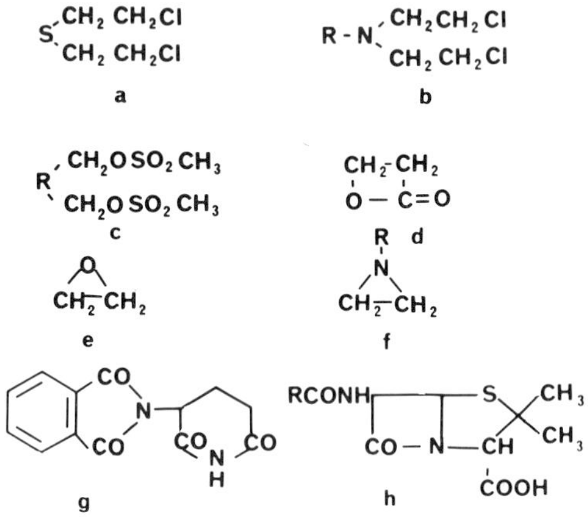

Fig. 1.1.   Examples of chemically reactive drugs (*a*) sulphur mustards, (*b*) nitrogen mustards, (*c*) methylsulphonyl esters, (*d*) propiolactone, (*e*) ethylene oxide, (*f*) ethyleneimines, (*g*) thalidomide, (*h*) penicillanic acid.

Most of the toxic compounds to which we are exposed consist of carbon in combination with a hetero atom, usually oxygen, nitrogen or sulphur, and during metabolism either the carbon, nitrogen or sulphur is attacked. It is worth considering toxic metabolites produced by these processes separately.

Toxic metabolites produced via metabolic attack on carbon

Due to the potent carcinogenic properties of a number of polycyclic aromatic hydrocarbons, this group of compounds have been extensively studied over nearly half a century, Kennaway (1930) having isolated and characterized the first pure carcinogens as aromatic hydrocarbons. It was early recognized the dihydrodiols were formed as metabolites of aromatic hydrocarbons (Boyland & Levi, 1935; Young, 1947; Boyland & Wolf,

1950), a fact that led Boyland (1950) to suggest that aryl epoxides were intermediates in the metabolism of hydrocarbons. It was not until the successful synthesis of this type of compound had been accomplished by Newman & Blum (1964) that aryl epoxides were shown to exist; this ultimately led to the direct detection of naphthalene-1,2-epoxide as a metabolite of naphthalene by Jerina *et al.* (1968).

Aryl epoxides, as predicted by Boyland, are compounds capable of several reactions; these are exemplified in Figure 1.2. Aryl epoxides can isomerize to give phenols, the phenol formed depending upon the electron density of the carbon atoms involved, they can react with water, as substrates for the enzyme epoxide hydrase, or they can react with nucleophiles.

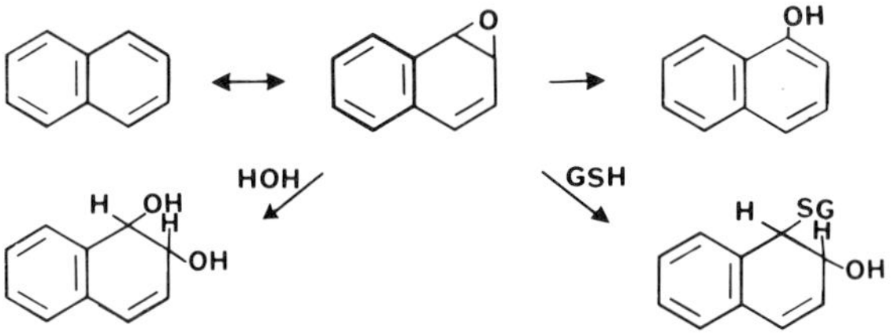

Fig. 1.2.   Metabolism of naphthalene.

Figure 1.2 shows reaction with glutathione, and this type of reaction is thought to occur when epoxides react with cellular macromolecules of protein, DNA or RNA. *In vivo* glutathione conjugates are ultimately excreted as mercapturic acids. Aryl epoxides can also be reduced to the parent hydrocarbon. The role of epoxides in aromatic hydrocarbon metabolism and carcinogenesis has been reviewed by Sims & Grover (1974).

The role of epoxides in hydrocarbon metabolism becomes even more complicated when one considers the number of possible sites available for epoxidation in the larger molecules which are of major toxicological interest. An example of this complexity is indicated in Figure 1.3, which shows the three primary sites of oxidation of benzanthracene. These epoxides, viz. 5:6, 8:9 and 10:11, all react with water to form dihydrodiols as well as form analogous products as described for naphthalene earlier. There have been many attempts to correlate the site of oxidation within the hydrocarbon with the initiation of carcinogenesis, the most widely accepted being the K region hypothesis (Pullman & Pullman, 1955). However there were always anomalies and it was a major breakthrough when Swaizland *et al.* (1974) established that further epoxidation of 8,9-dihydro-8,9-dihydroxybenzanthracene was involved in the reaction of the parent hydrocarbon with nucleic acids (Figure 1.3). A similar reaction was observed with benzpyrene (Sims *et al.*, 1974). These diol-epoxides which are produced are also substrates for epoxide hydrase, being converted to tetrahydrotetrols (Figure 1.3). Many diol-epoxides are now known to be intermediates in the reaction of hydrocarbons with nucleic acids. From Figure 1.3 it can be seen that several diol-epoxides could be formed from each hydrocarbon, and while this may be the case, it appears that epoxidation of a double bond in a

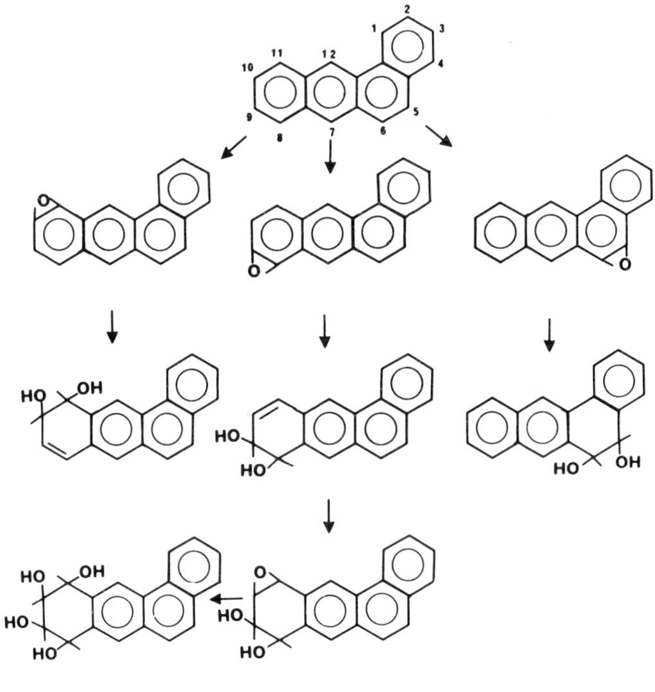

Fig. 1.3.   Metabolism of benzanthracene.

diol-containing ring which is adjacent to a 'bay' in the molecule (indicated ⤸ in Figure 1.4) produces the most reactive metabolite.

From a consideration of the data on the carcinogenicity of substituted hydrocarbons and quantum mechanical calculations, a theory has been developed predicting that bay region epoxides derived from non-K-region dihydrodiols would have the highest biological activity (Jerina & Daly, 1977; Jerina et al., 1977). Further examples of diol-epoxides derived from carcinogenic hydrocarbons are shown in Figure 1.4.

Epoxidation as a toxication process is not restricted to aromatic hydrocarbons and it has been suggested that they are formed during the metabolism of safrole (Figure 1.5A). In the case of this weak carcinogen, it is not certain whether hydroxylation of the methylene carbon is also required to produce the proximate carcinogen (Stilwell et al., 1974). Aflatoxin B_1, which is a potent naturally occurring carcinogen, is also thought to be activated via epoxidation of the distal furan ring (Figure 1.5B) (Swenson, Miller & Miller, 1974). Epoxidation may also be involved in the toxic effects produced by vinyl chloride.

From the foregoing it might be presumed that epoxidation was always associated with enhanced toxicity. However, studies using epoxides known to be formed as metabolites of carbamazepine, cyproheptadine and cyclobenzaprine (Figure 1.6) showed that they were fully devoid of mutagenic activity when tested in systems capable of detecting either frameshift or

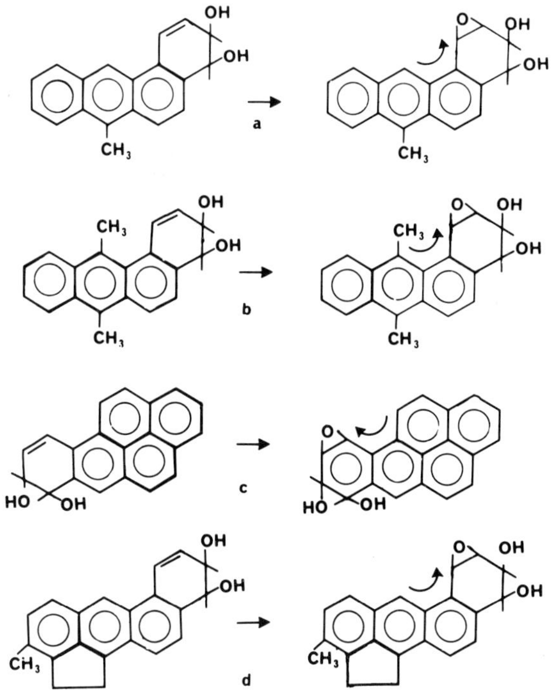

Fig. 1.4   Conversion of (*a*) 7-methylbenzanthracene, (*b*) 7, 12 dimethylbenzanthracene, (*c*) benzpyrene, (*d*) methylcholanthrene, to 'bay region' epoxides.

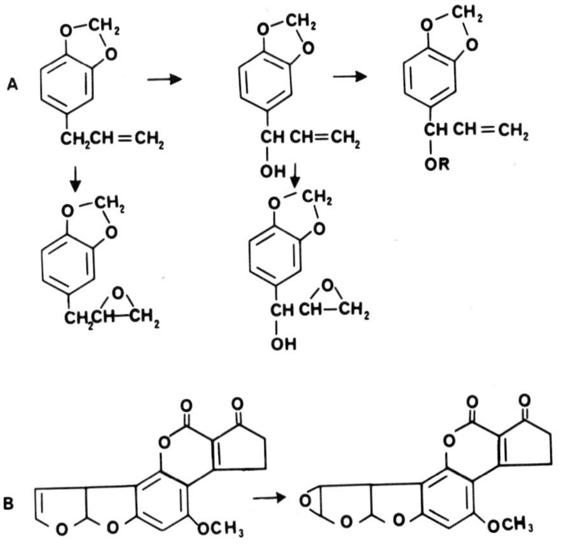

Fig. 1.5   Metabolism of (A) safrole and (B) of aflatoxin to form epoxides.

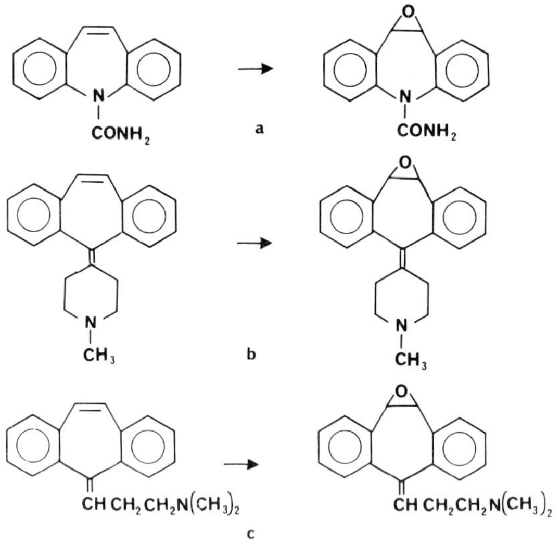

Fig. 1.6.   Epoxidation of drugs containing an aliphatic double band.

base substitution mutagens (Glatt *et al.*, 1975). Indeed, studies on the metabolism of the hepatotoxic agent bromobenzene (Figure 1.7) (Jollow & Smith, 1977) suggest that whereas pretreatment of experimental animals with phenobarbitone produces more bromobenzene-3,4-epoxide, leading to enhanced toxicity, pretreatment with methylcholanthrene leads to more 2,3-epoxide, leading to diminished toxicity as the toxic 3,4-epoxide is formed in

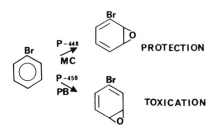

Fig. 1.7.   Possible metabolic conversion of bromobenzene to two different epoxides.

lower amounts. Clearly epoxidation can be a reaction which is involved in producing a toxic effect. However, the variety of further reactions which epoxides can undergo (Figure 1.2) and the rate at which these reactions proceed, will determine the role of epoxides in the metabolism and toxicity of any molecule. As the site of epoxidation and the properties of the epoxide formed are dependent upon the electron distribution within the molecule and the activity of the various P-450-type cytochromes and the environment within which they are formed, it may be that in many cases the potential toxic effect is never realized or only manifests itself under certain conditions.

The administration of high doses of 7,12-dimethylbenzanthracene to rats leads to the production of adrenal necrosis (Huggins & Morri, 1961). Studies on the metabolism of this compound showed that both methyl groups could be separately oxidized to hydroxymethyl compounds (Figure 1.8) and that the toxic response seemed to be mediated via the 7-hydroxymethyl derivative (Wheatley *et al.*, 1966). Allison & Dingle (1966) showed that 7-hydroxymethylbenzanthracene had a powerful lytic effect on a rat adrenal lysosomal preparation, the 12-hydroxymethyl compound being far less active.

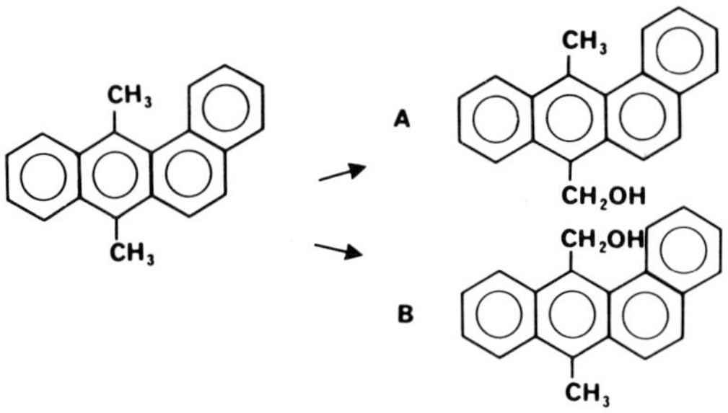

Fig. 1.8.   Conversion of 7, 12 dimethylbenzanthracene to isomeric hydroxymethyl derivatives.

Hydroxymethyl compounds are usually intermediates in the conversion of methyl groups to carboxylic acids and therefore may only be present at low concentrations in most situations. It is worth remembering that many drugs are administered explicitly to elicit a toxic reaction in an invading organism, ideally without harming the host. In this respect it is of interest that the active metabolite of the antischistosomicidal drugs Miracil D (Rosi *et al.*, 1967), Miradan (Rosi *et al.*, 1966) and the trichomonacidal drug, Metronidazole (Stambough, Feo & Manthei, 1967) are all hydroxymethyl metabolites (Figure 1.9).

Some years ago it was reported that direct hydroxymethylation of aniline (Sloane, 1964) and benzene (Sloane, 1965) could occur and that these compounds were intermediates in the production of the corresponding phenols (Figure 1.10). Flescher and Sydnor (1973) more recently showed that 6-hydroxymethylbenzpyrene was formed during the metabolism of benzpyrene by rat liver homogenates and suggested that as this compound is a potent carcinogen, this route of metabolism may play some role in carcinogenisis by aromatic hydrocarbons. From the foregoing it appears that hydroxymethyl compounds may be toxic metabolites, and in this respect they may be similar to the simpler compounds methanol and ethanol which are not without toxic properties!

Compounds with alkyl groups attached to hetero atoms are often dealkylated (McMahon, 1966), this metabolic reaction proceeding via an α-carbinolamine which usually spontaneously breaks down to produce an aldehyde and the parent compound. In certain cases, where the presence of an adjacent electron-withdrawing group delocalizes the electrons, the intermediate carbinolamines are stable enough to be isolated (Gorrod & Temple,

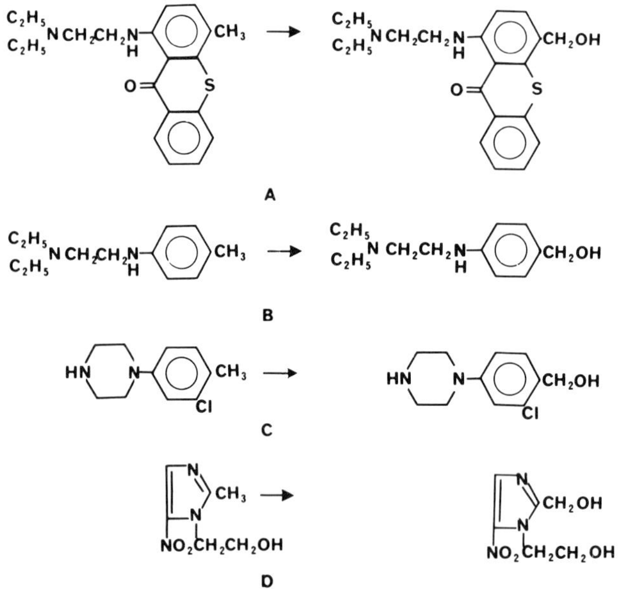

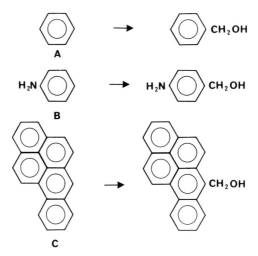

Fig. 1.9. Conversion of (A) Miracil D, (B) Mirasan, (C) *N*-(3-chloro-4 methylphenyl)-piperazine, (D) Metronidazole, to the corresponding hydroxymethyl derivatives.

1976). *N*-Methyl groups are converted into an *N*-hydroxymethyl function which may be involved as the active toxicant. Thus the choline esterase inhibitor octamethylpyrophosphoramide (Schradan) is thought to act via the *N*-hydroxymethyl compound (Figure 1.11A) (Spencer, O'Brian & White, 1957); as is the cytotoxic anticancer drug hexamethylmelamine

Fig. 1.10. Metabolic hydroxymethylation of (A) benzene, (B) aniline, (C) benzpyrene.

(Figure 1.11B) (Rutty & Connors, 1977). Roberts & Warwick (1964) had previously shown that incubation of 4-aminoazobenzene, in the presence of formaldehyde, with liver homogenates, produced a greater binding of the azo dye to cellular proteins than when formaldehyde was omitted from the system. It was suggested that this was due to the formation of an *N*-hydroxymethyl compound (Figure 1.11C).

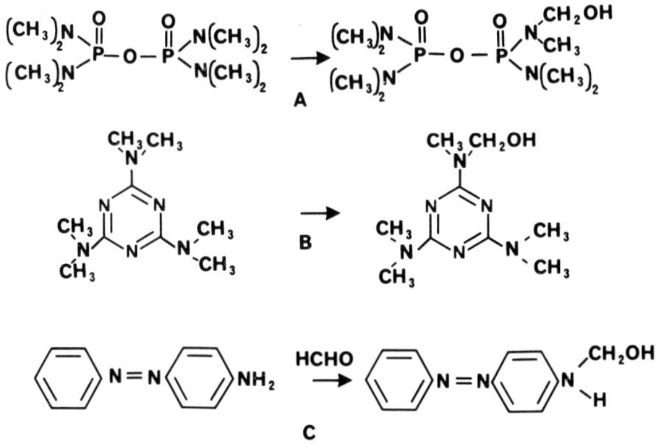

Fig. 1.11. Active hydroxymethyl compound formed from (A) Hexamethylmelamine, (B) Schradan and (C) 4-Aminoazobenzene.

A new type of reactive intermediate was implicated during studies on the metabolism of the tobacco alkaloid nicotine. This compound was early shown to be converted to cotinine *in vivo* (McKennis, Turnbull & Bowman, 1958) and *in vitro* (Hucker, Gillette & Brodie, 1960). The intermediates in this reaction have not been isolated but probably involve 5′-hydroxynicotine in equilibrium with nicotine-$\Delta^{1'(5')}$-iminium ion (Murphy, 1973) (Figure 1.12, route a). This iminium ion (Figure 1.12d) has been synthesized by Brandänge & Lindblom (1978) and shown to be converted to cotinine

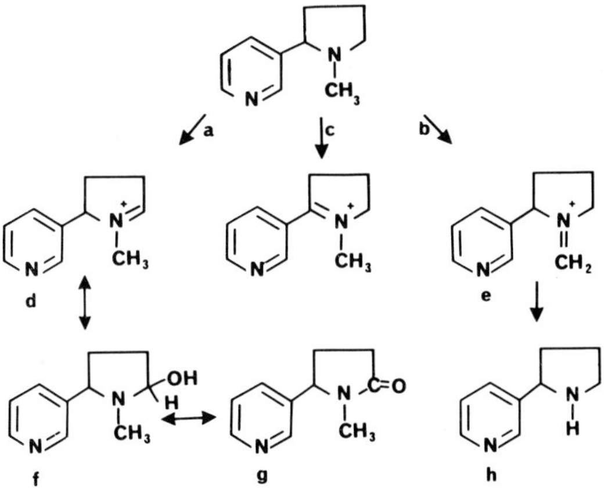

Fig. 1.12. Conversion of nicotine to isomeric iminium compounds.

both *in vitro* and *in vivo* (Hibberd & Gorrod, 1978). The isomeric nicotine $\Delta^{1'(2')}$-iminium ion has been implicated during the mercuric acetate dehydrogenation of nicotine (Figure 1.12, route c) by Sanders, De Bardeleben & Osdene (1975), but as yet no biological role has been assigned to it. Nicotine-Δ-$^{1'}$-methyliminium ion (Figure 1.12e) has been suggested as an intermediate in the metabolism of nicotine to nornicotine (Nguyen, Gruenke & Castagnoli, 1976).

All of these iminium ions are very reactive compounds and form stable nitriles in the presence of cyanide, and this has led Gorrod & Jenner (1975) to suggest that they may react with nucleophilic centres occurring in biological systems. In support of this concept, Gorrod & Hibberd (1978) have obtained evidence for an adduct produced by reaction of nicotine-$\Delta^{1'5'}$-iminium ion with glutathione.

The suggestion that an iminium ion is involved in the formation of the pyrrolidine compound cotinine implies that analogous intermediates may be formed en route to other pyrrolidones. Examples of pyrrolidone formation occur during the metabolism of Tremorine (Figure 1.13A) (Cho, Haslett & Jenden, 1961) and Prolintane (Figure 1.13B) (Hucker, Staufer & Rhodes, 1972; Yoshihara & Yoshimura, 1972). In the case of Tremorine, both

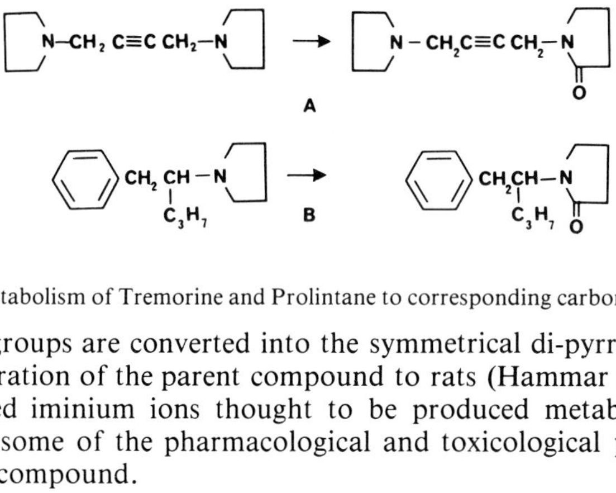

Fig. 1.13.   Metabolism of Tremorine and Prolintane to corresponding carbonyl compounds.

pyrrolidine groups are converted into the symmetrical di-pyrrolidone after the administration of the parent compound to rats (Hammar *et al.*, 1969). The proposed iminium ions thought to be produced metabolically may account for some of the pharmacological and toxicological properties of this type of compound.

Toxic products produced via metabolic attack on constituent nitrogen

Early observations by Heubner (1913) and Lipschitz and Weber (1923) that phenylhydroxylamine could oxidize haemoglobin to ferrihaemoglobin led to the suggestion that this may be the toxic metabolite produced from aniline. However, it was not until Kiese (1959a) detected nitrosobenzene and phenylhydroxylamine in the blood of dogs receiving aniline that biological *N*-oxidation of aromatic amines was established. Kiese (1959b) also showed that perfusion of dogs with phenylhydroxylamine to produce the same plasma levels as found after a dose of aniline, produced about the same level of ferrihaemoglobin.

Since then, numerous aromatic amines have been shown to be metabolized to the corresponding hydroxylamine, and these hydroxylamines are probably the major route to ferrihaemoglobic formation (Kiese, 1974). Recent results from our laboratory are shown in Figure 1.14 where it can be

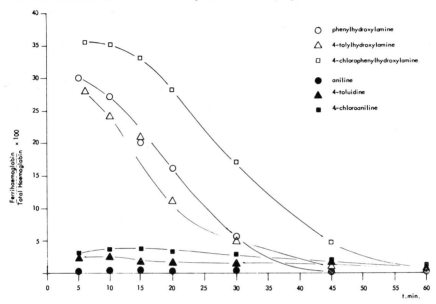

Fig. 1.14. Formation of ferrihaemoglobin from aromatic amines and the corresponding aryl hydroxylamines. Rabbits were injected intravenously with 0.025 mmol/kg of the base or the hydroxylamine.

seen that when equimolar doses of aromatic amines and hydroxylamines are given to rabbits the hydroxylamines produce far greater amounts of ferrihaemoglobin than the corresponding amine. During the oxidation of haemoglobin by arylhydroxylamines, the corresponding nitroso compound is formed (Figure 1.15). As the cell has a mechanism to convert the nitroso compound back to the hydroxylamine, a cyclic system is produced (Figure 1.15), which is able to generate about forty molecules of ferrihaemoglobin from each molecule of phenylhydroxylamine. Thus the toxicity of aromatic amines will depend not only upon the extent that they are N-hydroxylated but also upon the rate of regeneration of the hydroxylamine from the nitroso derivative. This will depend upon the nutritional status and co-enzyme levels within the cell (Wagner, 1968; Burger *et al.*, 1967). A further comparison of aromatic amines and their N-hydroxylated derivatives is shown in Table 1.2. A similar activating effect on ferrihaemoglobin formation by N-hydroxylation has been observed with alkylcarbamates (Nery, 1971). Smith *et al.* (1978) showed that N-hydroxyaliphatic amines, tertiary aromatic amine-N-oxides and heterocyclic aromatic N-oxides were without effect on ferrihaemoglobin levels when they were administered to rabbits.

When ferrihaemoglobin is further oxidized, it leads to production of precipitated haemoglobin which becomes attached to the red cell

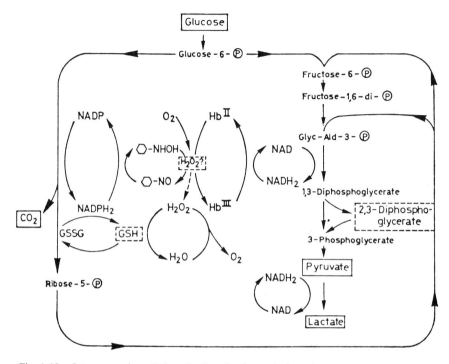

Fig. 1.15. Interconversion of phenylhydroxylamine and nitrosobenzene during ferrihaemo-globin formation, and relationship to glucose metabolism. (From Burger, A., Wagner, J., Uehleke, H., & Gotz, E. (1967), *Arch. Pharmak. exp. Path.*, 256, 333.)

membrane, causing gross deformities (Figure 1.16) (Allen & Jandl, 1961). These deformed cells are rapidly removed by the reticulo-endothelial system. Arylhydroxylamines can also produce Heinz bodies, as was shown in a study utilizing several possible metabolites of Dapsone (Figure 1.17) where only those metabolites which were *N*-hydroxylated had any effect on haemoglobin.

Table 1.2. Comparison of ferrihaemoglobin formation by aromatic amines and hydroxylamines in the rabbit.

Compound	Maximal $HbFe^{3+}\%$ of Total Hb after amine	Time (min)	Maximal $HbFe^{3+}\%$ of Total Hb after hydroxylamine	Time (min)
Aniline	<1.0	–	30	5
4-Fluoroaniline	<1.0	–	22	10
4-Chloroaniline	3.0	10	35	10
4-Bromoaniline	6.0	10	36	10
4-Iodoaniline	12.0	10	30	10
4-Toluidine	2.5	10	30	10
4-Ethylaniline	4.0	10	24	10
4-Aminoacetophenone	<1.0	–	27	10
4-Nitroaniline	8.0	15	53	10
4-Aminobiphenyl	15.0	5	44	10

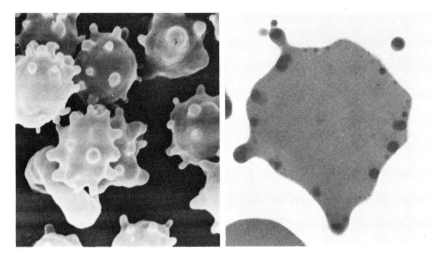

Fig. 1.16.   Electron micrographs of erythrocytes containing Heinz bodies. (*a*) Transmission micrograph (Philips 301G Microscope, x 13500; (*b*) Scanning micrograph (Jeol 50A Microscope) x 11250. (From Le Blond, C.B. (1977), *Proc. R. Micr. Soc.*, 12, 220.)

The metabolism of several aromatic amines has been extensively studied owing to their carcinogenic activity in man and experimental animals (Boyland, 1963; Gorrod, 1964; Miller & Miller, 1969; Miller, 1970; Weisburger & Weisburger, 1973; Kriek, 1974). In addition certain acetylated amines were also shown to be carcinogenic, notably 2-acetylaminofluorene, which produces tumours at several sites (Wilson, De Eds & Cox, 1941)

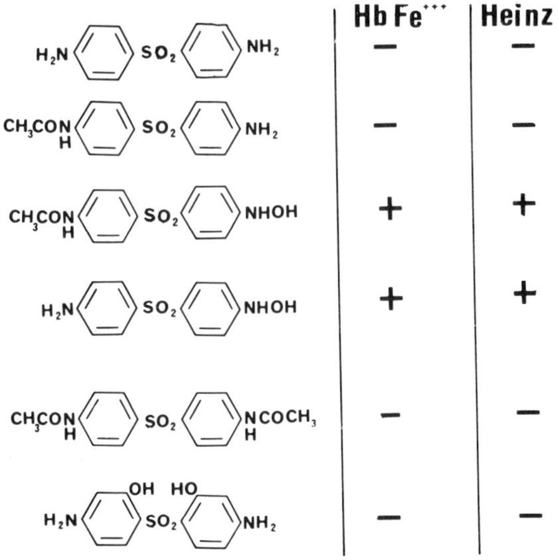

Structure	Hb Fe$^{\cdots}$	Heinz
H_2N—⬡—SO_2—⬡—NH_2	—	—
$CH_3CON(H)$—⬡—SO_2—⬡—NH_2	—	—
$CH_3CON(H)$—⬡—SO_2—⬡—$NHOH$	+	+
H_2N—⬡—SO_2—⬡—$NHOH$	+	+
$CH_3CON(H)$—⬡—SO_2—⬡—$NCOCH_3(H)$	—	—
H_2N—⬡(OH)—SO_2—(HO)⬡—NH_2	—	—

Fig. 1.17.   Toxic derivatives of dapsone produced via *N*-hydroxylation, and ferrihaemoglobin and Heinz body formation.

and 2-acetylaminophenanthrene which produces leukaemia in mice (Miller *et al.*, 1955). It was from a study of 2-acetylaminofluorene metabolism that Cramer, Miller & Miller detected a new metabolite which was characterized as the *N*-hydroxy derivative (hydroxamic acid). Subsequently *N*-hydroxy derivatives have been detected as metabolites of other carcinogenic amides (Figure 1.18) and have been shown to be more active than the parent

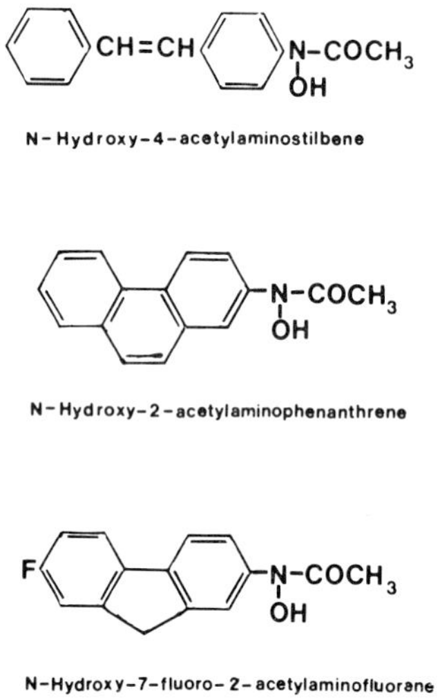

N-Hydroxy-4-acetylaminostilbene

N-Hydroxy-2-acetylaminophenanthrene

N-Hydroxy-7-fluoro-2-acetylaminofluorane

Fig. 1.18. *N*-Hydroxyamides detected as metabolites of carcinogenic amides.

amides. Not all species are susceptible to the carcinogenic action of 2-acetyl-aminofluorene and further evidence for the carcinogenic role of the hydroxamic acids came when it was shown that resistant species failed to *N*-hydroxylate this amide to any significant extent (Table 1.3).

Parallel studies *in vivo* showed that whereas hydroxamic acids were reactive with nucleophiles, this activity could be greatly enhanced by

Table 1.3. Conversion of 2-acetylaminofluorene to the *N*-hydroxy derivative by various species. (From Weisburger & Weisburger, 1973.)

Species	Carcinogenic effect of 2AAF	% dose excreted as *N*-hydroxy derivative
Rabbit	+	13-20
Rat	+	0.3-15
Dog	+	5.2
Hamster	+	5.0
Mouse	+	1.8-2.3
Cat	+	1.5
Steppe-lemming	−	trace
Guinea-pig	−	0
Rainbow trout	−	0

esterification of the hydroxyl group. Model experiments used the relatively stable *O*-acetyl derivative which was shown to react with tryptophan, cysteine, tyrosine and methionine (Miller & Miller, 1969). Figure 1.19 shows the reaction with methionine and indicates that binding to cellular proteins

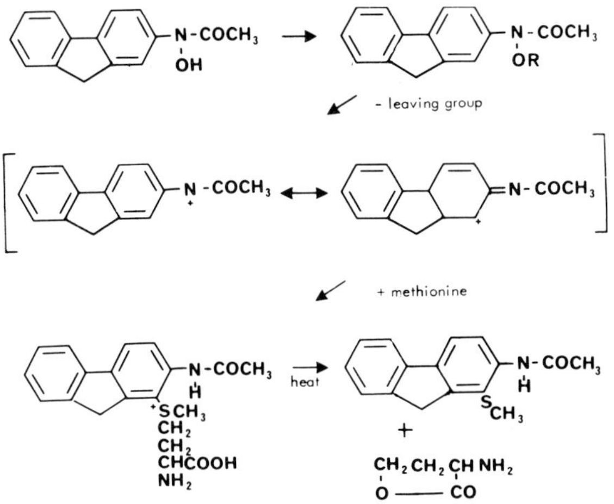

Fig. 1.19.   Reaction of *N*-hydroxyacetylaminofluorene with methionine.

may involve the formation of an onium linkage which is able to break down releasing the 3-methylmercapto derivative. There is no evidence for the formation of the *O*-acetyl derivative *in vivo*, but extensive studies by Lotlikar (1968), Lotlikar & Luha (1971), and by Irving (1970, 1973) have shown that under certain conditions a variety of groups can esterify hydroxamic acids and lead to their greater reactivity (Figure 1.20). Experiments in which acetanilide plus or minus sodium sulphate were incorporated into the diet of rats fed either 2-acetylaminofluorene or the *N*-hydroxy derivative

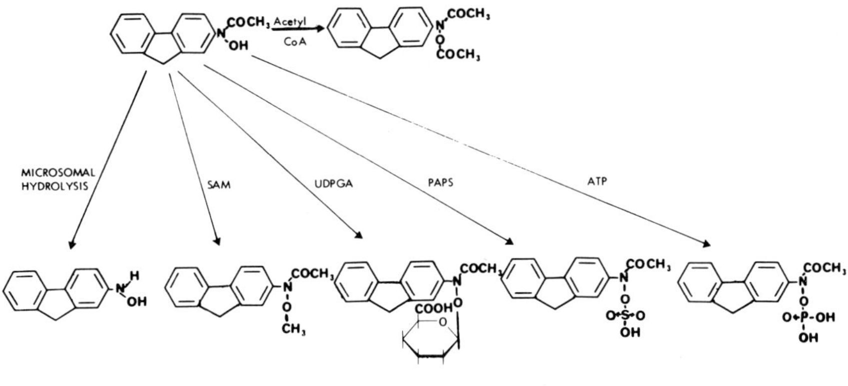

Fig. 1.20.   Possible routes to the formation of reactive esters of hydroxamic acids.

(Table 1.4) indicated that tumour yield varied depending upon the additives. This was interpreted as acetanilide inhibiting the N-hydroxylation of the parent amide and depleting sulphate (by conjugating with p-hydroxyacetanilide formed as a metabolite) in the case of the N-hydroxy compound. The sulphate ions, which restored carcinogenic activity, were

Table 1.4.   Influence of added acetanilide and sulphate on the induction of tumours by 2-acetylaminofluorene and its N-hydroxy derivative. (From Weisburger & Weisburger, 1973.)

Diet		% Animals with liver neoplasms
2-Acetylaminofluorene	0.03%	100
2-Acetylaminofluorene plus acetanilide	0.03% 0.8%	10
2-Acetylaminofluorene plus acetanilide plus sodium sulphate	0.03% 0.8% 0.84%	0
N-Hydroxy-2-acetylaminofluorene	0.032%	100
N-Hydroxy-2-acetylaminofluorene plus acetanilide	0.032% 0.8%	10
N-Hydroxy-2-acetylaminofluorene plus acetanilide plus sodium sulphate	0.032% 0.8% 0.84%	60

thought to act by forming the reactive ester (Weisburger & Weisburger, 1973). More recent experiments (Weisburger et al., 1973; Yamamoto et al., 1973) in which the effects of p-hydroxyacetanilide on amide carcinogenesis were investigated have failed to fully substantiate this concept and the authors suggest that other esters play some role in initiating the carcinogenic process. N-Hydroxylation is also the activation step in the metabolism of methylaminazobenzene (Kadlubar, Miller & Miller, 1976).

Another group of compounds which can be chemically N-oxidized to produce potent oncogens are the purines (Brown, 1968). The structures of some of these compounds are shown in Figure 1.21.

Stöhrer & Brown (1970) isolated 8-chloroxanthine (Figure 1.22,4) and 8-methylmercaptoxanthine (Figure 1.22,5) from the urine of rats receiving 3-hydroxyxanthine (Figure 1.22,1) and suggested that a reactive ester was formed, as the acetoxy derivative (2a) produced the same products *in vitro*. By analogy with the hydroxamic acids, discussed earlier, it might be thought that the sulphate ester would be a likely candidate as the proximate carcinogen. However, studies of sulphotransferase activity using a number of N-oxidized purines as substrates showed no correlation between sulphate conjugation and tumour-producing ability (Table 1.5) (McDonald, Stöhrer & Brown 1973).

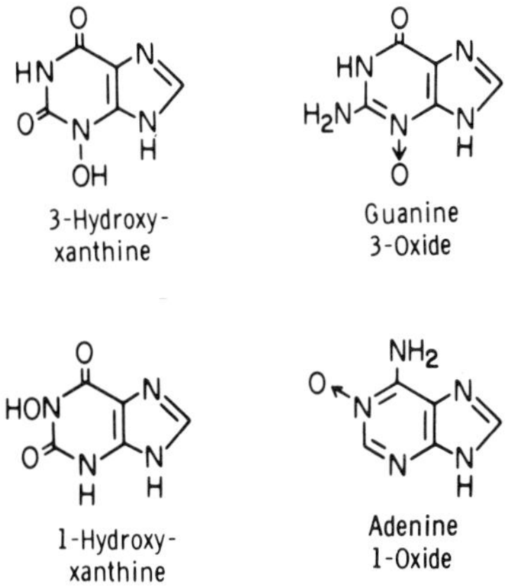

Fig. 1.21. Structures of carcinogenic *N*-hydroxypurines.

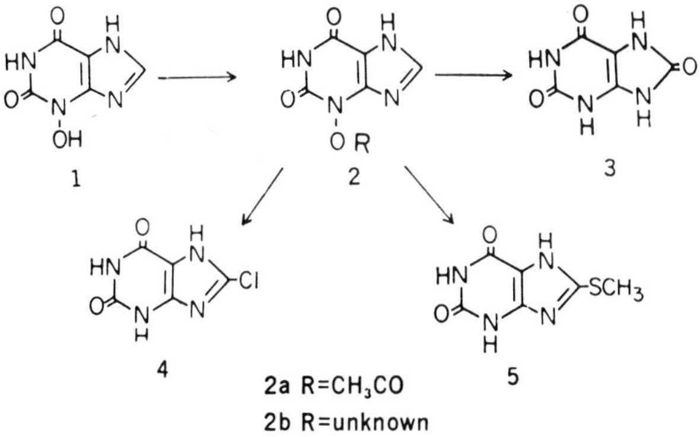

2a R=CH₃CO
2b R=unknown

Fig. 1.22. Conversion of 3-hydroxyxanthine to 8-chloroxanthine and
8-methylmercaptoxanthine.

As mentioned earlier, many aromatic amines are carcinogenic and these are *N*-oxidized to form more carcinogenic aryl hydroxylamines (as opposed to hydroxamic acids). Current evidence suggests that the active agent in bladder tumour formation is a urine-borne conjugate and recently Radomski *et al.* (1977) have isolated an *N*-glucuronide conjugate of 4-hydroxylaminobiphenyl. These authors have also shown that this compound is a mutagen when tested against *Salmonella typhimurium* strains TA1538 and TA98. Many *N*-oxidized compounds are mutagenic to microorganisms (Pai *et al.*, 1978) and whilst it is current practice to attempt to relate this activity to mammalian carcinogenic activity, to the microorganism it is far from a toxication reaction as it allows growth in media which was hitherto anutrient.

Two further examples serve to illustrate that *N*-oxidation can be a toxication reaction. The first involves the analgesic agents phenacetin and

Table 1.5. Relationship between sulphate conjugation and carcinogenicity of *N*-oxidized purines. (Constructed from McDonald *et al.*, 1973.)

Purine	% conversion	Oncogenic activity
3-Hydroxyxanthine	44	+++
3-Hydroxy-1-methylxanthine	45	+++
3-Hydroxy-7-methylxanthine	41	0
3-Hydroxy-8-methylxanthine	28	+?
3-Hydroxy-9-methylxanthine	7	0
3-Hydroxy-7,9-dimethylxanthine	3	0
3-Hydroxy-8-azaxanthine	27	+
1-Hydroxyxanthine	43	0
7-Hydroxyxanthine	47	0
3-Hydroxyguanine	12	+++
1-Methylguanine-3-oxide	3	+++
3-Hydroxy-7-methylguanine	17	0
3-Hydroxy-8-methylguanine	17	0
3-Hydroxy-9-methylguanine	10	0
Hypoxanthine-3-oxide	26	++
Adenine-1-oxide	0	+
Purine-3-oxide	0	++

paracetamol; both these materials can produce toxic effects when given in large doses to man or laboratory animals. Numerous studies have been carried out showing that the major pathway of phenacetin metabolism leads to paracetamol. More recently, the minor pathways of phenacetin metabolism and the further metabolism of paracetamol have been examined in greater detail. Both compounds are able to generate active arylating species which can react with glutathione. In the absence of glutathione, these metabolites react with cellular macromolecules and thereby produce the toxic response. Utilizing radio-isotope techniques to investigate the reaction with glutathione, Hinson, Nelson & Mitchell (1977) showed that the evidence obtained supported the idea that whereas paracetamol was activated via the *N*-hydroxy metabolite, the structurally similar compound phenacetin was converted to the epoxide (Figure 1.23).

In separate experiments it has been confirmed that phenacetin can be *N*-hydroxylated metabolically (Hinson & Mitchell, 1976) supporting the data of Nery (1971). In this case it also appears that conjugation of *N*-hydroxy-phenacetin with either sulphuric or glucuronic acid produces more reactive metabolites (Mulder, Hinson & Gillette, 1977).

The last examples are the hydrazine-containing drugs, isoniazid and iproniazid, two substances which under certain conditions become hepato-toxic agents. These are both metabolized to active compounds, which are produced by initial hydrolysis followed by *N*-hydroxylation of the released hydrazines. These *N*-hydroxy compounds are thought to break down to carbonium ions which can then react with macromolecules (Nelson *et al.* 1975) (Figure 1.24).

Whilst it is now known that many different types of nitrogen-containing compound can be *N*-oxidized, in some cases the same type of product can

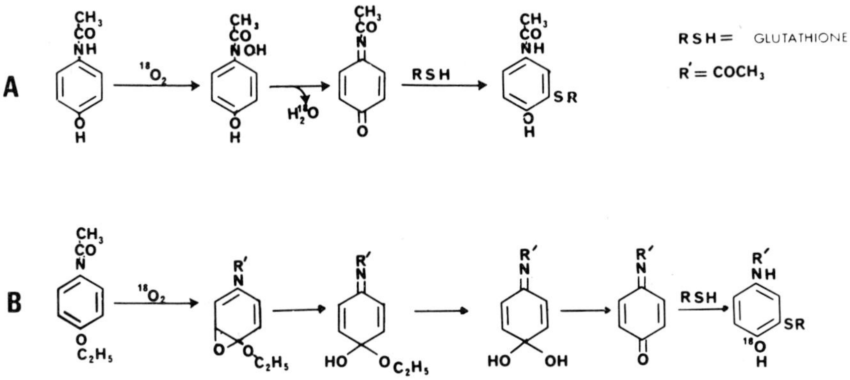

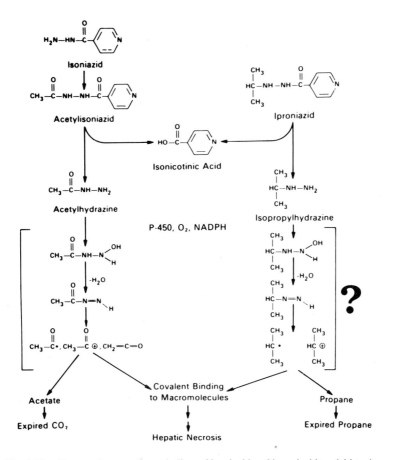

Fig. 1.23. Conversion of phenacetin and paracetamol to active arylating agents.

Fig. 1.24. Proposed routes of metabolism of isoniazid and iproniazid to yield toxic molecules. Reproduced from Nelson *et al.* (1975)

be produced by a reductive process. For example 4-nitroquinoline-*N*-oxide is a carcinogenic compound which is activated to the corresponding hydroxylamine by reduction (Figure 1.25). This reduction probably proceeds via the nitroso compound (Endo, Ono & Sugimura, 1971), although in common with other nitro compounds, nitro aromatic free radicals are

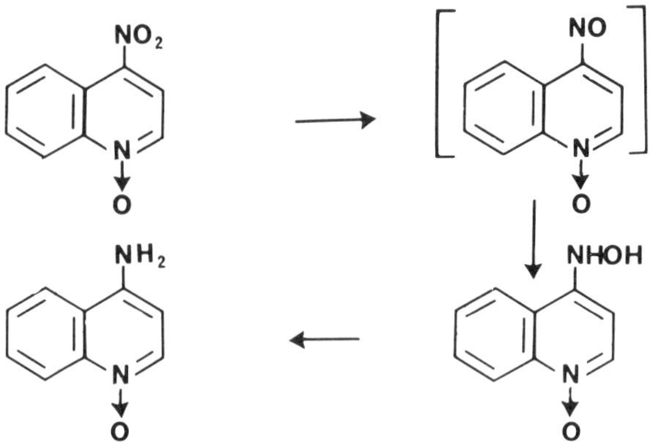

Fig. 1.25.   Reduction of 4-nitroquinoline-*N*-oxide.

also formed as intermediates (Mason & Holtzman, 1975). In view of the implication of radicals in many toxic reactions (see Chapter 6 and Slater, 1972), these intermediates may play some role in a toxic response to a nitro compound.

From the foregoing it might be assumed that *N*-oxidation is always associated with a toxic reaction. This is far from the case, as apart from a detergent effect on cells observed with long-chain alkyl dimethylamine-*N*-oxides (Subik *et al.*, 1977) tertiary amine oxides *per se* are usually devoid of pharmacological activity (Bickel, 1969). In fact the *N*-oxidation of nicotine, strychnine and the pyrrolizidine alkaloids must all be considered classical detoxication reactions.

Further examples of the complexity of *N*-oxidation in toxicology and pharmacology can be seen in Gorrod (1978a) and Buu-Hoi, Lambelin & Gillet (1970).

Toxic metabolites produced via metabolic attack on sulphur

Carbon disulphide causes a rapid loss of cytochrome P-450 when administered to starved rats without the appearance of a pathological lesion (Bond & De Matteis, 1969). This loss is markedly accelerated when carbon disulphide is given to rats which have been pretreated with phenobarbitone, and under these conditions produces a marked degenerative change in the centrilobular regions of the liver (Magos & Butler, 1972). These findings generated the idea that the toxicity was due to a metabolite rather than the parent compound. It has been shown by De Matteis and Seawright (1973) that carbon disulphide is converted to carbon dioxide by the rat *in vivo*, indicating that desulphuration takes place. Studies using radio-labelled sulphur (De Matteis, 1974) showed that during the metabolism of carbon disulphide, the sulphur produced becomes covalently bound to the liver microsomes and that the extent of binding was related to the activity of the microsomal enzymes (Figure 1.26). The nature of the bound material was investigated by Catignani & Neal (1975), who suggested that the sulphur

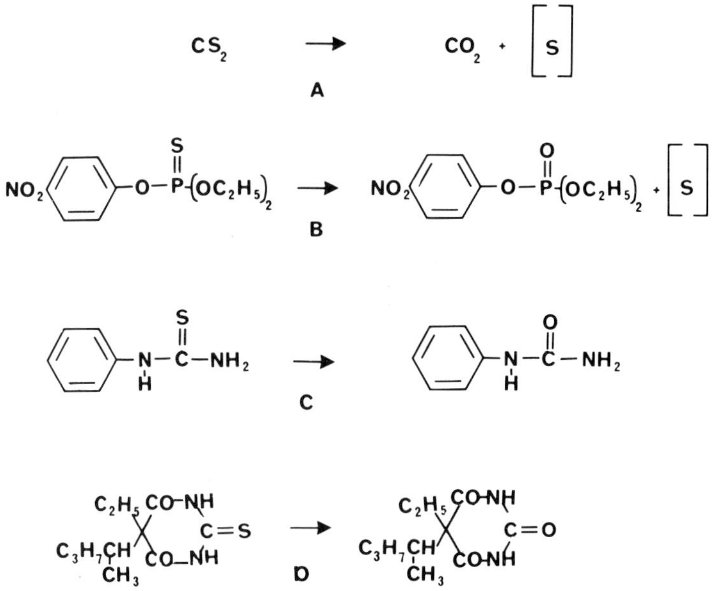

Fig. 1.26. Examples of some desulphurations known to occur during metabolism.

portion of the carbon disulphide was bound to the microsomal protein as hydrodisulphide, the majority of this bound material being released in the form of thiocyanate upon further incubation of the treated microsomes with cyanide.

An analogous reaction has also been shown to occur in the case of the phosphorothionate triester, Parathion. This substance, which is widely used as an insecticide, has been extensively studied by Neal and his coworkers (Norman, Poore & Neal, 1974; Ptashne, Wolcott & Neal, 1971; Ptashne & Neal, 1972). Thus the oxygen analogue, Paraoxon, is formed during metabolism, with the concomitant release of sulphur from the molecule (Figure 1.26). The sulphur formed is then bound to the microsomal protein in the form of a hydrodisulphide. The mechanism of this reaction appears to involve a primary attack upon the constituent sulphur to yield a sulphine-like intermediate, which rearranges to form a cyclic phosphorus-sulphur-oxygen product which then eliminates sulphur (Ptashne & Neal, 1972).

Other metabolic desulphurations are well established, although the enzymology of the reactions has never been fully studied nor the nature of the released sulphur elucidated. Phenylthiourea (Figure 1.26) and many related compounds are converted into phenylureas *in vivo* (Smith & Williams, 1961; Scheline, Smith & Williams, 1961). This reaction occurs with a number of thioureas, some of which have useful properties as rodenticides. It was earlier thought that the toxicity of these compounds was related to their ability to release hydrogen sulphide *in vivo*. However, in the light of the results from carbon disulphide and Parathion, this mechanism requires further investigation. An example of desulphuration occurring in a drug molecule is seen with the short-acting barbiturate, thiopentone (Figure 1.26). This substance is converted into pentobarbitone *in vivo* (Winters *et al.*, 1955). Thiouracil is converted to uracil by rat hepatic minces and by the intact animal (Spector & Shideman, 1959). It may be that some of the pharmacological and toxicological effects observed with these compounds are produced via release of a reactive form of sulphur.

Conclusions

From the foregoing it can be seen that the body has the ability to produce molecules which are more toxic than the parent compounds during metabolic processes. In many cases these routes may only be minor pathways and yet they may be responsible for the production of the biochemical lesion responsible for initiating the toxic process. In other cases these minor pathways may not be important until some other factor, which may be chemical (i.e. another drug) or biological, i.e. a change in physiological status or viral infection, produces a change in either the amount of toxic metabolite formed or a change in the susceptibility of the tissue to the toxic metabolite.

It should also be remembered that whereas the major proportion of drug metabolic reactions (both in quantity and diversity) are carried out by the liver, many other tissues have some drug-metabolizing activity (Gorrod, 1978b) and the presence or absence of an enzyme in a particular tissue may ensure that effective levels of the toxicant or its active metabolites are maintained.

References

Allen, D.W. and Jandl, J.H. (1961). *J. clin. Invest.* 40, 454.
Allison, A.C. and Dingle, J.T. (1966). *Nature, Lond.*, 209, 303.
Bickel, M.H. (1969). *Pharmac. Rev.*, 21, 325.
Bond, E.J. and De Matteis, F. (1969). *Biochem. Pharmac.*, 18, 2531.
Boyland, E. (1950). *Biochem. Soc. Symp.*, 5, 40.
Boyland, E. (1963). *The Biochemistry of Bladder Cancer*. Springfield, Ill.: Charles C. Thomas
Boyland, E. and Levi, A.A. (1935). *Biochem. J.*, 29, 2679.
Boyland, E. and Wolf, G. (1950). *Biochem. J.*, 47, 64.
Brandänge, S. and Lindblom, L. (1978). *Acta chem. Scand.* (in the press).
Brown, G.B. (1968). *Progr. Nucleic Acid Res.*, 8, 209.
Burger, A., Wagner, J., Uehleke, H. and Gotz, E. (1967). *Arch. Pharmak exp. Path.,* 256, 333.
Buu-Hoi, N.P., Lambelin, G. and Gillet, C. (1970). *Res. Progr. in Org. Biol. & Med. Chem.*, 2, 2.
Catignani, G.L. and Neal, R.A. (1975). *Biochem. Biophys. Res. Commun.*, 65, 629.
Cho, A.K., Haslett, W.L. and Jenden, D.J. (1961). *Biochem. Biophys. Res. Commun.*, 5, 276.
Cramer, J.W., Miller, J.A. and Miller, E.C. (1960). *J. biol. Chem.*, 235, 885.

De Matteis, F. and Seawright, A.A. (1973). *Chem.-Biol. Interact.*, 7, 375.
De Matteis, F. (1974). *Molec. Pharmac.*, 10, 849.
Endo, H., Ono, T. and Sugimura, T. (1971). *Chemistry and Biological Actions of 4-Nitro-quinoline N-Oxide*. Berlin: Springer, Verlag.
Erlanger, B.F. (1973). *Pharmac. Rev.*, 25, 271.
Flescher, J.W. and Sydnor, K.L. (1973). *Int. J. Cancer*, 11, 433.
Glatt, H.R., Oesch, F., Frigerio, A. and Garattini, S. (1975). *Int. J. Cancer*, 16, 787.
Gorrod, J.W. (1964). *Atti del Seminario Studi Biologici*, Università da Bari, 1, 207.
Gorrod, J.W. (ed.) (1978a) *Biological Oxidation of Nitrogen*. Amsterdam: Elsevier/North Holland.
Gorrod, J.W. (1978b). In *Drug Metabolism in Man*, Editors: J.W. Gorrod and A.H. Beckett, p. 157, London: Taylor & Francis.
Gorrod, J.W. and Hibberd, A.R. (1978). Unpublished observations.
Gorrod, J.W. and Jenner, P. (1975). *Essays in Toxicology*, 6, 35.
Gorrod, J.W. and Temple, D.J. (1976). *Xenobiotica*, 6, 265.
Hammar, C.G., Hammer, W., Holmstedt, B., Karlin, B., Sjöqvist, F. and Vessman, J. (1969). *Biochem. Pharmac.*, 18, 1549.
Heubner, W. (1913). *Naunyn-Schmiedebergs Arch. Exp. Path. Pharmak.*, 72, 241.
Hibberd, A.R. and Gorrod, J.W. (1978). *Proc. Intern. Pharmac. Conf.* Paris (Abstract No. 2082).
Hinson, J.A. and Mitchell, J.R. (1976). *Drug Metab. Disp.*, 4, 430.
Hinson, J.A., Nelson, S.D. and Mitchell, J.R. (1977). *Molec. Pharmac.*, 13, 625.
Hucker, H.B., Gillette, J.R. and Brodie, B.B. (1960). *J. Pharmac. exp. Ther.*, 129, 94.
Hucker, H.B., Staufer, S.C. and Rhodes, R.E. (1972). *Experientia*, 28, 430.
Huggins, C. and Morri, S. (1961). *J. exp. Med.*, 114, 741.
Irving, C.C. (1970). In *Metabolic Conjugation and Metabolic Hydrolysis*, Editor, W. Fishman, p. 53. New York: Academic Press.
Irving, C.C. (1973). *Methods in Cancer Res.*, 7, 189.
Jerina, D.M. and Daly, J.W. (1977a). In *Drug Metabolism — From Microbe to Man*, Editors D.V. Parke and R.L. Smith, p. 13. London: Taylor & Francis.
Jerina, D.M., Daly, J.W., Witkop, B., Zaltzman-Nirenberg, P. and Udenfriend, S. (1968). *J. Am. chem. Soc.*, 90, 6525.
Jerina, D.M., Lehr, R., Schaefer-Ridder, M., Yagi, H., Karle, J.M., Thakker, D.R., Wood, A.W., Lu, A.Y.H., Ryan, D., West, S., Levin, W. and Conney, A.H. (1977). In *Origins of Human Cancer*, Editors J.D. Watson and H. Hiatt, p. 639. New York: Cold Spring Harbor Laboratories.
Jollow, D.J. and Smith, C. (1977). In *Biological Reactions Intermediates*, Editors Jollow, D.J., Kocsis, J.J., Snyder, R. and Vario, H. New York: Plenum Press.
Kadlubar, F.F., Miller, J.A. & Miller, E.C. (1976). *Cancer Res.*, 36, 1196.
Kennaway, E.L. (1930). *Biochem. J.*, 24, 497.
Kiese, M. (1959a). *Naunyn-Schmiedebergs Arch. Exp. Path. Pharmak.*, 235, 354.
Kiese, M. (1959b). *Naunyn-Schmiedebergs Arch. Exp. Path. Pharmak.*, 235, 360.
Kiese, M. (1974). *Methemoglobinemia: A Comprehensive Treatise*. Cleveland, Ohio. C.R.C. Press.
Kriek, E. (1974). *Biochem. Biophys. Acta*, 355, 177.
Lipschitz, W. and Weber, J. (1923). *Hoppe-Seylers Z. Physiol. Chemie*, 132, 251.
Lotlikar, P.D. (1968). *Biochem. Biophys. Acta*, 170, 468.
Lotlikar, P.D. and Luha, L. (1971). *Biochem. J.*, 124, 69.
Magos, C. and Butler, W.H. (1972). *Br. J. indust. Med.*, 29, 95.
Mason, R.P. & Holtzman, J.L. (1975). *Biochemistry*, 14, 1626.
McDonald, J.J., Stöhrer, G. and Brown, G.B. (1973). *Cancer Research*, 33, 3319.
McKennis, H., Turnbull, L.B. and Bowman, E.R. (1958). *J. Am. chem. Soc.*, 80, 6597.
McMahon, R.E. (1966). *J. Pharm. Sci.*, 55, 457.
Miller, J.A. (1970). *Cancer Res.*, 30, 559.
Miller, J.A. and Miller, E.C. (1969). *Progr. exp. Tumour Res.*, 11, 273.
Miller, J.A., Sandin, R.B., Miller, E.C. and Rusch, H.P. (1955). *Cancer Res.*, 15, 188.
Mulder, G.J., Hinson, J.A. and Gillette, J.R. (1977). *Biochem. Pharmac.*, 26, 189.
Murphy, P.J. (1973). *J. biol. Chem.*, 248, 2796.

Nelson, S.D., Snodgrass, W.R. and Mitchell, J.R. (1975). *Fedn. Proc.,* 34, 784.

Nery, R. (1971). *Br. J. Haemat.*, 21, 507.

Nery, R. (1971). *Xenobiotica*, 1, 339.

Newman, M.S. and Blum, S. (1964). *J. Am. chem. Soc.*, 86, 5598.

Nguyen, T.L., Gruenke, L.D. and Castagnoli, N. (1976). *J. med. Chem.*, 19, 1168.

Norman, B.J., Poore, R.E. and Neal, R.A. (1974). *Biochem. Pharmac.*, 23, 1733.

Pai, V., Bloomfield, S.F., Jones, J. and Gorrod, J.W. (1978). In *Biological Oxidation of Nitrogen*, Editor: J.W. Gorrod, p. 375. Amsterdam: Elsevier/North Holland.

Ptashne, K.A., Wolcott, R.M. and Neal, R.A. (1971). *J. Pharmac. exp. Ther.*, 179, 380.

Ptashne, K.A. and Neal, R.A. (1972). *Biochemistry*, 11, 3224.

Pullman, A. and Pullman, B. (1955). *Cancerisation par les substances chimiques et structure moléculaire*. Paris: Masson.

Radomski, J.L., Hearn, W.L., Radomski, T., Moreno, H. and Scott, W.E. (1977). *Cancer Research*, 37, 1757.

Roberts, J.J. and Warwick, G.P. (1963). *Nature*, 197, 87.

Roberts, J.J. and Warwick, G.P. (1964). *Biochem. J.*, 93, 18P.

Rosi, D., Merola, A.J. and Archer, S. (1967). *Life Sciences*, 6, 1433.

Rosi, D., Peruzzotti, G., Dennis, E.W., Berberian, D.A., Freele, H., Tullar, B.F. and Archer, S. (1967). *J. med. Chem.*, 10, 867.

Rutty, C.J. and Connors, T.A. (1977). *Biochem. Pharmac.*, 26, 2385.

Sanders, E.B., De Bardeleben, J.F. and Osdene, T.S. (1975). *J. org. Chem.*, 40, 2848.

Scheline, R.R., Smith, R.L. and Williams, R.T. (1961). *J. med. Chem.*, 4, 109.

Sims, P. and Grover, P.L. (1974). *Advn. Cancer Res.*, 20, 165.

Sims, P., Grover, P.L., Swaizland, A.J., Pal, K. and Hewer, A. (1974). *Nature (Lond.)*, 252, 326.

Slater, T.F. (1972). *Free Radical Mechanisms in Tissue Injury*. London: Pion.

Sloane, N.H. (1964). *Biochem. Biophys. Acta*, 81, 408.

Sloane, N.H. (1965). *Biochem. Biophys. Acta*, 107, 599.

Smith, R.L. and Williams, R.T. (1961). *J. med. Chem.*, 4, 137.

Smith, M.R., Damani, L.A., Disley, L.G., Gorrod, J.W., Marsden, J.T., Patterson, L.H. and Rhenius, S.T. (1978). In *Biological Oxidation of Nitrogen*, Editor: J.W. Gorrod, p. 363. Amsterdam: Elsevier/North Holland.

Spector, E. and Shideman, F.E. (1959). *Biochem. Pharmac.*, 2, 182.

Spencer, E.Y., O'Brien, R.D. and White, E.W. (1957). *J. agric. Fd Chem.*, 5, 123.

Stambaugh, J.E., Feo, L.G. and Manthei, R.W. (1967). *Life Sciences*, 6, 1811.

Stilwell, W.G., Carman, M.J., Bell, L. and Horning, E. (1974). *Drug Metab. Disp.*, 2, 489.

Stöhrer, G. and Brown, G.B. (1970). *Science*, 167, 1622.

Subik, J., Takacsova, G., Psenak, M. and Devinsky, F. (1977). *Antimicrob. Agents Chemother.*, 12, 139.

Swaizland, A.J., Hewer, A., Pal, K., Keysell, G.R., Booth, J., Grover, P.L. and Sims, P. (1974). *F.E.B.S. Letters*, 47, 34.

Swenson, D.H., Miller, E.C. and Miller, J.A. (1974). *Biochem. Biophys. Res. Commun.*, 60, 1036.

Wagner, J. (1968). *F.E.B.S. Proceedings*, 16, 161.

Weisburger, J.H. and Weisburger, E.K. (1973). *Pharmac. Rev.*, 25, 1.

Weisburger, J.J., Weisburger, E.K., Madison, R.M., Wenk, M.L. and Klein, D.S. (1973). *J. natl. Cancer Inst.*, 51, 235.

Wheatley, D.N., Hamilton, A.G., Currie, A.R., Boyland, E. and Sims, P. (1966). *Nature (Lond.)*, 211, 1311.

Wilson, R.H., De Eds, F. and Cox, A.J.C. (1941). *Cancer Res.*, 1, 595.

Winters, W.D., Spector, E., Wallach, D.P. and Shideman, F.E. (1955). *J. Pharmac. exp. Ther.*, 114, 343.

Yamamoto, R.S., Williams, G.M., Richardson, H.L., Weisburger, E.K. and Weisburger, J.H. (1973). *Cancer Research*, 33, 454.

Yoshihara, S. and Yoshimura, H. (1972). *Biochem. Pharmac.*, 21, 3205.

Young, L. (1947). *Biochem. J.*, 41, 417.

2. Developmental aspects of the metabolism and toxicity of drugs

W. Robert Jondorf

Introduction

Despite the fact that there have been quite a number of recent reviews on developmental and perinatal pharmacology (Done, 1966; Sereni & Principi, 1968; Mirkin, 1970; Ginsburg, 1971; Eriksson & Yaffe, 1973; Pomerance & Yaffe, 1973; Boréus, 1973; Dancis & Hwang, 1974; Hänninen, 1975; Morselli, Garattini & Sereni, 1975; Netter, 1976; Dutton *et al.*, 1977), what follows will not be merely a review of reviews. The subject of the influence of age on the metabolism and toxicity of drugs is here integrated with a number of significant factors that are not usually considered.

Brodie (1956) established various generalizations that characterized the special nature of the non-specific enzymes responsible for the biotransformation of foreign compounds in experimental vertebrates.

At that time, it was already known that these enzymes were localized in the liver, that they had unusual co-factor requirements, and that they did not metabolize normally occurring substrates. Further, it was appreciated that there were species differences in drug metabolizing enzyme activity. Dealkylation and oxidation reactions, readily measured when liver homogenates of normally available laboratory mammals were incubated with test drugs under the appropriate conditions, were not observed in corresponding experiments with turtle, frog or goldfish liver preparations. It was suggested that the drug-metabolizing enzymes might be absent in lower animals because such animals had the ability to excrete drugs unchanged.

When it became clearer that lipid solubility of drugs was a rate-limiting factor in urinary excretion (Brodie & Hogben, 1957) and that the drug-metabolizing enzymes converted relatively hydrophobic foreign compounds to more polar, more readily excretable derivatives, the absence of drug metabolism in fish or amphibian species could be understood. Lipid solubility of drugs or foreign compounds is not a barrier to their excretion in these aquatic species, which can eliminate them by continuous dialysis through the lipoidal membranes of their gills or skin.

The drug-metabolizing enzymes can be considered in terms of biochemical evolution accompanying the transition from aquatic to terrestrial life (Brodie, Maickel & Jondorf, 1958). This required ways of disposing of non-polar foreign compounds compatible with water-retention priorities for the organism.

This idea was put to the test by studying drug metabolism in the toad (Gaudette, Maickel & Brodie, 1958; Maickel, Jondorf & Brodie, 1958, 1959; Jondorf, Maickel & Brodie, 1959; Brodie & Maickel, 1962). When test drugs were administered to toads which in their adult form lead a primarily terrestrial existence, recoveries of unchanged drugs were low. The toad had the ability to excrete exogenous phenols as glucuronide and ethereal sulphate conjugates. Incubations of dialysed toad liver preparations showed that drug-metabolizing enzyme activity was localized in the supernatant fraction and was activated by NADP. The end products of monomethyl-4-aminoantipyrine metabolism were 4-hydroxyantipyrine and methylamine. The sub-cellular localization, co-factor requirements and route of metabolism were different from those in reptiles, birds and mammals (Brodie & Maickel, 1962).

Another remarkable feature was that the tadpoles of toads did not metabolize foreign compounds; the drug-metabolizing enzymes appeared during metamorphosis of the aquatic larvae to terrestrial adults. Developmental and evolutionary considerations arising from this kind of experimentation led to the suggestion that in the transition from foetal to neonatal life, mammals undergo a transition from an aquatic to a terrestrial environment, reminiscent of the evolutionary development of the lower vertebrate.

Mammals

Although some drugs and environmental chemicals are excreted from the body unchanged, they are more generally converted to metabolites by non-specific enzymes before excretion, unless they resemble endogenous intermediates to such an extent that they serve as substrates for enzymes of intermediary metabolism and become incorporated into cellular macromolecules. The fate of most drugs undergoing metabolic transformation in the higher vertebrates, as shown in Figure 2.1, was conveniently classified into Phase I and Phase II reactions by Williams (1959). He pointed out that Phase I reactions were those that converted one functional group into another or introduced polar groups into non-polar compounds. He included the various synthetic reactions that conjugate existing or newly introduced polar groups with endogenous entities, as glucuronides, sulphates or mercapturic acids in the Phase II classification.

The oxidative Phase I reactions tend to occur primarily in liver endoplasmic reticulum, and they are catalysed by mixed-function oxidases consisting of NADPH-cytochrome c reductase and CO-sensitive haemoproteins making up what is known as cytochrome P-450 (Gillette, 1966). The elaboration of the original Williams (1959) scheme for understanding the patterns of drug metabolism took place in consequence of a greater understanding of the complexities of cytochrome P-450 interactions with hydrophobic, relatively non-polar substrates. The current concepts of drug-metabolizing events in the liver are perhaps best illustrated by

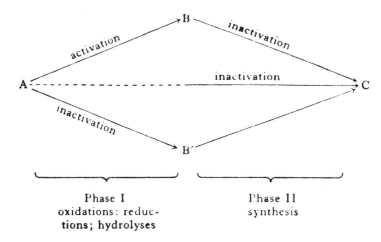

Fig. 2.1. Schematic summary of hepatic drug metabolism according to Williams (1959). Drug or foreign compound A is converted into a more active compound B or a less active intermediate B¹ by Phase I reactions. The intermediates B or B¹ may be further metabolized by Phase II synthetic reactions to form inactive water-soluble conjugate(s) C excretable into urine or bile. Depending on the nature of the compound A, it may also be conjugated directly without modification by Phase I reactions.

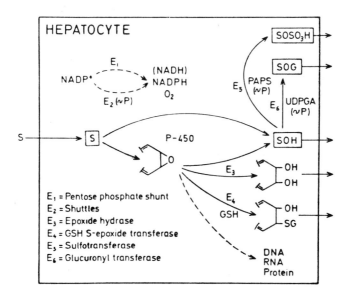

Fig. 2.2. Schematic representation of drug-metabolizing events in the hepatocyte, according to Orrenius (1976). Drug substrate S undergoes cytochrome-P450 catalysed monooxygenation, requiring NADPH and molecular O_2', and subsequently undergoes energy-requiring ($\sim$P) conjugation reactions. Aromatic compounds give rise to intermediate epoxides which may bind to macromolecular cell components, but more usually undergo further transformation to phenols, dihydrodiols and various conjugates.

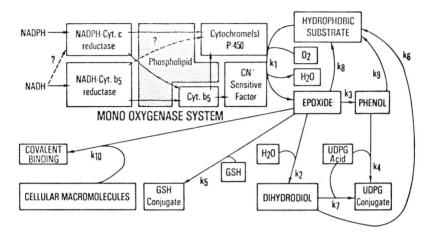

Fig. 2.3. Scheme according to Nebert *et al.* (1977), for membrane-bound multi-component
cytochrome P-450 mediated mono-oxygenase system, and possible metabolic pathway,
followed by hydrophobic drug substrates. For any given substrate, the relative reaction
rates k_1-k_{10} are not known, and would be expected to vary with factors related to age,
strain, species, hormonal and nutritional status.

Figure 2.2 (Orrenius, 1976) and Figure 2.3 (Nebert *et al.*, 1977).

As shown in Table 2.1, early experiments comparing the liver microsomal
drug-metabolizing ability of test substrates in foetal, neonatal and older
guinea-pigs *in vitro* (Jondorf, Maickel and Brodie, 1958) showed that the
Phase I enzyme activities for *N*-dealkylation, (monomethyl-4-amino antipyrine), *O*-dealkylation (phenacetin), side-chain oxidation (hexobarbital),
and Phase II glucuronide conjugation (phenolphthalein) were all lacking at
birth, and had not attained their adult level even 21 days after birth. A
similar pattern of gradual post-natal development of liver microsomal drug-
metabolizing activity was observed in rabbits (Fouts & Adamson, 1959).
Brown & Zuelzer (1958) ascribed the virtual absence of glucuronide
conjugation mechanism in foetal and neonatal guinea-pig liver preparations

Table 2.1. Effect of age on metabolism of drugs by equivalent amounts of guinea-pig liver
preparations (9000 *g* supernatant fractions) incubated *in vitro* with 2 μmole of substrate
in the presence of appropriate co-factors. Figures represent range of values obtained.

Age (days)	Number of experiments	Amount of substance metabolized (in μmol/h)				
		Monomethyl Aminopyrine	Amido- pyrine	Phenacetin	Hexobarbi- tal	Phenol phthalein
−2 (foetus)	(1)	0	–	–	–	0
1	(3)	0	0	0	0	0
7	(3)	0.23-0.35	0.11-0.16	0.16-0.27	0.05-0.07	0.04-0.05
21	(3)	0.37-0.47	0.38-0.55	0.56-0.86	0.26-0.42	0.13-0.18
Adults (3 months old)	(5)	0.69-0.94	0.62-0.88	0.96-1.08	0.57-0.78	0.44-0.57

Data from Jondorf, Maickel & Brodie (1958).

(phenolphthalein and *o*-aminophenol substrates) to deficient glucuronyl transferase and uridine-diphosphate-glucose dehydrogenase activities. They related these findings quite convincingly to the phenomenon of transient neonatal jaundice in paediatrics, emanating from the failure to form the bilirubin glucuronide conjugates. However, such an explanation ignored the possibilities that a number of progestational agents inhibiting glucuronyl transferase (Hsia *et al.*, 1960) or enhancing β-glucuronidase activity associated with human milk (Takimoto & Matsuda, 1971) could accentuate neonatal jaundice in the nursing period.

In experiments with neonatal and more mature mice injected with hexobarbital (Jondorf *et al.*, 1958), the assay of unchanged drug recoverable after a given time was correlated with the duration of the hexobarbital-induced hypnosis (Quinn, Axelrod & Brodie, 1958), a measure of the duration of drug action *in vivo*. Deficiency in drug-metabolizing ability was related to the prolongation of the drug-induced hypnosis. The toxicity of hexobarbital to neonatal mice was thought to be related not only to the inability to metabolize the drug, but to the permeability to drugs of the blood-brain barrier at that stage of development (Driscoll & Hsia, 1958).

Although the absence of drug-metabolizing activity in the neonate can enhance the toxicity of other drugs, as in the case of urethane (Mirvish, Cividalli & Berenblum, 1964) or chloramphenicol (Weiss, Glazko & Weston, 1960), some drugs are rather less toxic to the neonate than to the adult. It has been known for a long time (Whipple, 1912) that young pups are not susceptible to chloroform poisoning, and that new-born rats are similarly protected from hepatotoxic effects of carbon tetrachloride (Dawkins, 1963). More mature rats with drug-metabolizing activity inhibited by pretreatment with SKF-525A (Marchand *et al.*, 1971) are protected against the hepatotoxic effects of carbon tetrachoride which are thought to be due to formation of active metabolites (Butler, 1961; Glende & Recknagel, 1969) (see chapter 6).

Similarly, neonatal rats are not susceptible to the poisonous principles of amanita mushrooms (Fiume, 1965; Wieland, 1968) or to bromobenzene (Mitchell *et al.*, 1971) which are normally metabolized to more toxic metabolites.

However, there would appear to be more instances where the lack of drug-metabolizing enzyme activity demonstrably prolongs the action of drugs in the neonate. Thus, in their experiments with rats ranging in age from 1 to 250 days, Kato *et al.* (1964) showed that the duration of observable pharmacological effects *in vivo* after administrations of barbiturate, strychnine or carisoprodol (isopropyl meprobamate), was inversely related to the liver microsomal metabolizing activity of these drugs measured *in vitro*. The liver microsomal enzymes were at peak activity at 30 days of age and declined thereafter. It was established in a series of cross-over experiments that the differences in liver microsomal drug-metabolizing activities at different ages were not due to the presence of activators or inhibitors.

In a comprehensive series of experiments with pigs, Short, Maines and Westfall (1972) showed that some pathways of drug metabolism, though deficient, were nonetheless present in foetal and neonatal liver and other tissues. Post-natal development of drug-metabolizing activity was most pronounced in liver. In experiments with guinea-pigs, Bend *et al.* (1975) demonstrated glutathione-dependent transferase activity in foetal and neo-natal tissues which was most precociously developed in the lung. These animal experiments, when taken in conjunction with the literature that has grown around the discovery that human foetal tissue also has drug metabolizing capability (Yaffe *et al.*, 1970; Hänninen, 1975; Pelkonen *et al.*, 1975), gave rise to speculation about the toxicological implications of drug metabolism on the foetal side of the placenta during gestation (Pelkonen *et al.*, 1975). An example to illustrate that not all might be well in precociously developed drug-metabolizing activity in the guinea-pig foetus is provided by the experiments of Schenker, Dawber and Schmid (1964). They showed that unconjugated [^{14}C]bilirubin injected intravenously to the exteriorized guinea-pig foetus crossed the placenta and was excreted via the maternal liver. [^{14}C]Bilirubin glucuronide, when similarly injected, did not cross the placenta.

The deficiencies in measurable liver microsomal drug-metabolizing activities in the new-born mammal focused attention on the nature of post-natal structural and functional induction of the deficient enzyme activities (Dallner, Siekevitz & Palade, 1965; Greengard, 1974) and on the possibili-ties of premature induction with chemical inducers (Hart *et al.*, 1962) administered either to the pregnant animal before term or to the neonate. However, before dealing with these topics and the related question of the inducibility of drug-metabolizing enzyme activity of embryonic cells in tissue culture (Gelboin, Kinoshita & Wiebel, 1972; Pelkonen *et al.*, 1975) it is necessary to consider some features of pregnancy which are relevant to drug metabolism and toxicity.

Pregnancy

In placental mammals, life does not begin at birth; before birth, embryo-genesis proceeds in a predetermined sequence of cell proliferation, differ-entiation, migration and morphogenesis, regulated by a subtly synchronized complex of biochemical events. These events, linked with the physiological unity of the mother, can be the unintended target of therapeutic or adverse effects of drugs during pregnancy.

Maternal exposure to environmental chemicals (Nelson, 1969; Sparschu, Dunn & Rowe, 1971) or maternal needs unrelated to the maintenance of pregnancy could give rise to side effects of drugs which in extreme cases could cause severe malformations in the progeny, as with thalidomide (McBride, 1961; Lenz, 1961; Fabro & Smith, 1966) or with antiepileptic compounds such as diphenylhydantoin (Mirkin, 1971; Hill, Horning & Horning, 1973).

The maternal-embryonic exchange mechanisms from the point of view of pharmacology and drug metabolism begin even before implantation at the blastocyst stage of development. A variety of isotopically labelled drugs including caffeine, nicotine and isoniazid administered to six-day pregnant rabbits (Sieber & Fabro, 1971) were identified in the uterine secretion and in the blastocyst, together with certain of their metabolites. In analogous experiments with |[^{14}C]thalidomide, Fabro *et al.* (1964) identified thalidomide and a number of its spontaneous hydrolysis products (Schumacher, Smith & Williams, 1965) in the blastocyst. Lutwak-Mann (1973) correlated the uptake of thalidomide by pre- and post-implantation blastocysts with characteristic cytological disorganization. It was also found (Lutwak-Mann, Schmid & Keberle, 1967) that [^{14}C]thalidomide administered to male rabbits penetrated into the semen and was bound to the spermatozoa, which suggested that progeny could conceivably be affected adversely by drugs even by the paternal route at the time of fertilization.

In a review on drug distribution in pregnancy, Mirkin (1973) evaluated the effects of drugs on foetal development. What emerged was that the administration of a pharmacologically active compound early in gestation was more likely to have teratological consequences than administration shortly before parturition, where effects on the progeny would tend to be relatively transient. Evidently the irreversible toxicological risks are compounded when a potential teratogen or antimetabolite at the critical dosage interferes with essential intermediary metabolism. This could happen through deprivation of appropriate vitamins by competing analogues, or blockage of their utilization in co-enzyme systems (Landauer & Clark, 1964) at those characteristic times in embryonic development when, according to the genetic constitution of a particular species, its organogenesis may be disturbed (Larsson, 1973).

Factors which determine transplacental passage of drugs and metabolites are thought to be related to lipid solubility and degree of ionization (Maickel & Snodgrass, 1973), blood flow in the placenta (Finster & Mark, 1971; Asling & Way, 1971) placental drug-metabolizing competence (Juchau, Symms & Zachariah, 1974; Juchau, 1975; Netter & Bergheim, 1975) and indirectly, the concomitant potentiating effects from inducing substances taken in from the environment (Nebert & Gelboin, 1969); Welch *et al.*, 1972; Oesch, 1975; Nebert *et al.*, 1977).

After passage across the placenta, drugs and metabolites may be distributed in the foetus, excreted into the amniotic fluid, possibly be metabolized to a limited extent as in human and non-human primates (Rane *et al.*, 1973a; Dvorchik, Stenger & Quattropani, 1974; Pelkonen *et al.*, 1975) or returned to the maternal circulation via retrograde placental transfer as illustrated by Netter (1976).

Distribution studies have been helped by autoradiographic techniques (Waddell, 1972; Ullberg, 1973) which have shown that a great variety of isotopically labelled compounds of pharmacological interest administered to pregnant mice a few days before parturition localize in the same tissues of mother and foetuses (Waddell, 1972). Even when labelled [^{14}C]thalidomide and [^{14}C]diphenylhydantoin were administered under these conditions, there were few indications to suggest the cause of teratogenic anomalies from examination of the autoradiographs (Waddell, 1972). However from the work of Ullberg's group (Ullberg, 1973), it became clear that some physiologically important substances such as ^{58}Co-labelled vitamin B$_{12}$ are not evenly distributed between target organs in pregnant mouse and foetuses, but tend to concentrate in the placenta, whence they are distributed to the foetuses where they subsequently accumulate. The placenta exerts a similar selective function for trace elements such as iodine and iron, and for vitamin B_1 and ascorbic acid, but the lipid-soluble vitamins A and E have restricted passage through the placenta. With regard to drugs, [^{35}S]chlorpromazine and [^{14}C]chloroquine accumulate in the foetal eye and [^{14}C]thiourea in the foetal thyroid.

By analysis of foetal body fluids after administration of drugs to the mother, a clearer differentiation between drug and metabolites becomes possible. An example of this is the administration of thalidomide to pregnant rabbits (Keberle *et al.*, 1965) followed by electrophoresis of plasma and amniotic fluid with metabolite standards. The distribution in the foetus of these compounds at critical times in the gestation period can thus be thoroughly evaluated and compared by injecting any or all of the identifiable metabolites under corresponding conditions. The method has general application once the critical days for various stages of development in different species are tabulated (Wilson, 1971; Waddell, 1972).

Greater problems arise where a pharmacological agent may be teratogenic for one species when administered to pregnant females, and carcinogenic for the progeny of another under the same circumstances. Urethane is teratogenic for Syrian hamsters and induces precocious lung tumours in mice (Di Paolo & Elis, 1967); depending on the treatment regimen, urethane can produce these tumours as early as three days after birth (Smith & Rous, 1948). What is disturbing is the realization that the lung tumour incidence in mice is increased when urethane is administered to the pregnant mice on the day before parturition (Larsen, 1947; Klein, 1952, 1954), for this kind of major toxicological effect is not expected from the criteria discussed by Mirkin (1973). However, an attempt will be made in a later section to establish some rationale for such findings.

A cause-and-effect relationship between adenocarcinoma of the vagina in adolescent girls and the administration of diethylstilboestrol to their mothers during pregnancy (Herbst & Scully, 1970; Herbst, Ulfelder & Poskanzer, 1971) appears to extend the period of vigilance for such carcinogenic effects.

The placenta

In some reviews on the placental transfer of drugs (Asling & Way, 1971; Finster & Mark, 1971; Ginsburg, 1971; Pomerance & Yaffe, 1973) it is not clear that the placenta may have drug-metabolizing enzyme activity, although Telegdy (1973) in assessing the complementary roles of foetus and placenta in steroidogenesis left no doubt that the placenta was intimately concerned with biotransformations involving steroid substrates. The function of the placenta in biosynthetic steroid reactions was also well documented by Juchau *et al.* (1973) and by Pelkonen *et al.* (1975).

It is now well established that in the animal placenta (Nebert & Gelboin, 1969; Welch *et al.*, 1972; Schlede & Merker, 1972; Rane *et al.*, 1973b; Bend *et al.*, 1975), several of the Phase I drug-metabolizing pathways can be measured *in vitro*, in incubations of microsomal preparations with suitable substrates. Activities of human placental preparations (Pelkonen, Arvela and Kärki, 1971; Juchau, 1971; Juchau *et al.*, 1973, 1974) also indicated that they were dependent on the typical components of the drug-oxidizing mono-oxygenase system.

Several characteristic features of placental drug-metabolizing activity emerged from what is obviously an intensely studied subject. The placental drug-metabolizing activity is lower and relatively more specific than that of the liver. There are only a few pathways (Juchau *et al.*, 1974; Pelkonen *et al.*, 1975) of Phase I drug metabolism. This appears to be a reflection of the low content, different spectral properties and binding characteristics of placental cytochrome P-450 (Netter & Bergheim, 1975; Netter, 1976) which has unusual affinities for endogenous substrates (Netter & Bergheim, 1975). No doubt this ensures appropriate specificity for positional hydroxylations of the relevant steroid substrates (Juchau, 1975) and thus exerts an appropriate co-ordinating influence on foetal steroidogenesis (Telegdy, 1973).

Contrary to expectation, placental NADPH-cytochrome c reductase activity in placenta is not rate-limiting for drug-metabolizing activity (Rane *et al.*, 1973b; Pelkonen *et al.*, 1975), but apparently this enzyme is regulated by thyroid hormonal factors (Tata, Ernster & Lindberg, 1962; Tata *et al.*, 1963) and is therefore critically geared to developmental functions.

Placental drug-metabolizing activity is inducible by polycyclic hydrocarbons (Nebert & Gelboin, 1969; Welch *et al.*, 1969; Schlede & Merker, 1972). As shown in Table 2.2, induction of benzpyrene hydroxylation in rat placenta can be brought about by various polycyclic hydrocarbons regardless of whether they are carcinogenic or not.

Table 2.2. Effect of pretreating pregnant rats (18th day of gestation) with polycyclic hydrocarbons (40mg/kg, orally), on induction of benzpyrene hydroxylase activity in the placenta.

Polycyclic hydrocarbon	8-Hydroxybenzpyrene formed (ng/g/h)
Control	218 ± 81
1,2-Benzanthracene	4 034 ± 519
1,2,5,6-Dibenzanthracene	3 577 ± 494
3,4-Benzpyrene	3 543 ± 114
Chrysene	3 267 ± 147
3,4-Benzofluorene	1 939 ± 98
Anthracene	1 377 ± 346
Pyrene	1 232 ± 306
Fluoranthene	1 123 ± 129
Phenanthrene	721 ± 155

Data from Welch *et al.* (1969).

In human placenta, some pathways of Phase I drug metabolism are not normally detectable and become measurable only in placental preparations from smoking mothers (Pelkonen *et al.*, 1975) although other pathways specifically related to steroid metabolism are not induced in this way by smoking (Juchau *et al.*, 1973).

Induction of drug-metabolizing activity by administration of compounds to the pregnant females of a number of species (Nebert & Gelboin, 1969; Schlede & Merker, 1972) induces not only placental drug-metabolizing activity, but transplacental activity in specific foetal tissues.

Despite the obvious toxicological value of the type of study shown in Table 2.2, an extended, systematic appraisal of drugs known to induce or inhibit a variety of steroid-specific hydroxylations (Telegdy, 1973) for effects they might exert on steroid metabolism in the placenta and in the foetus does not appear to have been undertaken.

In rabbit, placental Phase II conjugation reactions, particularly with respect to mercapturic acid formation (Bend *et al.*, 1975), have been measured and considered in the context of protecting the foetal tissues from adverse effects of epoxides (Oesch, 1975) formed as obligatory intermediates in the metabolism of polycyclic aromatic hydrocarbons (Daly, Jerina & Witkop, 1972). In the guinea-pig, the glutathione-dependent *S*-transferase activity in the placenta declines with the gestation period as a compensating increase in such activity comes into play in the foetus (Bend *et al.*, 1975). Unlike the Phase I drug-metabolizing reactions in the placenta, the glutathione *S*-transferases are known to have very broad overlapping substrate specificities (Grover, 1977).

In view of some of the difficulties experienced in assessing adverse effects of drugs on the foetus when compounds are administered to the maternal side of the placenta, and when inducing substances can affect placental factors differently according to species, it is a curious oversight that little attention has been paid to the suggestion that work with marsupials could be very rewarding (Schmidt-Nielsen, 1967) in the general context of developmental biology. The foetus in these non-placental species is exteriorized at an early stage of development (Sharman & Pilton, 1964) and would lend itself to rather more elaborate work in the realm of drug metabolism than has hitherto been reported (Marsh, 1969; Renfree & Heap, 1977; Cooley & Janssens, 1977) particularly if the elegant techniques requiring only very small plasma samples (Caldwell *et al.*, 1977) were applied for monitoring maternal-foetal exchange systems.

Induction during mammalian development

Drug-metabolizing enzyme activity in placental mammals is altogether absent or deficient in the foetus and the neonate. This was confirmed particularly elegantly by Rane *et al.* (1973b) who measured the various components of the mixed-function oxidase system in rabbit liver from the 20th day of gestation to the 14th day after parturition and correlated these not only with the electron microscopic appearance of the livers, with particular reference to the endoplasmic reticulum, but with measurements of microsomal drug-metabolizing activities.

There are ways in which the normal developmental pattern can be manipulated by exogenous inducers (Conney, 1967). An early example of this was the work of Hart *et al.* (1962) which showed that the administration of phenobarbital to pregnant rabbits near the end of the gestation period induced hepatic drug-metabolizing enzyme activity in the foetal livers at term, and in the neonates after parturition. Hart *et al.* (1962) noted that the induction could not be evoked in less mature foetal livers taken from pre-treated does, and that the transplacental inductive effects on the neonate were not as great as those seen when the neonates were treated with the barbiturate.

From this latter observation, it was scarcely surprising that when Yaffe *et al.* (1966) applied the principle of neonatal induction and treated infants with phenobarbital, they could show that the glucuronide conjugation of bilirubin was induced to relieve the symptoms of neonatal jaundice.

Induction mechanisms were studied more extensively by Nebert & Gelboin (1969), who treated pregnant hamsters and neonates with 3-methyl-cholanthrene (Table 2.3) and monitored aryl hydrocarbon hydroxylase,

Table 2.3. Effect of 24 h pretreatment with 3-methylcholanthrene (MC) on aryl hydrocarbon hydroxylase activity in tissues from pregnant hamster, foetus and newborn.
MC administration (100mg/kg, intraperitoneally) on 15th day of gestation or on day of birth. Tissues prepared from 2 adults or 5-20 foetuses or newborns were assayed for experiments (figures in parentheses refer to number of experiments).

Tissue	Aryl hydrocarbon hydroxylase specific activity (units/mg tissue protein)					
	Mother		Foetus		Newborn	
	Control	MC	Control	MC	Control	MC
Liver	2430-3555(3)	3435-3945(3)	14-27(3)	174-426(3)	500-620(2)	2505-2835(2)
Lung	< 6-11(3)	33-48(3)	< 6(3)	18-45(3)	21-23(2)	63-98(2)
Small intestine	< 6-18(3)	75-83(3)	< 6(3)	9-20(3)	< 6-17(2)	134-155(2)
Kidney	14-33(3)	162-207(3)	< 6(3)	32-33(3)	12-15(2)	132-144(2)

Data from Nebert and Gelboin (1969).

previously shown to be an inducible enzyme (Conney *et al.*, 1959), in maternal, foetal and neonatal tissues. They found that enzyme activity was inducible transplacentally not only in the liver where the effect was pre-dominant, but also in other tissues such as lung and kidney. Further, the control neonatal enzyme activity in the liver was greater than the induced foetal enzyme level and far greater than the foetal baseline activity. The liver enzyme activity at birth was only 20% of that of the untreated maternal controls but could be induced by 3-methylcholanthrene treatment to attain the maternal value in 24 hours. In other tissues the enzyme activity at birth, though low, appeared to be the same as that of the corresponding maternal tissue, and was equally inducible in mother and neonate. No extra-hepatic inducibility was detected in similar experiments involving adminis-tration of phenobarbital to pregnant hamsters.

Welch *et al.* (1972) administered benzpyrene to pregnant rats and found that relatively small doses of the polycyclic hydrocarbons induced drug-metabolizing enzyme activity in the maternal liver and in the placenta, but that much larger doses were required to induce the drug-metabolizing activity of the foetal liver. In complementary experiments, Schlede &

Merker (1972) showed that the benzpyrene-induced benzpyrene hydroxylase activity in pregnant rats was more pronounced in the maternal liver than in the placenta, and the foetal effects depended on the age of the foetus. Oesch (1975) dissociated benzpyrene hydroxylation into separate enzyme activities that took into account the metabolic formation of epoxide intermediates (Daly *et al.*, 1972), and determined that 3-methylcholanthrene administered to pregnant rats selectively induced foetal hepatic mono-oxygenase activity (which could lead to an adverse accumulation of mutagenic epoxide intermediates in the foetus), whereas phenobarbital administration under similar circumstances differentially induced the epoxide hydrase in foetal liver. Conclusions from this type of experiment could be drawn only if the other variables in the overall picture (Figures 2.2 and 2.3) could be assessed.

With regard to endogenous induction, the striking differences in hepatic benzpyrene hydroxylase activity in pre-natal and neonatal hamsters shown in Table 2.3 (Nebert & Gelboin, 1969), the equally striking delayed post-natal differentiation according to sex, of hepatic *N*-demethylating activity in the rat (Henderson, 1971), and the effect on the duration of hexobarbital-induced hypnosis brought about in female rats by pretreating them with testosterone (Quinn *et al.*, 1958) or other anabolic steroids (Booth & Gillette, 1962), have implicated hormonal factors in induction phenomena. What has not been so readily appreciated is that thyroid hormones have quite distinctive effects on drug-metabolizing activities. Thus Kato & Takahashi (1968) showed convincingly that thyroxine administered to female rats induced their liver microsomal capacity for metabolizing aminopyrine and hexobarbital, but inhibited these activities in male rats. NADPH-cytochrome c reductase and related liver enzyme activities were induced in rats of either sex by thyroxine, inhibited by thyroidectomy and restored to pre-thyroidectomy levels by thyroxine or tri-iodothyronine.

Vesell (1977) and Fishman & Barlow (1977) demonstrated that thyroid hormones were also inducers of drug-metabolizing enzymes in humans in certain medical conditions.

For reasons that will become apparent later when amphibia are discussed, prolactin secretion (Meites *et al.*, 1972) must also play a part as an endogenous factor in the developmental aspects of drug-metabolizing activity.

Yet another consideration with regard to induction is the inducibility of drug-metabolizing enzyme activity in foetal cells in tissue culture (Nebert & Gelboin, 1969; Gelboin *et al.*, 1972; Nebert & Gielen, 1972; Poland & Glover, 1974, 1975; Niwa, Kumaki & Nebert, 1975).

Benzpyrene hydroxylase activity is inducible in foetal cell cultures from whole hamster, mouse or rat grown in the presence of 1,2-benzanthracene in the medium (Nebert & Gelboin, 1969; Nebert & Gielen, 1972). The enzyme activity is also inducible in foetal cell cultures obtained from specific organs of the hamster (Nebert & Gelboin, 1969). Apparently, the induction requires continuous protein synthesis after an initial burst of RNA synthesis. The enzyme activity is not simply a detoxication mechanism but also has cytotoxic consequences, since polycyclic hydrocarbons are covalently bound to cellular macromolecules (Gelboin *et al.*, 1972). By inhibiting the induction process (with 7,8-benzoflavone), the cytotoxic consequences of concurrent exposure to 7,12-dimethylbenzanthracene are reduced.

This finding is very important since it contrasts with the increased susceptibility of new-born mice to carcinogenic polycyclic hydrocarbons (Domsky *et al.*, 1963) which allegedly is related to the slower rate of elimination from the neonate of administered polycyclic hydrocarbons like dimethylbenzanthracene. This suggests that regulatory factors which determine the response to the carcinogenic action of polycyclic hydro-carbons are not comparable for cells in tissue culture and for the neonate. Alternative explanations involving neonatal appearance of some 'cluster of enzymes' (Greengard, 1974) or prolactin-related factors (Meites & Nicoll, 1966) may be needed.

The work on foetal cells in tissue culture revealed that 2,3,7,8-tetra-chlorodibenzo-*p*-dioxin (TCDD) was a much more potent inducer of aryl hydrocarbon hydroxylase activity than 'conventional' inducers such as 3-methylcholanthrene. TCDD was found to be about 30000 times more potent as an inducer in rat liver (Poland & Glover, 1974), but in foetal cell cultures from hamster, rat, rabbit, mouse and in human lymphocytes in cell cultures, TCDD-mediated inductions were only 250-900 times as potent as those brought about by 3-methylcholanthrene (Niwa *et al.*, 1975). The differential in inducing activities between TCDD and 3-methylcholanthrene *in vivo* in the rat and *in vitro* in cell culture in the studies cited, again points to some regulatory factors which are not evoked in both sets of experi-ments.

Despite the fact that TCDD and 3-methylcholanthrene effects on enzyme induction in rats produce similar maximal stimulation although at greatly different pretreatment levels (Poland & Glover, 1974), the TCDD-mediated inductions are much more persistent, lasting well over one month. It would be interesting to know how the induction of benzpyrene hydroxylase activity and the sustained increase in *N*-demethylation and the NADPH-cytochrome c reductase activity are compatible with the apparent resistance of TCDD to metabolic biotransformation and excretion.

Lastly, benzpyrene hydroxylase is inducible in human foetal liver cells in culture medium in the presence of polycyclic hydrocarbons, provided that the cells are taken from foetuses nine weeks or more after conception (Pelkonen *et al.*, 1975). The more alarming mutagenic (Oesch, 1975) or carcinogenic (Gelboin *et al.*, 1972) possibilities for the foetus implicit in maternal exposure to benzpyrene or cigarette smoking (Conney, 1972; Robinson *et al.*, 1975) should be balanced against the reassuring concept that the highly reactive epoxide intermediates formed in the benzpyrene hydroxylase system could be removed by concomitant selective induction of glutathione *S*-transferase (Robinson *et al.*, 1975; Grover, 1977) leading to mercapturic acid conjugation (Figure 2.3) rather than covalent binding to self-replicating macromolecules in cells that are proliferating and differ-entiating.

Avian species

Liver microsomal preparations from avian species can metabolize a variety of drug substrates under appropriate conditions *in vitro* (Brodie & Maickel, 1962; Debackere & Uehleke, 1964; Hitchcock & Murphy, 1971; Gutman & Kidron, 1971; Patterson & Roberts, 1971; Drummond, McCall & Jondorf, 1972; Wit, 1977). Conjugation mechanisms have been well characterized in the chick in particular, in terms of endogenous and exogenous induction (Burchell, Dutton & Nemeth, 1972; Dutton, 1973; Fyffe & Dutton, 1975; Dutton *et al.*, 1977).

There are indications that the developmental aspects of Phase I drug-metabolizing activity (Brodie & Maickel, 1962; Jondorf, MacIntyre & Powis, 1973; Powis *et al.*, 1976), and Phase II conjugation with glucuronide formation (Dutton & Ko, 1966; Dutton, 1973; Dutton *et al.*, 1977) differ in important details from those of more usually studied mammalian laboratory species (Jondorf *et al.*, 1958; Fouts & Adamson, 1959; Brodie & Maickel, 1962; Eriksson & Yaffe, 1973; Netter, 1976).

When liver microsomal preparations from chick embryos (1 day before hatching) and from 1-7 day-old chicks were essayed *in vitro* for oxidative drug-metabolizing activity with aminopyrine, aniline and naphthalene as substrates (Powis *et al.*, 1976), the metabolizing activity for all these substrates was highest in preparations from 1 day-old chicks (Figure 2.4). This was more than twice the activity in preparations from 7 day-old or more mature chicks, and about three times that of the pre-hatched embryos. The post-hatching surge in drug-metabolizing activities was the same for either sex and persisted for three days before declining towards the 7 day levels.

The developmental time-course of drug-metabolizing activity was independent of any factor in the 105 000 g supernatant fractions and of such microsomal parameters as cytochrome b_5 and cytochrome P-450 content or NADPH-cytochrome c reductase activity, but was related, as might have been expected (Holtzman *et al.*, 1968; Davies, Gigon & Gillette, 1969), to changes in NADPH-cytochrome P-450 reductase activity.

When 7 day-old chicks are treated with exogenous inducers of drug-metabolizing enzyme activity (Powis *et al.*, 1976), the time-course of the inductions is related to both cytochrome P-450 content and NADPH-cytochrome P-450 reductase activity, which suggests that there may be quite distinctive features in endogenous post-hatching induction of drug metabolism attendant on the resorption of the residual egg yolk, which are not mimicked in exogenous induction brought about by such agents as sodium phenobarbital or 3-methylcholanthrene. In any case, the parameters of the electron transport system in the newly-hatched chick liver preparations (Powis *et al.*, 1976) differ from those in developing rat (Dallner *et al.*, 1965) or rabbit liver (Rane *et al.*, 1973b).

The liver microsomal pre-hatching competence to perform Phase I oxidative drug metabolism by the pigeon and the chick (Brodie & Maickel, 1962) is reflected also by the ability of chick embryo liver cells growing in tissue culture to metabolize a variety of substrates (Poland & Kappas, 1971). Testosterone inhibits such metabolizing activity, presumably because

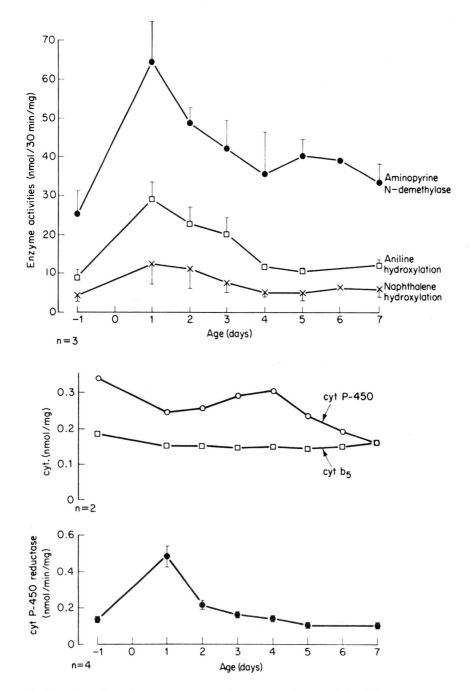

Fig. 2.4.   Some liver microsomal parameters in the perinatal period of the chick (Powis *et al.*, 1976), showing how the peak drug-metabolizing activity on the first day after hatching is related to elevated cytochrome P-450 reductase activity.

the androgenic steroid is an embryonic regulator substance (Mainwaring, 1977) implicated in foetal differentiation after undergoing characteristic pre-ordained NADPH-dependent metabolic conversions. The pre-hatching drug-metabolizing activity is also manifest as Phase II conjugations with sulphate (Spencer & Raftery, 1966), and glucuronide by glucuronyl transfer from UDP-glucuronic acid to acceptors such as *o*-aminophenol (Dutton & Ko, 1966).

The UDP-glucuronyl transferase activity in the developing chick is observed early in incubation *in ovo* in embryo liver and kidney, and on hatching, in the intestinal mucosa (Dutton & Ko, 1966). If embryo liver is cultured *in vitro* (Ko, Dutton & Nemeth, 1967; Burchell *et al.*, 1972), there is precocious development of UDP-glucuronyl transferase activity requiring different diffusible factors from the incubation media, which appear to be dependent on the embryonic age of the incubate.

It is thought, from grafting experiments, that endogenous regulatory factors in modulating UDP-glucuronyl transferase activity implicate certain trophic pituitary secretions (Wishart & Dutton, 1975a; Dutton *et al.*, 1977), and that exogenous inducers such as sodium phenobarbital can, when injected into eggs override the endogenous regulatory factors and induce the conjugation mechanism (Wishart & Dutton, 1975b). The remarkable findings on the rise and fall of the enzymes required for glucuronidation, and the changes occurring in endogenous regulatory controls with embryonic age in the chick, emphasize the advantages of using the avian embryo for studies on biochemical metamorphosis.

Embryo extracts (Kuru, Kosaki & Watanabe, 1962; Kagen & Linder, 1972) can affect the overall integrity of the developing chick. Different anti-metabolites such as spermine (Butros, 1972) or deoxyguanosine (Karnofsky & Lacon, 1962; Karnofsky & Young, 1967) when applied to the developing avian embryo at certain time points can cause not only dramatic teratogenic defects, but afford relatively straightforward opportunities for studying ways of overcoming them. Thus the teratogenic effects of deoxyguanosine can be prevented by deoxycytosine (Karnofsky & Young, 1967). Similarly, teratogenic effects of hydroxythalidomide derivatives in chick embryos (Boylen, Horne & Johnson, 1963) produced on injection into the yolk sac could be overcome by simultaneous administration of *L*-glutamine.

It is as if these experiments, beyond the aspirations of Holtfreter (1933) or Waddington, Needham & Needham (1933) were related to the older definitions of the organizer links between developmental biochemistry and morphology, and to the amazing unfolding in sequence of a succession of appropriate plasma protein constituents (Grieninger & Granick, 1975) that could produce the predetermined if incompletely understood events which for example activate the embryonic heart with catecholamines (Shideman & Ignarro, 1967).

Amphibia

Returning now to the work on amphibians mentioned in the introduction, we found originally that tadpoles of toads or certain kinds of frog (Brodie *et al.*, 1958) could not metabolize drugs either by oxidation or conjugation, but that after adaptation to terrestrial environment by metamorphosis, the toad could metabolize test substrates (Maickel *et al.*, 1958; Brodie & Maickel, 1962) and conjugate test phenols. Adult frogs also had some capacity for sulphate and glucuronide conjugation.

What was significant was that metamorphosis of free-living aquatic larval forms to terrestrial adults was accompanied by a biochemical metamorphosis with respect to drug-metabolizing enzyme activity which was as dramatic as that of the sequential changes of nitrogen excretion patterns (Munro, 1939, 1953) and plasma protein, visual pigment and haemoglobin characteristics reviewed by Wald (1958) and Bennett & Frieden (1962).

Because of the profound implications for mammalian developmental toxicology, it is worthwhile to consider how the changes in amphibian metamorphosis occur. When it was discovered that feeding tadpoles on mammalian thyroid tissue induced precocious metamorphosis (Gudernatsch, 1912) that thyroidectomy prevented metamorphosis (Allen, 1916; Hoskins & Hoskins, 1917) and that surviving thyroidectomized tadpoles given thyroxine in their environment could metamorphose, it was established that amphibian metamorphosis was responsive to regulation by mammalian hormones. Later, it was discovered that metamorphosis could be expedited by other specific chemically defined substances such as iodine and tyrosine (Hoffmann and Gudernatsch, 1933), thyroxine analogues, and tri-iodothyronine (Roth, 1953). Morphogenetic events responsive to the thyroid stimulus were diverse and yet quite specific, as illustrated by the tail resorption phenomena in Figure 2.5.

The biochemical events studied by Munro (1953) in amphibia with different degrees of aquatic and terrestrial organization were connected with the end products of nitrogen metabolism (for which there existed a model in the developing chick (Needham, 1931)). Ammonia excretion was predominant in the early larval stage, and urea predominated after metamorphosis in those species that became terrestrial. The biochemical and physical metamorphosis of the axolotl could be manipulated with thyroxine. *Xenopus* underwent an apparent second metamorphosis and remained aquatic. This was characterized by a reversion to the original larval ammonia excretion pattern after the development of an intermediate transient urea excretion phase (Underhay & Baldwin, 1955).

Compounds like thiourea and 2-thiouracil can interfere with the metamorphosis pattern of *Xenopus* larvae (Gasche & Druey, 1946). It was also realized that prolactin exerted a juvenilizing effect on tadpoles (Bern & Nicoll, 1968) which overcame the thyroxine-induced metamorphosing 'terrestrial drive', and instead induced a prolongation of the aquatic phase of growth. Moreover, prolactin induced secondary metamorphosing changes in adult terrestrial newts, enabling them to return to the aquatic habitat for spawning.

As part of a series of classical experiments on enzyme activities during tadpole metamorphosis, Brown, Brown & Cohen (1959), Paik & Cohen (1960, 1961) and Metzenberg *et al.* (1961) found that thyroxine induced the synthesis of specific enzymes such as carbamyl phosphate synthetase in

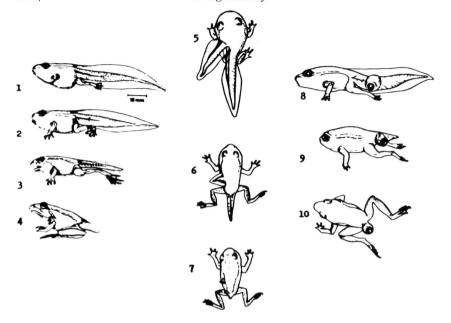

Fig. 2.5. Metamorphosis undergone by *Rana pipiens* showing gradual appearance of frog-like organization (1-4). Organ specificity of the metamorphosing responses in the tadpoles is illustrated by atrophy of tail tip grafted on trunk region (5-7), which undergoes resorption simultaneously with host tail tissue (Geigy, 1941). In related experiments with eye-cup grafted on tail (Schwind, 1933), the eye-cup is not resorbed, and is only affected positionally by the resorption of the host tail tissue (8-10). Illustrations adapted from Weber (1967).

tadpole liver, and that this remarkable induction could be blocked as shown in Table 2.4 by antithyroid drugs such as 2-thiouracil and other thiouracil derivatives, by thiourea, and by certain nitrobenzotriazoles which were known to delay amphibian development (Liedke, Engelman & Graff, 1955).

Table 2.4. Effect of various inhibitory compounds (dissolved in 2.6 x 10^{-8}M thyroxine solution at the concentrations indicated) on the induction of carbamyl phosphate synthetase in tadpole liver.

Agents added to thyroxine solution (2.6 × 10^{-8}M)	Final concentration (M)	Specific activity of carbamyl-phosphate synthetase after 12-day treatment
None	–	11.8
2-Thiouracil	3.5 × 10^{-3}	6.0
2,6-Dithiouracil	8.7 × 10^{-4}	4.5
2,4-Dithiouracil	6.9 × 10^{-4}	8.1
2,4-Dihydroxypyrimidine	3.9 × 10^{-3}	4.0
5-Nitrobenzotriazole	1.5 × 10^{-4}	3.2
6-Chloro-4-nitrobenzotriazole	5.0 × 10^{-5}	2.1
Thiourea	6.6 × 10^{-3}	7.8

Data from Paik & Cohen (1961).

Carbamyl phosphate synthetase is the key enzyme not only in the urea cycle, but also in the molecular events leading to the biosynthesis of monomeric precursors required for nucleic acid synthesis (Mahler & Cordes, 1971). The synthesis *de novo* of this Mg^{2+} and biotin-dependent enzyme, which can utilize either ammonia or glutamine as amino-group donor, is induced in the tadpole by thyroxine, the hormone which also induces the observable developmental changes towards the froglet stage (Figure 2.5).

$$\text{Glutamine} + 2ATP + HCO_3^- \xrightarrow{Mg^{2+}/\text{biotin}} NH_2-\overset{\overset{\displaystyle O}{\|}}{C}-OPO_3H^- + 2ADP + P_i$$
$$+ \text{ glutamic acid}$$

$$NH_3 + 2ATP + HCO_3^- \longrightarrow NH_2-\overset{\overset{\displaystyle O}{\|}}{C}-OPO_3H^- + 2ADP + P_i$$
$$\text{Carbamyl phosphate}$$

On the assumption that this is a primordial event in response to the metamorphosing stimulus provided by thyroid hormones, it is critical to the economy of the developing animal whether the appropriate glutamine or ammonia is utilized and whether the precursor carbamyl phosphate is switched to urea or pyrimidine synthetic pathways.

Without going into exhaustive detail, or getting too speculative about 3',5'-cyclic AMP-mediated cellular responses to hormonal stimulation (Jost & Rickenberg, 1971), there are morphogenetic considerations in simple experimental systems like that used by Schindler & Sussman (1977), which are worth considering in the context of amphibian metamorphosis and developmental biochemistry in general. The stationary phase cells of the slime mould *Dictostelium discoideum* with their capacity for aggregation and choice of morphogenetic pathways between slug migration and fruit body construction have that choice regulated by interaction between locally accumulated ammonia and 3',5'-cyclic AMP.

It is conceivable that in the earliest zygotic subdivisions, cyto-differentiation and translocation in the higher forms of life are critically determined by appropriate ammonia concentrations. It is a possible interpretation for the maintenance of mechanisms in early life that ensure the catabolic production of ammonia.

Compounds that interfere with embryonic or larval development could do so by interfering with locally generated appropriate ammonia concentrations, by competing with glutamine-dependent reactions, by blocking the effects of biotin in the carbamyl phosphate synthetase reaction, by causing aberrations in the utilization of Mg^{2+} or carbamyl phosphate, and by virtue of any antithyroid activity.

It could be predicted that drugs which interfered with prolactin release or feedback control (Grant and Cooper, 1965) would also have profound toxicological effects on development.

Although in our own early work on drug metabolism in the toad (Brodie, Maickel & Jondorf, 1958; Brodie & Maickel, 1962) the threshold appearance of drug-metabolizing activity was not precisely mapped with the stage of tadpole development, the implication of the rapid onset of thyroxine-induced urea cycle enzyme activity indicates that the onset of related phenomena, whether they be tail resorption or drug-metabolizing enzyme activity, is also ultimately under thyroid control. This ought to bring about a major reassessment of what constitutes a threat to primordial events, because in the last analysis a great deal may depend on the maintenance of locally generated ammonia in the environment of proliferating and differentiating cells. This probably means that the balance between prolactin and thyroid hormones is more important than either alone.

Lastly, in considering amphibia, what emerges from comprehensive reviews on the biochemistry of metamorphosis (Bennett & Frieden, 1962; Weber, 1967) is the need to integrate our later knowledge, techniques and resources with the earlier profoundly important observations based in great measure on histology and tissue-grafting experiments (Needham, 1942) which delved into the morphogenetic substratum in a quest for the organizing principles.

Some implications for mammalian developmental pharmacology

In view of the critical importance of thyroid hormones in the metamorphosis and biochemical sequential development of amphibians, and their direction of tissue-specific events, and bearing in mind the balance that must exist between thyroid-mediated (Weber, 1967; Tata, 1971) and prolactin-mediated effects (Meites & Nicoll, 1966; Bern & Nicoll, 1968), some reorientation in research in mammalian developmental pharmacology may be required.

No longer should thyroid effects on Phase I (Kato & Takahashi, 1968; Vesell, 1977; Fishman & Bradlow, 1977) and Phase II drug metabolism (Miettinen & Leskinen, 1970) be regarded as incidental curiosities. One of the features of the largely descriptive catalogues of drugs which penetrate the placenta during gestation (Ginsburg, 1971; Mirkin, 1973; Pomerance & Yaffe, 1973; Hathway, 1975), is that they provide clues to side effects exerted on maternal central nervous system, endocrine system, temperature regulation, plasma protein binding and kidney function.

These clues should be re-evaluated in the context of recent authoritative reviews of thyroid function and developmental competence (Gilman & Murad, 1975; Fisher *et al.*, 1977) and thyroid hormone synthesis (Taurog, 1970) in placental mammals. Further, these clues should be reassessed in the light of what is known about dopaminergic and oestrogenic controls of prolactin release, which have also been well documented in connection with mammalian development and function (Meites *et al.*, 1972; Frantz, Kleinberg & Noel, 1972).

Whilst it is beyond the scope of this review to deal with all the complex interrelationships that exist for integrating the pathways of iodine metabolism (Gilman & Murad, 1975), it is instructive to compare the effects of various drugs on the iodination of bovine serum albumin with thyroid peroxidase (Taurog, 1970), a model system for the iodination of tyrosyl residues in protein in the presence of hydrogen peroxide (Table 2.5). Compounds that interfere include not only overtly anti-thyroid compounds

Table 2.5.   Effect of various compounds on iodination of bovine serum albumin with thyroid peroxidase.
Thyroid peroxidase, ^{131}I-labelled iodide, bovine serum albumin and added compound in buffer were preincubated. Reaction started with H_2O_2 was analysed after further incubation under standard conditions.

Compound added	Concentration (M)	Iodination (% of control)
None	—	100
1-Methyl-2-mercaptoimidazole	5×10^{-5}	0.76
Thiouracil	5×10^{-5}	0.95
Thiourea	5×10^{-5}	1.3
Thiocyanate	5×10^{-5}	27.5
Reduced glutathione	5×10^{-5}	17.8
Cysteine	5×10^{-5}	103.7
Resorcinol	5×10^{-6}	1.5
Phloroglucinol	5×10^{-6}	1.1

Data from Taurog (1970).

like thiouracil and thiourea, but resorcinol, phloroglucinol, aminotriazole and reduced glutathione.

The generation of hydrogen peroxide in thyroid cells, required for the iodination of tyrosine residues in thyroglobulin and their subsequent coupling to form tri-iodothyronine and thyroxine, further emphasizes the importance of the NADPH-cytochrome c reductase enzyme link with thyroid function established by Tata *et al.* (1962, 1963) and Kato & Takahashi (1968).

Although the precise details of interconversion of thyroxine, tri-iodothyronine and mono- and di-iodotyrosines are not known, it does seem probable that drugs and environmental chemicals that can be dehalo-genated, or others that can bind to thyroglobulin or covalently sequester iodide, may turn out to be hitherto unsuspected thyroid antimetabolites needing reassessment in terms of developmental toxicology. Other drugs and environmental chemicals that prevent thyroxine-mediated effects on carbamyl phosphate synthetase activity ought to be re-examined, for their value in developmental pharmacology would be likely to become restricted to that of research tools.

With regard to control of anterior pituitary prolactin secretion in mammals (Meites *et al.*, 1972), it is known that in females, prolactin secretion rises at the time of puberty, rises at mating, and then declines during pregnancy. Before parturition, and after parturition in response to the suck-ling stimulus there is a surge in prolactin release. The pituitary prolactin secretion appears to be under dopaminergic inhibitory control of the hypo-thalamus, and is directly stimulated by oestrogens. Again, it is beyond the scope of this review to analyse the function of prolactin in both sexes in detail.

Nevertheless some comments are necessary, since prolactin is involved in mammary growth, mammary tumour induction, and quite specific modula-tion of tumour induction brought about by dimethylbenzanthracene

(Meites & Nicoll, 1966). Hypothalamic inhibitory control of prolactin release from the pituitary can be depressed (with resultant increase in prolactin secretion) with phenothiazines and other drugs used in psychiatric disorders (Byck, 1975), or increased with ergot alkaloids (Meites *et al.*, 1972). It is of considerable toxicological interest that dibenzanthracene-induced tumour incidence can be increased in experimental animals with haloperidol, and decreased with ergot alkaloids.

Drugs used in psychiatric disorders such as phenothiazines, tricyclic anti-depressants, butyrophenones and rauwolfia alkaloids, could, because of their action on the hypothalamus affect the maintenance of appropriate prolactin levels in pregnancy. Perhaps, in view of the as yet incompletely understood antipodal effects of prolactin and thyroid function at the time of birth (Fisher *et al.*, 1977), more research into the effects of these drugs during pregnancy is needed.

Lastly, prolactin control is also involved in foetal lung maturation (Hauth *et al.*, 1978), and prolactin secretion is responsive to thyroid releasing hormone (Tashijan, Barowsky & Jensen, 1971). Since, as was discussed in an earlier section, urethane (ethyl carbamate) is not only teratogenic, but transplacentally carcinogenic to the new-born, depending on species (Mirvish, 1968), it would seem possible that the exceptional developmental toxicity of urethane was in some way related to a prolactin factor, or to a combined aberration of thyroid- and prolactin-mediated developmental control mechanisms.

References

Allen, B.M. (1916). *Science*, 44, 755.
Asling, J.L. and Way, E.L. (1971). In *Fundamentals of Drug Metabolism and Disposition*, Editors: La Du, B.N., Mandel, H.G. and Way, E.L., p. 88. Baltimore: Williams and Wilkins.
Bend, J.R., James, M.O., Devereux, T.R. and Fouts, J.R. (1975). In *Basic and Therapeutic Aspects of Perinatal Pharmacology*, Editors: Morselli, P.L., Garattini, S. and Sereni, F., p. 229. New York: Raven Press.
Bennett, T.P. and Frieden, E. (1962). In *Comparative Biochemistry*, Editors: Florkin, M. and Mason, H.S., Vol. 4, p. 483. New York: Academic Press.
Bern, H.A. and Nicoll, C.S. (1968). *Recent Progr. Hormone Res.*, 24, 681.
Booth, J. and Gillette, J.R. (1962). *J. Pharmac. exp. Ther.*, 137, 374.
Boréus, L.O. (1973). *Fetal Pharmacology*. New York: Raven Press.
Boylen, J.B., Horne, H.H. and Johnson, W.J. (1963). *Lancet*, 1, 552.
Brodie, B.B. (1956). *J. Pharm. Pharmac.*, 8, 1.
Brodie, B.B. and Hogben, C.A.M. (1957). *J. Pharm. Pharmac.*, 9, 345.
Brodie, B.B. and Maickel, R.P. (1962). In *Proceedings of the First International Pharmacology Meeting, Vol. 6*, Editors: Brodie, B.B. and Erdös, E.G., p. 299. London: Pergamon Press.
Brodie, B.B., Maickel, R.P. and Jondorf, W.R. (1958). *Fedn. Proc.*, 17, 1163.
Brown, G.W., Brown, W.R. and Cohen, P.P. (1959). *J. biol. Chem.*, 234, 1775.
Brown, A.K. and Zuelzer, W.W. (1958), *J. clin. Invest.*, 37, 332.
Burchell, B., Dutton, G.J. and Nemeth, A.M. (1972). *J. Cell Biol.*, 55, 448.
Butler, T.C. (1961). *J. Pharmac. exp. Ther.*, 134, 311.
Butros, J. (1972). *Teratology*, 6, 181.
Byck, R. (1975). In *The Pharmacological Basis of Therapeutics*, Editors: Goodman, L.S. and Gilman, A., 5th edition, p. 152. New York: Macmillan.

Caldwell, J., Moffatt, J.R., Smith, R.L., Lieberman, B.A., Beard, R.W., Snedden, W. and Wilson, B.W. (1977). *Biomed. Mass Spectrom.*, 4, 322.
Cooley, H. & Janssens, P.A. (1977). *Gen. comp. Endocrinol.*, 33, 352.
Conney, A.H. (1967). *Pharmac. Rev.*, 19, 317.
Conney, A.H. (1974). In *The Biochemistry of Disease*, Editors: T'So, P. and Di Paolo, J.A., p. 353. New Yolrk: Marcel Dekker.
Conney, A.H., Gillette, J.R., Inscoe, J.K., Trams, E.H. and Posner, H.S. (1959). *Science*, 130, 1478.
Dallner, G., Siekevitz, P. and Palade, G.E. (1965). *Biochem. Biophys. Res. Commun.*, 20, 135.
Daly, J.W., Jerina, D.M. and Witkop, B. (1972). *Experientia*, 28, 1129.
Dancis, J. and Hwang, J.C. (1974). *Perinatal Pharmacology: Problems and Priorities.* New York: Raven Press.
Davies, D.S., Gigon, P.L. and Gillette, J.R. (1969). *Life Sciences*, 8 (II), 85.
Dawkins, M.J.R. (1963). *J. Path. Bact.*, 85, 189.
Debackere, M. and Uehleke, H. (1964). *Proc. Eur. Soc. Study Drug Toxicity*, 4, 40.
Di Paolo, J.A. and Elis, J. (1967). *Cancer Res.*, 27, 1696.
Domsky, I.I., Lijinsky, W., Spencer, K. and Shubik, P. (1963). *Proc. Soc. exp. Biol. Med.*, 113, 110.
Done, A.K. (1966). *Ann. Rev. Pharmac.*, 6, 189.
Driscoll, S.G. and Hsia, D.Y.-Y. (1958). *Pediatrics*, 22, 785.
Drummond, A.H., McCall, J.M. and Jondorf, W.R. (1972). *Biochem. J.*, 130, 73P.
Dutton, G.J. (1973). *Enzyme*, 15, 304.
Dutton, G.J. and Ko, V. (1966). *Biochem. J.,* 99, 550.
Dutton, G.J., Wishart, G.J., Leakey, J.E.A. and Goheer, M.A. (1977). In *Drug Metabolism —from Microbe to Man*, Editors: Parke, D.V. and Smith, R.L., p. 71. London: Taylor & Francis.
Dvorchik, B.H., Stenger, V.G. and Quattropani, S.L. (1974). *Drug Metab. Disp.*, 2, 539.
Eriksson, M. and Yaffe, S.J. (1973). *Ann. Rev. Med.*, 24, 29.
Fabro, S., Schumacher, H., Smith, R.L. and Williams, R.T. (1964). *Nature*, 201, 1125.
Fabro, S. and Smith, R.L. (1966). *J. Path. Bact.*, 91, 511.
Finster, M. and Mark, L.C. (1971). In *Concepts in Biochemical Pharmacology Part I*, Editors: Brodie, B.B. and Gillette, J.R., p. 276. New York: Springer Verlag.
Fisher, D.A., Dussault, J.H., Sack, J. and Chopra, I.J. (1977). *Recent Progr. Hormone Res.*, 33, 59.
Fishman, J. and Bradlow, H.L. (1977). *Clin. Pharmac. Ther.*, 22, 721.
Fiume, L. (1965). *Lancet*, 1, 1284.
Fouts, J.R. and Adamson, R.H. (1959). *Science*, 129, 897.
Frantz, A.G. Kleinberg, D.L. and Noel, G.L. (1972). *Recent Progr. Hormone Res.*, 28, 527.
Fyffe, J. and Dutton, G.J. (1975). *Biochim. Biophys. Acta*, 411, 41.
Gasche, P. and Druey, J. (1946). *Experientia*, 2, 26.
Gaudette, L.E. Maickel, R.P. and Brodie, B.B. (1958). *Fedn Proc.*, 17, 370.
Geigy, R. (1941). *Rev. Suisse Zool.*, 48, 483.
Gelboin, H.V., Kinoshita, N. and Wiebel, F.J. (1972). *Fedn Proc.*, 31, 1298.
Gillette, J.R. (1966). *Adv. Pharmac.*, 4, 219.
Gilman, A.G. and Murad, F. (1975). In *The Pharmacological Basis of Therapeutics*, Editors: Goodman, L.S. and Gilman, A., 5th Edition, p. 1398. New York: Macmillan.
Ginsburg, J. (1971). *Ann. Rev. Pharmac.*, 11, 387.
Glende, E.A. and Recknagel, R.O. (1969). *Exp. Molec. Path.*, 11, 172.
Grant, W.C. and Cooper, G. (1965). *Biol. Bull.*, 129, 510.
Greengard, O. (1974). In *Perinatal Pharmacology: Problems and Priorities*, Editors: Dancis, J. and Hwang, J.C., p. 15. New York: Raven Press.
Grieninger, G. and Granick, S. (1975). *Proc. Nat. Acad. Sci.*, 72, 5007.
Grover, P.L. (1977). In *Drug Metabolism — from Microbe to Man*, Editors: Parke, D.V. and Smith, R.L., p. 105. London: Taylor & Francis.
Gudernatsch, J.F. (1912). *Arch. Entwicklings Mech. Organismen*, 35, 457.
Gutman, Y. and Kidron, M. (1971). *Biochem. Pharmac.*, 20, 3547.
Hänninen, O. (1975). *Acta Pharmac. Tox.* 36, Suppl. II, 3.

Hart, L.G., Adamson, R.H., Dixon, R.L. and Fouts, J.R. (1962). *J. Pharmac. exp. Ther.*, 137, 103.

Hathway, D.E. (1975). In *Foreign Compound Metabolism in Mammals, Vol. 3*, Editor: Hathway, D.E., p. 631, London: The Chemical Society.

Hauth, J.C., Parker, C.R., MacDonald, P.C., Porter, J.C. and Johnston, J.M. (1978). *Obstet. Gynecol.*, 51, 81.

Henderson, P.T. (1971). *Biochem. Pharmac.*, 20, 1225.

Herbst, A.L. and Scully, A.E. (1970). *Cancer*, 25, 745.

Herbst, A.L., Ulfelder, H. and Poskanzer, D.C. (1971). *New Engl. J. Med.*, 284, 878.

Hill, R.M., Horning, M.G. and Horning, E.C. (1973). In *Fetal Pharmacology*, Editor: Boréus, L.O., p. 375, New York: Raven Press.

Hitchcock, M. and Murphy, S.D. (1971). *Toxic. appl. Pharmac.*, 19, 37.

Hoffmann, O. and Gudernatsch, F. (1933). *Endocrinol.*, 17, 239.

Holtfreter, J. (1933). *Naturwiss.*, 21, 766.

Holtzman, J.L., Gram, T.E., Gigon, P.L. and Gillette, J.R. (1968). *Biochem. J.*, 110, 407.

Hoskins, E.R. and Hoskins, M.M. (1917). *Proc. Soc. Exp. Biol. Med.*, 14, 74.

Hsia, D.Y.-Y., Dowben, R.M., Shaw, R. and Grossman, A. (1960). *Nature*, 187, 693.

Jondorf, W.R., Maickel, R.P. and Brodie, B.B. (1958). *Biochem. Pharmac.*, 1, 352.

Jondorf, W.R., Maickel, R.P. and Brodie, B.B. (1959). *Fedn Proc.*, 18, 407.

Jondorf, W.R., MacIntyre, D.E. and Powis, G. (1973). *Br. J. Pharmac.*, 47, 624P.

Jost, J.-P. and Rickenberg, H.V. (1971). *Ann. Rev. Biochem.*, 40, 741.

Juchau, M.R. (1971). *Toxic. appl. Pharmac.*, 18, 665.

Juchau, M.R. (1975). In *Basic and Therapeutic Aspects of Perinatal Pharmacology*, Editors: Morselli, P., Garattini, S. and Sereni, F., p. 29. New York: Raven Press.

Juchau, M.R., Lee, Q.H., Louviaux, G.L., Symms, K.G., Krasner, J. and Yaffe, S.J. (1973). In *Fetal Pharmacology*, Editor: Boréus, L.O., p. 321. New York: Raven Press.

Juchau, M.R., Symms, K.G. and Zachariah, P.K. (1974). In *Perinatal Pharmacology: Problems and Priorities*, Editors: Dancis, J. and Hwang, J.C., p. 89. New York: Raven Press.

Kagen, L.J. and Linder, S. (1972). *Proc. Soc. exp. Biol. Med.*, 140, 1325.

Karnofsky, D.A. and Lacon, C.R. (1962). *Fedn Proc.*, 21, 379.

Karnofsky, D.A. and Young, C.W. (1967). *Fedn Proc.*, 26, 1139.

Kato, R. and Takahashi, A. (1968). *Molec. Pharmac.*, 4, 109.

Kato, R., Vassanelli, P., Frontino, G. and Chiesara, E. (1964). *Biochem. Pharmac.*, 13, 1037.

Keberle, H., Loustalot, P., Maller, R.K., Faigle, J.W. and Schmid, K. (1965). *Ann. N.Y. Acad. Sci.*, 123, 252.

Klein, M. (1952). *J. Nat. Cancer Inst.*, 12, 1005.

Klein, M. (1954). *Cancer Res.*, 14, 438.

Ko, V., Dutton, G.J. and Nemeth, A.M. (1967). *Biochem. J.*, 104, 991.

Kuru, M., Kosaki, G. and Watanabe, H. (1962). *Gann*, 54, 119.

Landauer, W. and Clark, E.M. (1964). *Nature*, 203, 527.

Larsen, C.D. (1947). *J. Nat. Cancer Inst.*, 8, 63.

Larsson, K.S. (1973). In *Fetal Pharmacology*, Editor: Boréus, L.O., p. 401. New York: Raven Press.

Lenz, W. (1961). *Deutsch. Med. Wschr.*, 86, 2555.

Liedke, K.B., Engelman, M. and Graff, S. (1955). *Anat. Record*, 123, 359.

Lutwak-Mann, C. (1973). In *Fetal Pharmacology*, Editor: Boréus, L.O., p. 419. New York: Raven Press.

Lutwak-Mann, C., Schmid, C. and Keberle, H. (1967). *Nature*, 214, 1018.

Mahler, H.R. and Cordes, E.H. (1971). *Biological Chemistry*, 2nd Ed., p. 774. New York: Harper and Row.

Maickel, R.P., Jondorf, W.R. and Brodie, B.B. (1958). *Fedn Proc.*, 17, 390.

Maickel, R.P., Jondorf, W.R. and Brodie, B.B. (1959). *Fedn Proc.*, 18, 418.

Maickel, R.P. and Snodgrass, W.R. (1973). *Toxic. appl. Pharmac.*, 26, 218.

Mainwaring, W.I.P. (1977). In *The Mechanism of Action of Androgens*, p. 23. Heidelberg: Springer.

Marchand, C., McLean, S., Plaa, G.L. and Traiger, G. (1971). *Biochem. Pharmac.*, 20, 869.

Marsh, C.A. (1969). *Proc. Aust. Biochem. Soc.*, 2, 69.

McBride, W.G. (1961). *Lancet*, 2, 1358.
Meites, J., Lu, K.H., Wuttke, W., Welsch, C.W., Nagasawa, H. and Quadri, S.K. (1972). *Recent Progr. Hormone Res.*, 28, 471.
Meites, J. and Nicoll, C.S. (1966). *Ann. Rev. Physiol.*, 28, 57.
Metzenberg, R.L., Marshall, M., Paik, W.K. and Cohen, P.P. (1961). *J. biol. Chem.*, 236, 162.
Miettinen, T.A. and Leskinen, E. (1970). In *Metabolic Conjugation and Metabolic Hydrolysis*, Vol. 1, Editor: Fishman, W.H., p. 157. New York: Academic Press.
Mirkin, B.L. (1970). *Ann. Rev. Pharmac.*, 10, 255.
Mirkin, B. (1971). *J. Pediatr.*, 78, 329.
Mirkin, B.L. (1973). In *Fetal Pharmacology*, Editor: Boréus, L.O., p. 1. New York: Raven Press.
Mirvish, S.S. (1968). *Adv. Cancer Res.*, 11, 1.
Mirvish, S. Cividalli, G. and Berenblum, I. (1964). *Proc. Soc. exp. Biol. Med.*, 116, 265.
Mitchell, J.R., Reid, W.D., Christie, B., Moskowitz, J., Krishna, G. and Brodie, B.B. (1971). *Res. Commun. Chem. Path. Pharmac.*, 2, 877.
Morselli, P.L., Garattini, S. and Sereni, F. (1975). *Basic and Therapeutic Aspects of Perinatal Pharmacology*. New York: Raven Press.
Munro, A.F. (1939). *Biochem. J.*, 33, 1957.
Munro, A.F. (1953). *Biochem. J.*, 54, 29.
Nebert, D.W. and Gelboin, H.V. (1969). *Arch. Biochem. Biophys.*, 134, 76.
Nebert, D.W. and Gielen, J.E. (1972). *Fedn Proc.*, 31, 1315.
Nebert, D.W., Levitt, R.C., Orlando, M.M. and Felton, J.S. (1977). *Clin. Pharmac. Ther.*, 22, 640.
Needham, J. (1931). *Chemical Embryology*, p. 1082. Cambridge: Cambridge University Press.
Needham, J. (1942). *Biochemistry and Morphogenesis*. Cambridge: Cambridge University Press.
Nelson, B.T. (1969). *Science*, 166, 977.
Netter, K.J. (1976). In *Proceedings of the Sixth International Congress of Pharmacology*, Editor: Kärki, N.T., Vol. 6, p. 3. Oxford: Pergamon Press.
Netter, K.J. and Bergheim, P. (1975). In *Basic and Therapeutic Aspects of Perinatal Pharmacology*, Editors: Morselli, P., Garattini, S. and Sereni, F., p. 39. New York: Raven Press.
Niwa, A., Kumaki, K. and Nebert, D.W. (1975). *Molec. Pharmac.*, 11, 399.
Oesch, F. (1975). In *Basic and Therapeutic Aspects of Perinatal Pharmacology*, Editors: Morselli, P.L., Garattini, S. and Sereni, F., p. 53. New York: Raven Press.
Orrenius, S. (1976). In *Proceedings of the Sixth International Congress of Pharmacology*, Editor: Kärki, N.T., Vol. 6, p. 39. Oxford: Pergamon Press.
Paik, W.K. and Cohen, P.P. (1960). *J. gen. Physiol.*, 43, 683.
Paik, W.K. and Cohen, P.P. (1961). *J. biol. Chem.*, 236, 531.
Patterson, D.S.P. and Roberts, B.A. (1971). *Biochem. Pharmac.*, 20, 3377.
Pelkonen, O., Arvela, P. and Kärki, N.T. (1971). *Acta Pharmac. Tox.*, 30, 385.
Pelkonen, O., Korhonen, P., Jouppila, P. and Kärki, N.T. (1975). In *Basic and Therapeutic Aspects of Perinatal Pharmacology*, Editors: Morselli, P.L., Garattini, S. and Sereni, F., p. 65. New York: Raven Press.
Poland, A. and Glover, E. (1974). *Molec. Pharmac.*, 10, 349.
Poland, A. and Glover, E. (1975). *Molec. Pharmac.*, 11, 389.
Poland, A. and Kappas, A. (1971). *Molec. Pharmac.*, 7, 697.
Pomerance, J.J. and Yaffe, J.J. (1973). *Current Problems in Pediatrics*, Vol. 4, Part 1, p. 1. Chicago: Year Book Medical Publishers.
Powis, G., Drummond, A.H., MacIntyre, D.E. and Jondorf, W.R. (1976). *Xenobiotica*, 6, 69.
Quinn, G.P., Axelrod, J. and Brodie, B.B. (1958). *Biochem. Pharmac.*, 1, 152.
Rane, A., von Bahr, C., Orrenius, S. and Sjöqvist, F. (1973a). In *Fetal Pharmacology*, Editor: Boréus, L.O., p. 287. New York: Raven Press.
Rane, A., Berggren, M., Yaffe, S. and Ericsson, J.L.E. (1973b). *Xenobiotica*, 3, 37.
Renfree, M. and Heap, R.B. (1977). *Theriogenol.*, 8, 164.
Robinson, J.R., Felton, J.S., Thorgeirsson, S.S. and Nebert, D.W. (1975). In *Basic and Therapeutic Aspects of Perinatal Pharmacology*, Editors: Morselli, P.L., Garattini, S. and Sereni, F., p. 155. New York: Raven Press.

Roth, P.C.J. (1953). *Compt. Rend. Soc. Biol.*, 147, 1140.

Schenker, S., Dawber, N.H. and Schmid, R. (1964). *J. clin. Invest.*, 43, 32.

Schindler, J. and Sussman, M. (1977). *Biochem. Biophys. Res. Commun.*, 79, 611.

Schlede, E. and Merker, H.-J. (1972). *Naunyn Schmiedebergs Arch. Pharmac.*, 272, 89.

Schmidt-Nielsen, K. (1967). *Fedn Proc.,* 26, 981.

Schumacher, H., Smith, R.L. and Williams, R.T. (1965). *Br. J. Pharmac. Chemother.*, 25, 324.

Schwind, J.L. (1933). *J. exp. Zool.*, 66, 1.

Sereni, F. and Principi, N. (1968). *Ann. Rev. Pharmac.*, 8, 453.

Sharman, G.B. and Pilton, P.E. (1964). *Proc. Zool. Soc. (Lond.)*, 142, Pt. I, 29.

Shideman, F.E. and Ignarro, L.J. (1967). *Fedn Proc.*, 26, 1137.

Short, R.C., Maines, M.D. and Westfall, B.A. (1972). *Biol. Neonate*, 21, 54.

Sieber, S.M. and Fabro, S. (1971), *J. Pharmac. exp. Ther.*, 176, 65.

Smith, W.E. and Rous, P. (1948). *J. exp. Med.*, 88, 520.

Sparschu, D.L., Dunn, F.L. and Rowe, V.K. (1971). *Fd Cosmet. Toxic.*, 9, 405.

Spencer, B. and Raftery, J. (1966). *Biochem. J.*, 99, 35P.

Takimoto, M. and Matsuda, I. (1971). *Biol. Neonate*, 18, 66.

Tashijan, A.H., Barowsky, N.J. and Jensen, D.K. (1971). *Biochem. Biophys. Res. Commun.*, 43, 516.

Tata, J.R. (1971). *Current Topics Dev. Biol.*, 6, 79.

Tata, J.R., Ernster, L. and Lindberg, O. (1962). *Nature*, 193, 1058.

Tata, J.R. Ernster, L., Lindberg, O., Arrhenius, E., Pedersen, S. and Hedman, R. (1963). *Biochem. J.*, 86, 408.

Taurog, A. (1970). *Recent Progr. Hormone Res.*, 26, 189.

Telegdy, G. (1973). In *Fetal Pharmacology*, Editor: Boréus, L.O., p. 335. New York: Raven Press.

Ullberg, S. (1973). In *Fetal Pharmacology*, Editor: Boréus, L.O., p. 55. New York: Raven Press.

Underhay, E.E. and Baldwin, E. (1955). *Biochem. J.*, 61, 544.

Vesell, E.S. (1977). *Clin. Pharmac. Ther.*, 22, 659.

Waddington, C.H., Needham, J. and Needham, D.M. (1933). *Naturwiss.*, 21, 771.

Waddell, W.J. (1972). *Fedn Proc.*, 31, 52.

Wald, G. (1958). *Science*, 128, 1481.

Weber, R. (1967). In *The Biochemistry of Animal Development*, Vol. 2, Editor: Weber, R., p. 227. New York: Academic Press.

Weiss, C.F., Glazko, A.J. and Weston, J.K. (1960). *New Engl. J. Med.*, 262, 787.

Welch, R.M., Gommi, B., Alvares, A.P. and Conney, A.H. (1972). *Cancer Res.*, 32, 973.

Whipple, G.H. (1912). *J. exp. Med.*, 15, 259.

Wieland, T. (1968). *Science*, 159, 946.

Williams, R.T. (1959). *Detoxication Mechanisms*, 2nd Ed., p. 717. London: Chapman and Hall.

Wilson, J.G. (1971). *Fedn Proc.,* 30, 104.

Wishart, G.J. and Dutton, G.J. (1975a). *Biochem. J.*, 152, 325.

Wishart, G.J. and Dutton, G.J. (1975b). *Biochem. Pharmac.*, 24, 451.

Wit, J.G. (1977). In *Drug Metabolism — from Microbe to Man*, Editors: Parke, D.V. and Smith, R.L., p. 247. London: Taylor & Francis.

Yaffe, S.J., Levy, G., Matsuzawa, T. and Baliah, T. (1966). *New Engl. J. Med.*, 275, 1461.

Yaffe, S.J., Rane, A., Sjöqvist, F., Boréus, L.O. and Orrenius, S. (1970). *Life Sci.*, 9 (II), 1189.

3. Genetic factors affecting side effects of drugs

A. R. Boobis

Introduction

Every drug will produce side effects in all members of the population if given at a sufficiently high dose. These side effects may be an exaggeration of the desired pharmacological effect of the drug, or may result from a different pharmacological action altogether; e.g., clonidine is used as a centrally-acting hypotensive agent but produces sedation as a common side effect (Connolly *et al.*, 1972). Some drugs at a normal dose, however, will produce a side effect in certain subjects, and some subjects may show marked differences in sensitivity to the drug. Such abnormal responses, occurring at therapeutic doses, have been termed idiosyncratic drug reactions.

The effect of a drug will depend, in most instances, on the tissue concentration of the drug, which in turn, will depend upon absorption, distribution, metabolism and excretion of the drug. Furthermore, most drug effects depend upon interaction of that drug with receptor sites, such as enzyme active sites or membrane-bound receptors. At each of these points, in the complex sequence of events determining a particular response to a drug, specific proteins are involved and each of these proteins is the product of a single structural gene (the 'one gene-one enzyme' concept). Genetic differences in the formation of any one of these proteins could lead to idiosyncratic drug reactions. This frequently occurs and is the basis of pharmacogenetics (Motulsky, 1957). However, this realization still leaves the problem of identifying these idiosyncratic reactions from normal variation within the population. Although it could be argued that many such variations within the normal range are a reflection of subtle genetic differences within a complex, multifactorial system, drug idiosyncrasy is usually regarded as a discontinuity from the normal range of drug responses. Such a definition can lead to significant differences in the contribution of a small number of genes being overlooked. For example, in a study on red cell acid phosphatase activity Eze *et al.* (1974) found that the distribution of this enzyme activity was unimodal and Gaussian in the members of 50 British families (Figure 3.1(*a*)). However, when the population was analysed for the frequencies of each of the five possible electrophoretic phenotypes of the enzyme known (Hopkinson, Spencer & Harris, 1963), a distinct polymorphism was found to exist (Figure 3.1(*b*)) as the enzyme is controlled by three alleles at a single locus.

Observation of pharmacogenetic sub-groups within the population may come about in two different ways. If genetic differences in one aspect of the response to a drug become of paramount importance, then sub-groups may be identified due to a discontinuity in that response. The observation

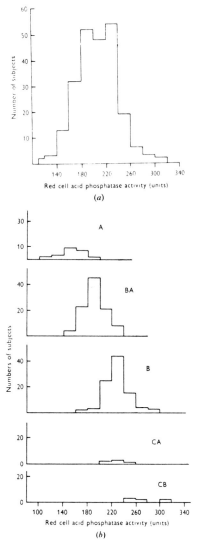

Fig. 3.1.   Frequency distribution histogram of red-cell acid phosphatase activites (*a*) in 234 subjects, and (*b*) in individuals of the five phenotypic categories. The five phenotypes in Figure 1(*b*) are denoted (from top to bottom) A, BA, B, CA and CB. (Data from Eze *et al.* (1974). From Atlas & Nebert (1977) by permission of the authors and Taylor & Francis Ltd.)

that some subjects responded to succinylcholine with a prolonged apnoea revealed the existence of atypical cholinesterase (Kalow & Genest, 1957). Alternatively, identification of sub-groups may occur when some parameter being observed is closely associated with an interaction of the drug and the gene product in which genetic differences exist. Recording rates of isoniazid acetylation revealed the polymorphism for drug acetylation (Evans & White, 1964).

In pharmacogenetic studies, some response to a drug administered to a population is measured and a frequency histogram is plotted. When the population falls within one curve, the response being measured is probably regulated by a number of genes and hence is said to be under polygenic or multifactorial control. The population is said to be unimodal. If the histogram is discontinuous, i.e. there are two or more modes, there may only be one gene regulating the response and each mode is said to represent a single phenotype. The existence of more than one phenotype represents a polymorphism and control is monogenic.

The possibility that a polymorphism exists in the response to a drug can be investigated in a number of ways. One could analyse existing clinical data on an empirical basis but the frequent occurrence of polygenic regulation by a small number of genes as for acid phosphatase means that a number of polymorphisms would be missed. A better approach is by twin studies. Variation in drug response is determined in fraternal and identical twins and this enables the genetic contribution to such variation to be determined. Family studies, in addition to providing evidence for possible genetic differences in drug response, may also enable the type of inheritance to be determined. There are a number of sophisticated mathematical approaches that may be used in the analysis of population or family data to determine the contribution of genetic factors to variation in drug response. The reader is referred to an article by Evans (1977) for details of such approaches. Finally, animal models, using highly inbred strains, have enabled the identification of several genetic polymorphisms in drug effect that would have been difficult to demonstrate otherwise. However, the cause of such a polymorphism in an animal model may not be the cause of a similar polymorphism in man. Animal models do enable the consequences of genetic polymorphism to be investigated on a mechanistic basis rarely possible in man.

Normal man has 22 pairs of autosomes and one pair of sex chromosomes. The basic unit of the chromosome is the gene, each one of which codes for a single polypeptide. Mutation of such structural genes may lead to alterations in the amount or structure of the polypeptide coded for. Mutation of regulator genes, which control the activity of structural genes, may lead to altered amounts of the proteins coded for by the genes they regulate, but rarely would the structure of such proteins be affected. In diploid cells, the synthesis of each protein is governed by a single locus at the same position on the corresponding chromosome from each parent. There are thus two genes involved, known as alleles or allelic genes. Theoretically, in a completely inbred strain, at every locus the two alleles would be identical to each other. The net expression of a pair of allelic genes is known as the phenotype, whereas the actual nature of the two genes involved is known as the genotype. When the two alleles at a locus are identical, the genotype is homozygous, whereas when the two alleles are different, the genotype is heterozygous. Although, obviously, there can never be more than two alleles at the same locus in a single individual there may be several possible alleles at that locus within the population.

When there is full expression of a trait in the heterozygote, that trait is said to be dominant, and when expression of a trait occurs only in the homozygote for that trait, it is said to be recessive. Autosomally-linked traits are those determined by any of the non-sex chromosomes, whereas X-linked traits are those determined by the X-chromosomes. Since males have only one X-chromosome, all X-linked traits, whether dominant or recessive, will be expressed in male subjects. For many dominant traits expression of one gene in the heterozygote is sufficient to produce the trait fully, and thus the heterozygote cannot be identified. However, in autosomal recessive conditions the heterozygote may produce altered amounts or type of protein due to expression of both genes, thus enabling detection of the heterozygote.

Classification of genetic disorders affecting drug side effects

Pharmacogenetic disorders may be classified in numerous ways, e.g. according to the mode of inheritance, the drug involved, or the lesion produced. None is ideal. Some disorders may fit equally well into different divisions within a particular classification. For example, altered excretion of a compound may be due to a disorder of tubular reabsorption, thus enabling such a trait to be classified as either an excretion defect or an absorption defect.

For this review, the various disorders have been classified as shown in Figure 3.2. The major division is into disorders of drug handling and those of drug response. Disorders of drug handling are those in which a normal dose of a drug produces an abnormal response because there is an

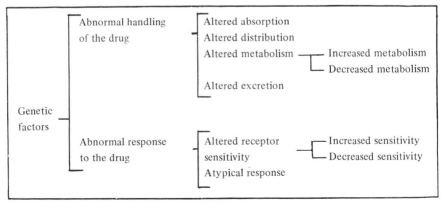

Fig. 3.2.   Classification of genetic factors affecting side effects of drugs.

inappropriate concentration of drug at the receptor site. In such disorders there is a normal response to a dose of drug adjusted such that an appropriate concentration is achieved at the active site. These disorders have been further divided into those that may be attributed to changes in absorption, distribution, metabolism and excretion of the drugs. Disorders of drug response are those in which there is an abnormal response to a concentration of drug at the receptor site that would produce a normal response at a normal receptor site. These disorders have been further divided into those in which there is altered receptor sensitivity and those in which the response is atypical.

Of necessity this classification is somewhat arbitrary. For example, a defect in one of the enzymes of drug metabolism would be classified as an alteration in drug metabolism. However, it could be argued that it also represents a disorder with decreased receptor affinity or perhaps with altered enzyme response. Thus any classification serves merely as a convenient framework from which to operate.

Altered absorption of drugs

Most drugs are given orally and are absorbed into the systemic circulation from the small intestine and, to a lesser extent, from the stomach. Drug absorption is affected by a variety of factors such as gastro-intestinal pH, gastric emptying time, and active transport processes in the small intestine. Almost nothing is known about genetic factors affecting drug absorption, although there are considerable inter-individual differences. Thus there is a 15-20-fold variation in phenacetin absorption among fasting healthy volunteers (Prescott, Steel & Ferrier, 1970) probably due to differences in the first-pass effect.

Juvenile pernicious anaemia. One example of a genetic abnormality in absorption is juvenile pernicious anaemia, which is caused by defective absorption of vitamin B_{12} from the terminal ileum (McIntyre *et al.*, 1965). Absorption of vitamin B_{12} is facilitated by a gastric glycoprotein called intrinsic factor (Herbert & Castle, 1964) and in juvenile pernicious anaemia this glycoprotein is absent or defective. Thus, subjects with this disorder are resistant to pharmacological doses of vitamin B_{12} given orally, but they may be successfully treated with intra-muscular vitamin B_{12} (McIntyre *et al.*, 1965). Several variants of the disorder have been described. There may be an hereditary absence of intrinsic factor (McIntyre *et al.*, 1965) in which absorption of vitamin B_{12} from the intestine is normal if exogenous intrinsic factor is supplied. In a second form there is production of immunologically normal intrinsic factor but this is unable to promote absorption of vitamin B_{12} (Katz, Lee & Cooper, 1972) and in a third form there is normal intrinsic factor production but absorption of the vitamin B_{12}-intrinsic factor complex is impaired. All variants are characterized by megaloblastic anaemia and neurological disturbances. The very high incidence of the disorder among siblings indicates a genetic basis, and although the mode of inheritance is not known, the frequency of consanguinity among the parents of affected individuals suggests autosomal recessive inheritance.

Altered distribution of drugs

Drug distribution may be affected by changes in regional tissue blood flow, cardiac output, pH gradients across biomembranes, plasma protein binding and cell membrane permeability. Of these, protein binding is of considerable importance since drug effect is proportional to free drug concentration. Increasing protein binding will, therefore, reduce the pharmacological effect. The corollary of this is that for highly protein-bound drugs any decrease in binding may result in toxic effects. Several drug side-effects may be directly attributable to hereditary differences in protein binding. In hereditary analbuminaemia, a disorder in which plasma albumin is virtually absent, drugs that are normally highly protein bound will have exaggerated effects. In Down's syndrome, a congenital defect in which there is an extra chromosome, i.e. trisomy 21, altered protein binding results in increased free salicylate levels (Ebadi & Kugel, 1970). Low serum albumin concentrations, whether hereditary or acquired, have been shown to correlate with adverse reactions in patients treated with prednisolone (Lewis *et al.*, 1971).

Thyroid-binding globulin. Hereditary abnormalities of the α-globulin thyroxine-binding globulin (TBG) have been reported. Autosomal dominant inheritance of a form of TBG that binds twice as much thyroxine as normal TBG has been found in a small group of subjects (Beierwaltes & Robbins, 1959) (Figure 3.3). Ingbar (1961) has reported a disorder of TBG

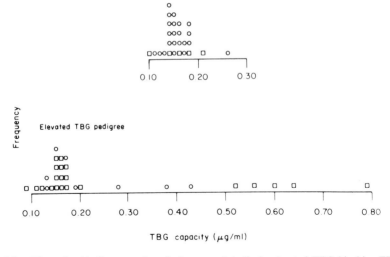

Fig. 3.3. Thyroxine-binding capacity of plasma α-globulin in elevated TBG kinship. TBG capacity is expressed as μg thyroxine bound per ml serum. Binding capacity in normal subjects (upper) and in subjects related to patient with elevated TBG capacity (lower). Squares, males and circles, females. (From Beierwaltes, Carr & Hunter (1961). By permission of William J. Dornan Inc. and John Wiley & Sons Inc.).

in which levels of the globulin are normal but it has almost no affinity for thyroxine. The mode of transmission is X-linked. As a result of the abnormal TBG, thyroxine half-life was increased 50% and free thyroxine entry into tissues was increased (Cavalieri & Searle, 1966). Treatment of affected subjects with oestrogen, which normally increases TBG capacity for thyroxine, was without effect, providing further evidence that the TBG in this disorder has almost no affinity for the hormone. Disorders of TBG may have little or no clinical significance.

Altered metabolism of drugs

Most drugs are metabolized in the liver to more polar derivatives before excretion. There are a wide variety of pathways possible and these have been divided broadly into two main groups. In Phase I reactions there are modifications of existing functional groups in the molecule, whereas in Phase II reactions there is conjugation with endogenous small molecules such as sulphate, glucuronic acid and glutathione. Many of the enzymes of drug metabolism catalysing a particular reaction can exist in multiple forms, e.g. glucuronyl transferase, glutathione transferase and the cytochrome P-450 dependent mixed-function oxidases. Each specific form of these enzymes has a particular substrate specificity, sensitivity to inhibitors and inducers, and, for cytochromes P-450 at least, metabolizes the substrate at a particular position on the molecule (site-specific metabolism). The role of metabolism in drug toxicity has already been discussed in Chapter 1. If toxicity of a drug is due to formation of a particular metabolite, then any alteration in the formation of this metabolite will alter its toxicity. From a genetic viewpoint this could arise from deficiencies in alternative routes of metabolism of the parent compound (to metabolites a or e in Figure 3.4),

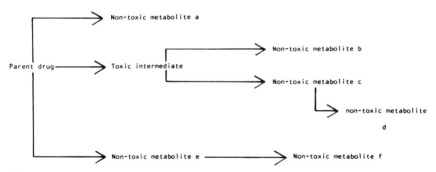

Fig. 3.4. Theoretical routes of metabolism of a model drug. The parent drug may be metabolized by oxidation to non-toxic product a, excreted unchanged, or non-toxic product e, conjugated to metabolite f before excretion. Activation of the drug by oxidation produces a toxic intermediate which may be inactivated to give product b, excreted unchanged, or product c, metabolized further before excretion.

deficiencies in routes of inactivation of the toxic metabolite (to metabolites b or c) or increased activity of the pathway generating the toxic intermediate. For toxic parent compounds, toxicity will be affected by the rate at which the drug is metabolized to inactive products (a or e in Figure 3.5). Since each individual form of the enzymes involved in these pathways is under the control of a single structural gene, mutation of any single gene could result theoretically in altered drug toxicity. Examples of such alterations in specific routes of metabolism leading to drug toxicity are listed below.

Increased drug metabolism

Plasma cholinesterase. Of 1029 male subjects studied, one had plasma cholinesterase (pseudocholinesterase or butyrylcholinesterase) activity 3-fold higher than normal (Neitlich, 1966). This subject showed decreased sensitivity to succinylcholine, a drug whose action is normally terminated by hydrolysis by plasma cholinesterase. Further studies showed that three other members of the subject's family showed a similar abnormality and that this was inherited under autosomal autonomous transmission. However, the trait is functionally dominant since expression of one allele is sufficient to give considerably increased enzyme activity (Neitlich, 1966).

Electrophoretic studies of plasma cholinesterase from affected subjects revealed the presence of a new component of the enzyme which has since been designated the Cynthiana variant. However, organophosphorus inhibitor (DFP) titrations and immunoinactivation studies were normal, so the abnormality may not be in the intrinsic activity of the enzyme, but may be the result of a regulator gene defect perhaps leading to an increased number of enzyme molecules (Yoshida & Motulsky, 1969).

Another variant in plasma cholinesterase, inherited as an autosomal dominant trait, has been found in 5-10% of British subjects studied (Harris *et al.*, 1963). There is an extra variant of plasma cholinesterase present on electrophoresis of plasma from these subjects, which has been designated C_5 (there are four normal components). Activity in the presence of this variant is increased 30% and as such does not influence sensitivity to succinylcholine.

Ethanol. Vesell, Page & Passananti (1971) have shown by twin studies that the rate of ethanol metabolism in normal volunteers is determined almost entirely by genetic factors, with an hereditability index of 0.98. In a study on ethanol metabolism *in vitro*, 20% of the livers from 59 subjects in Switzerland and 4% of those from 50 subjects in England had alcohol dehydrogenase activity 5-6 times higher than normal. However, *in vivo* the difference in ethanol metabolism in subjects with this 'atypical' enzyme was only 40-50% above normal (von Wartburg & Schürch, 1968). Thus the physiological effects of the genetic polymorphism remain unknown. In man, alcohol dehydrogenase is controlled by alleles at three separate structural loci ADH_1, ADH_2 and ADH_3, an allele at each locus producing a different polypeptide chain. It seems that it is an abnormality of the ADH_2 locus that gives rise to the atypical enzyme (Smith, Hopkinson & Harris, 1973).

Cytidine deaminase. Three different electrophoretic patterns of leucocyte cytidine deaminase have been observed in studying a large number of subjects (Teng, Anderson & Giblett, 1975). Homozygotes exhibit a single band that migrates either slowly or rapidly to the anode. In the third pattern, representing the heterozygote, five bands are observed; the two bands observed in the homozygotes plus three intermediate bands. These observations are consistent with cytidine deaminase existing as a tetramer with two possible monomeric forms. Homozygotes would thus possess either one of the two possible homotetramers, whereas the heterozygote would possess all five possible variants (two homotetramers and three heterotetramers). Transmission is as an autosomai autonomous trait. Cytidine deaminase metabolizes cytidine, deoxycytidine, and the nucleoside analogues used in cancer chemotherapy 5-azacytidine and cytosine arabinoside (Chabner *et al.*, 1974). A relative increase (or decrease) in the activity of the different forms of cytidine deaminase may result in altered effectiveness of these chemotherapeutics and alterations in their toxic side effects. Differences in the activity of the variants have yet to be demonstrated.

Acetylation. Isoniazid came into use as an effective antituberculous agent in the early 1950s (Grunberg *et al.*, 1952; Robitzek, Selikoff & Ornstein, 1952). It was soon observed that considerable interindividual differences in isoniazid metabolism exist (Hughes, 1953) and that the main excreted metabolites were acetylisoniazid, isonicotinic acid and the parent compound, although several minor derivatives were also detected (Hughes, Schmidt & Biehl, 1955). Although these large differences in metabolism were observed, urinary excretion of the free and acetylated drug always varied inversely with each other. Early studies in twins suggested a genetic component in acetylating capacity (Bönicke & Lisboa, 1957) and a bimodal distribution of percentage of drug excreted as acetylated metabolite was reported (Biehl, 1957). In 261 subjects from 53 Caucasian families plasma concentrations of isoniazid 6 hours after a normal oral dose were bimodally distributed, enabling subjects to be classified as either fast or slow inactivators (Evans, Manley & McKusick, 1960). It had already been shown that slow inactivation was inherited as an autosomal recessive trait (Knight, Selin & Harris, 1959). These differences were not due to differences in intestinal absorption, protein binding, renal glomerular filtration or renal tubular reabsorption (Jenne, McDonald & Mendoza, 1961). In 1964 it was established that differences in the rate of isoniazid inactivation are due to a polymorphism in the activity of the soluble liver enzyme acetyltransferase (Evans & White, 1964). Isoniazid half-life in fast acetylators is 45-80 min and in slow acetylators 140-200 min (Kalow, 1962). Acetyltransferase has been purified from fast and slow acetylators, but although the fast enzyme has twice the activity of the slow, there are no detectable physicochemical differences between the two forms (Jenne, 1965; Weber, Cohen & Steinberg, 1968). Acetyltransferase, which also exhibits a polymorphism for isoniazid acetylation, has been purified from rabbits, and recent electrophoretic studies suggest possible subtle differences between the two forms (La Du, 1972) although they are identical when compared on the same basis as the human enzymes were (Weber *et al.*, 1968). Acetylation polymorphism may thus be due to a structural defect in the enzyme. Acetyltransferase requires acetyl CoA and is located in liver and jejunal mucosa. In addition to isoniazid other monosubstituted hydrazines may serve as substrates. These include phenelzine, hydralazine, sulphamethazine, sulphapyridine, procainamide, dapsone and the amino metabolite of nitrazepam (Evans, 1965, 1977). The enzyme does not acetylate *p*-aminosalicylic acid, sulphanilamide or *p*-aminobenzoic acid, which are acetylated monomorphically and are probably substrates for another, extrahepatic, acetyltransferase (Weber, 1971).

There are considerable racial differences in the frequency of the slow acetylator phenotype (La Du, 1972) which ranges from 0.22 in Canadian Eskimoes to 0.91 in Egyptians. Orientals also have a low frequency of the phenotype, whereas Scandinavians have a high frequency (Motulsky, 1964). The natural substrate for the enzyme is unknown but the burden of naturally occurring hydrazine compounds is very low (Peters, Miller & Brown, 1965).

Many drug side effects can be directly attributed to differences in acetylator phenotype. Slow acetylators are much more prone to develop toxic peripheral neuropathy on isoniazid therapy (Hughes *et al.*, 1954; Devadatta *et al.*, 1960). This may be prevented by 'rescue' with pyridoxine (Carlson *et al.*, 1956) and is believed to be due to chemical inactivation of pyridoxine by isoniazid with subsequent depletion of this essential cofactor. There may also be competition between the drug and pyridoxal sulphate for apotryptophanase (Robson & Sullivan, 1963).

Since slow acetylation is a recessive trait, fast acetylation will be functionally dominant. In an analysis of almost 14 000 patients taking isoniazid in the United States, Orientals, 90% of whom are genetically fast acetylators, had a higher incidence of hepatic injury than other populations with a lower frequency of the fast acetylator phenotype (Smith *et al.*, 1972). In a follow-up study on 21 non-Oriental subjects who had recovered from isoniazid hepatitis Mitchell *et al.* (1975) found that 18 were fast acetylators. In common with all fast acetylators, these subjects excreted smaller amounts of isoniazid and larger amounts of isonicotinic acid than slow acetylators, yet when acetylisoniazid was administered it was converted to identical amounts of isonicotinic acid in the two groups (Mitchell *et al.*, 1975). The suggested explanation was that isoniazid is acetylated polymorphically to acetylisoniazid and this is then monomorphically hydrolysed to isonicotinic acid and acetylhydrazine. In rats, acetylhydrazine can be converted by cytochrome P-450 mediated *N*-hydroxylation to a potent acetylating agent capable of producing hepatic necrosis (Nelson, Snodgrass & Mitchell, 1975). The greater production of acetylhydrazine could thus explain the higher incidence of hepatic injury in these subjects. Unfortunately this elegant explanation cannot be the whole story. Ellard & Gammon (1977) have shown that the isoniazid metabolite acetylhydrazine is polymorphically acetylated in man, and thus fast acetylators, although producing more acetylhydrazine initially, rapidly convert it to diacetylhydrazine, an inactive product, and thus prevent accumulation of acetylhydrazine. This has been confirmed by Timbrell, Wright & Baillie (1977), who have also demonstrated that the presumptive metabolite, acetylhydrazine, is produced from isoniazid in man. The relationship between acetylation phenotype and isoniazid hepatitis is thus far from clear. Fast acetylators respond more poorly to once-weekly isoniazid therapy for tuberculosis than slow acetylators (Ellard, 1976). Isoniazid inhibits the hydroxylation of phenytoin. Thus inhibition of phenytoin metabolism occurs more frequently, with increased risk of phenytoin toxicity, in slow acetylators, who will have relatively higher concentrations of unchanged isoniazid (Kutt, Winters & McDowell, 1966). There is a higher incidence of antinuclear antibodies (Alarćon-Segovia, Fishbein & Alcala, 1971) and of systemic lupus erythematosus (SLE) like syndrome (Zingale, Minzer, Rosenberg & Lee, 1963) in slow acetylators than in fast acetylators taking isoniazid.

Almost all patients on procainamide therapy for over one year develop antinuclear antibodies. However, the mean duration of therapy to the development of antibodies in 50% of patients for slow acetylators was 2.9 months, whereas in fast acetylators it was 7.3 months (Woosley *et al.*, 1977). In addition, slow acetylators are more likely to develop SLE syndrome, and also to develop it more quickly than fast acetylators, the mean duration of therapy to the onset of SLE being 12 and 51 months respectively (Drayer & Reidenberg, 1977).

Slow acetylators are also more likely to develop SLE on hydralazine than fast acetylators (Perry, 1973). Out of 57 patients on long-term hydralazine therapy, all 12 who developed hydralazine toxicity were slow acetylators (Perry *et al.*, 1970). There also appears to be an association between 'idiopathic', or spontaneous, SLE and slow acetylation. In a survey of the literature, Drayer & Reidenberg (1977) found that 104 out of 132 subjects with spontaneous SLE were slow acetylators. It has been suggested that this provides evidence of a role for environmental compounds in the aetiology of so-called spontaneous SLE. These compounds would probably contain a free amino group, since this is the common feature of drugs that will cause SLE (Drayer & Reidenberg, 1977), and this would be inactivated by polymorphic acetylation. Fast acetylators required 58% higher dose of hydralazine for adequate control of blood pressure than did slow acetylators (Zacest & Koch-Weser, 1972) presumably because the parent drug is responsible for the hypotensive action.

Phenelzine is more likely to cause severe central side effects in slow acetylators than in fast acetylators (Evans, Davison & Pratt, 1965). The antidepressant effects and degree of monoamine oxidase inhibition by phenelzine are also greater in slow acetylators (Johnstone, 1976).

Salicylazosulphapyridine, which consists of sulphapyridine linked to 5-aminosalicylic acid through an azo group, is used in the treatment of ulcerative colitis. The azo group is split in the caecum by bacteria and free 5-aminosalicylic acid, the active constituent of the drug, has a local effect and is excreted unchanged. The sulphapyridine is absorbed into the systemic circulation and is subject to polymorphic acetylation. Side effects which include cyanosis and haemolysis, correlate well with plasma sulphapyridine levels. Thus, there is a higher incidence of side effects in slow acetylators (Das *et al.*, 1973).

Finally, it has been suggested that acetylation may play a role in protecting against bladder cancer caused by certain aromatic amines. Slow acetylators do have a higher incidence of bladder cancer from compounds such as 4-aminobiphenyl, 2-aminonaphthalene and benzidine than fast acetylators (Miller, 1970).

Decreased drug metabolism

Plasma cholinesterase. Plasma cholinesterase synthesis is controlled at two loci that have been designated E_1 and E_2 (Motulsky, 1964) and Ch_1 and Ch_2 (Goedde & Baitsch, 1964). Inheritance is by allelic codominance of the genes at the two loci (i.e. autosomal autonomous inheritance). The possible variants and their properties are shown in Table 3.1. In addition to the variants regulated at the E_2 and $E_{Cynthiana}$ loci that result in increased resistance to the depolarizing neuromuscular blockade of succinylcholine, a

Table 3.1.   Variants of plasma cholinesterase.

Type of enzyme	Genotype	Dibucaine number	Fluoride number	Enzyme activity	Response to succinylcholine	Frequency
Normal	$E_1^u E_1^u$	80	62	60-125	Rapid hydrolysis	(96/100) Normal population
Atypical	$E_1^u E_1^a$	60	50	26-90	Rapid hydrolysis	1/26
	$E_1^a E_1^a$	20	22	< 35	Apnoea	1/2800
Fluoride resistant	$E_1^u E_1^f$	75	52	60-125	Rapid hydrolysis	1/280
	$E_1^f E_1^f$	65	35	60-125	Apnoea	1/300 000
Silent gene	$E_1^u E_1^s$	80	62	Variably decreased	Rapid hydrolysis	1/190
	$E_1^s E_1^s$	–	–	0	Apnoea	1/140 000
Mixed	$E_1^a E_1^f$	50	35	26-90	Apnoea	1/29 000
	$E_1^a E_1^s$	20	22	20	Apnoea	1/20 000
	$E_1^f E_1^s$	65	35	61	Apnoea	1/200 000
C_5	$E_1^+ E_1^+$	80	62	30% above normal	Rapid hydrolysis	1/10 in UK
Elevated activity	$E_{Cynthiana}$ (locus not known)	80	62	2-3 × normal	Resistance	?

(Data from Harris *et al.* (1963); Lehmann & Liddell (1964). By permission of McGraw-Hill Book Corp. and John Wiley & Sons Inc.)

number of forms of the enzyme have been described that have a decreased capacity to metabolize the drug. The normal duration of action of succinylcholine is about 2 min but can increase to 2-3 hours in affected individuals. The prolonged neuromuscular blockade in such subjects leads to prolonged muscular relaxation and apnoea (Lehmann & Ryan, 1956).

Several different genetic abnormalities, all occurring at the E_1 locus, can cause succinylcholine sensitivity. The first was described soon after the drug was introduced and has been called atypical cholinesterase (Kalow & Lindsay, 1955; Kalow & Genest, 1957). The enzyme synthesized has considerably reduced affinity for all substrates (Davies, Marton & Kalow, 1960) and decreased sensitivity to inhibitors, including dibucaine and fluoride (Kalow & Davies, 1959). The defect is probably due to the $E_1{}^a$ allele, and is inherited as an autosomal autonomous trait. The incidence is about 2% evenly distributed throughout most ethnic groups but the allele appears absent in Japanese and Eskimoes and is very rare in Negroes and certain other groups (Lubin, Garry & Owen, 1971).

While studying the inhibition of plasma cholinesterase by dibucaine and fluoride, Harris and Whittaker (1963) found that some subjects exhibited almost normal sensitivity to dibucaine but were resistant to fluoride. The fluoride-resistant form of plasma cholinesterase is due to the presence of the $E_1{}^f$ allele at the E_1 locus.

Lehmann & Liddell (1964) have described a further variant in which there is a so-called silent gene at the E_1 locus, the $E_1{}^S$ allele. There is a very high incidence of this variant in Eskimoes, with 48 affected individuals from a population of 5000 studied (Scott, 1970). Two different forms of this variant have been described. In type 1 there is either total lack of enzyme production (Rubinstein *et al.*, 1970) or production of enzyme with absolutely no activity (Scott, 1973) and in type 2 there is production of 2% of normal enzyme (Rubinstein *et al.*, 1970).

Phenytoin hydroxylation. Defective metabolism of phenytoin was the first reported example of an hereditary abnormality of cytochrome P-450 dependent mixed-function oxidase activity (Kutt *et al.*, 1964b). In one family, the mother and two of four male offspring developed signs of phenytoin toxicity (nystagmus, ataxia and drowsiness) on a therapeutic dose of the drug. The symptoms were alleviated on reduction of the dose. The main route of elimination of phenytoin is by aromatic hydroxylation to 5-phenyl-5'-*p*-hydroxyphenylhydantoin (HPPH) which is then excreted in the urine as the glucuronic acid conjugate. In affected individuals, plasma concentrations of phenytoin were very high while urinary excretion of HPPH and its glucuronide was very low. The defect would seem to be a genetically determined deficiency in the ability to *p*-hydroxylate phenytoin. The resultant high plasma levels of phenytoin would explain the toxicity since there is an excellent correlation between plasma phenytoin and development of side effects to the drug (Kutt *et al.*, 1964a). Transmission is autosomal dominant. Interestingly, subjects with defective hydroxylation of phenytoin could still hydroxylate phenobarbitone and phenylalanine normally. Although the abnormality may represent a defect in the gene coding for a form of cytochrome P-450 specific for phenytoin *p*-hydroxylation and not phenobarbitone hydroxylation, the half-life of phenobarbitone is so long that it would have been difficult to see any defect in the metabolism of this compound if it were present.

Dicumarol hydroxylation. Another extremely rare example of a deficiency in mixed-function oxidase activity has been described for dicumarol (bishydroxycoumarin) (Solomon, 1968). A single patient being treated with dicumarol following myocardial infarction was found to have a plasma half-life for the drug of 82 h which is three times the normal half-life of about 27 h. Members of this patient's family were not studied but the patient's mother had previously become paraplegic due to a spinal cord haematoma while on low-dose warfarin therapy. It is thus possible that this family shared an hereditary defect in the ability to metabolize coumarin anti-coagulants, the predominant route of which is cytochrome P-450 mediated oxidation.

Phenacetin O-deethylation. There have been reports of a single pedigree in Switzerland in which phenacetin metabolism was impaired (Shahidi, 1967, 1968). The initial observation was in a 17 year-old girl who was found to suffer severe methaemoglobinaemia and haemolysis after ingestion of a normally non-toxic dose of phenacetin (2.5 g). The normal routes of phenacetin metabolism are shown in Figure 3.5. Comparison with normal subjects revealed that the patient converted only 30% of a dose of phenacetin to paracetamol and excreted large amounts of 2-hydroxyphenacetin and its deacetylated product (Table 3.2). A family study revealed that the only other member of the girl's family who developed phenacetin

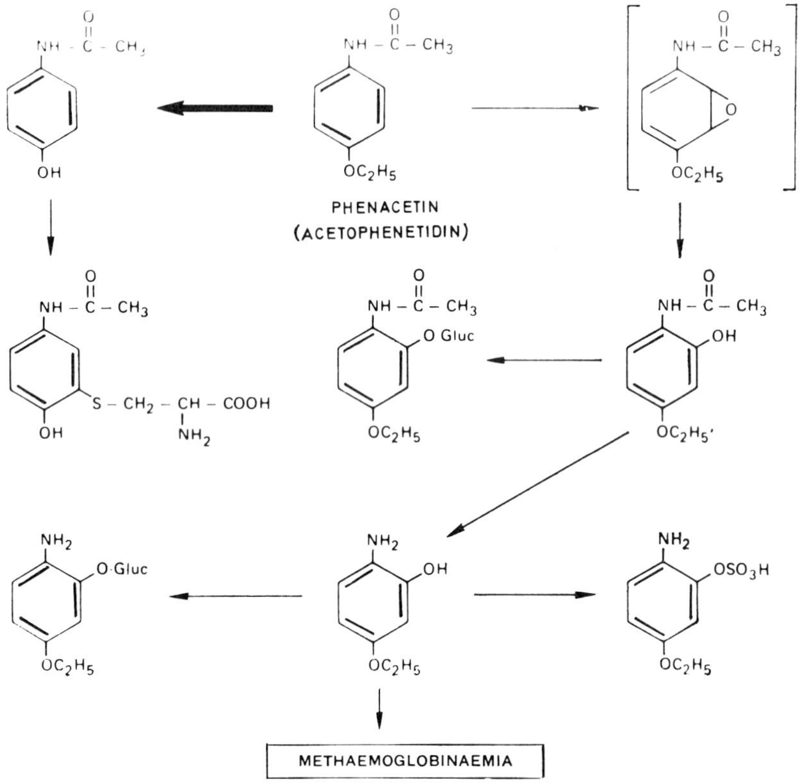

Fig. 3.5. Routes of phenacetin metabolism in man. Phenacetin is primarily *O*-deethylated by a cytochrome P-450 dependent reaction to paracetamol (upper left). This may be excreted as the mercapturic acid (centre left). A minor pathway, also cytochrome P-450 dependent, leads to 2-hydroxyphenacetin formation via a proposed epoxide intermediate (upper right). 2-Hydroxyphenacetin is excreted as the glucuronide conjugate (centre) or deacetylated to 2-hydroxyphenetidin (lower centre). The latter compound is a potent methaemoglobinaemic agent. (From data of Shahidi (1968). From Atlas & Nebert (1976), by permission of the authors and Taylor & Francis Ltd).

Table 3.2. Phenacetin metabolism.

Subject	Age	MetHb%		2-OH phenacetin glucuronide	2-OH phenetidin glucuronide	2-OH phenetidin sulphate	Paracetamol %
		Before	Max after				
Patient	17	0.2	11.4	++++	++++	++++	30
WB (F)	51	0.7	2.8	+	-	+	62
MH (F)	56	1.63	2.3	+	-	+	72
AK (M)	21	0.7	2.8	+	-	+	69
RB (M)	23	0.7	1.2	+	-	+	90
DF (F)	30	0.2	1.18	+	-	+	73
BR (M)	36	0.64	1.6	+	-	+	73
FR (M)	62	0	0.64	+	-	+	84

Modified from Shahidi (1968). By permission of the author and New York
Academy of Sciences.

toxicity, a sister, also excreted large quantities of 2-hydroxyphenacetin
(Table 3.3). Shahidi (1968) was able to show that 2-hydroxyphenetidin,
produced by deacetylation of 2-hydroxyphenacetin, readily produces
methaemoglobinaemia chemically. He concluded that the defect lay in an

Table 3.3. Family study of phenacetin metabolism.

Subject	Age	MetHb%		2-OH phenacetin glucuronide	2-OH phenetidin glucuronide	2-OH phenetidin sulphate	Paracetamol %
		Before	Max after				
Patient	17	0.2	11.4	++++	++++	++++	30
Sister	51?	0.4	0.4	+	-	+	72
Sister	38	0	5.4	++++	++++	++++	49
Brother	36	0.64	1.6	+	-	+	81
Father	62	1.1	1.9	+	-	+	68
Mother	61	0	0.64	+	-	+	80

Modified from Shahidi (1968). By permission of the author and New York
Academy of Sciences.

impaired ability to *O*-deethylate phenacetin, resulting in increased aromatic
hydroxylation, ultimately producing the toxic metabolite. Treatment with
phenobarbitone exacerbated the disorder, probably through induction of
aromatic hydroxylation. The defect appears to be autosomal recessive and
is possibly another example of a structural gene defect for a specific form of
cytochrome P-450.

Debrisoquine 4-hydroxylation. A polymorphism in the alicyclic
hydroxylation of debrisoquine to 4-hydroxydebrisoquine has recently been
reported (Mahgoub *et al.*, 1977). In a study of 94 subjects, 3 were defective
in 4-hydroxylating debrisoquine (Figure 3.6). These observations have been
confirmed by Tucker *et al.* (1977). Family studies suggested an autosomal
recessive mode of inheritance (Mahgoub *et al.*, 1977). In studies of a small
group of subjects (3 normal and 2 low 4-hydroxylators), 4-hydroxylation
was relatively more impaired than 5-, 6-, 7- or 8-hydroxylation (Angelo

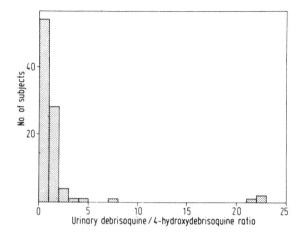

Fig. 3.6. Frequency histogram of urinary debrisoquine/4-hydroxydebrisoquine ratios in normal volunteers. The ratio of urinary debrisoquine/4-hydroxydebrisoquine is plotted for 94 subjects. (From Mahgoub *et al.* (1977). By permission of the authors and *The Lancet*.)

et al., 1977). More recently it has been shown that subjects with the 4-hydroxylation defect also have a reduced capacity to oxidize guanoxan and phenacetin (Smith *et al.*, 1978). However antipyrine 4-hydroxylation is unaffected (Tucker *et al.*, 1977). Whether this indicates a defect in a specific form of cytochrome P-450 remains to be established. Subjects with the defect require lower doses of debrisoquine for adequate control of blood pressure.

Amylobarbitone. It has been shown by means of twin studies that the metabolism of amylobarbitone, assessed by measuring its plasma half-life, is under multifactorial genetic regulation (Endrenyi, Inaba & Kalow, 1976). Recently, however, this group reported a polymorphism in the N-hydroxylation of amylobarbitone (Kalow *et al.*, 1977). There was a 20-fold difference in the excretion of the presumptive N-hydroxylated metabolite between affected and unaffected individuals but there was no difference in the formation of 3-hydroxyamylobarbitone between the groups. Inheritance of the defect is autosomal recessive (Kalow *et al.*, 1977). It now appears that the presumptive N-hydroxy metabolite was incorrectly identified (J. Gilbert & S. Murray, unpublished), the metabolite described by Kalow *et al.* (1977) more likely being a conjugate. Little or no N-hydroxyamylobarbitone is formed in man (J. Gilbert, & S. Murray, unpublished). Thus, this leaves unanswered the nature of the polymorphism described by Kalow *et al.* (1977).

Purine analogues. The purine analogues 6-mercaptopurine, 6-thioguanine, 8-azaguanine and azathioprine, normally used as chemotherapeutic agents, depend upon metabolism to their corresponding nucleotide analogues by the enzyme hypoxanthine guanine phosphoribosyl transferase (HGPRT) for their pharmacological effects. In Lesch-Nyhan syndrome, an X-linked recessive disorder, there is a total lack of HGPRT (Seegmiller, Rosenbloom & Kelley, 1967) and in one form of gout, also inherited by X-linked recessive transmission, HGPRT activity is reduced to 1% of normal (Kelley *et al.*, 1967). Subjects with either of these conditions would thus be expected to be resistant to the effects of these antimetabolites. This has been reported in one patient with leukaemia for 6-mercaptopurine (Davidson & Winter, 1964) and also for azathioprine (Brown, *et al.*, 1968).

Ethanol. Considerable inter-ethnic variations exist in ethanol susceptibility. More recently it has been shown that alcohol is metabolized polymorphically among different ethnic groups. In Caucasians the rate is 0.145 g/kg/h, in Eskimoes it is 0.110 g/kg/h and in Canadian Indians it is 0.101 g/kg/h (Fenna *et al.*, 1971). These genetically determined differences in the rate of ethanol metabolism correlate well with differences in susceptibility to the effects of ethanol.

Glucuronidation. There are several inherited disorders of bilirubin conjugation, all of which may result in side effects when drugs are given that are normally conjugated with glucuronic acid. The most severe of these is Crigler-Najjar syndrome inherited as an autosomal recessive trait (Childs, Sidbury & Migeon, 1959). Severe CNS disturbances occur due to excess unconjugated bilirubin and these may be fatal in early life (Schmid, 1972). The disorder is due to a total absence of functional UDP glucuronyltransferase responsible for bilirubin conjugation (Arias *et al.*, 1969). Conjugation of 4-methylumbelliferone and *o*-aminophenol *in vitro* is impaired but not absent (Arias *et al.*, 1969). *p*-Nitrophenol conjugation is normal (Crigler & Gold, 1969). *In vivo*, the conjugation of paracetamol, tetrahydrocortisol, tetrahydrocortisone, menthol (Figure 3.7), chloral hydrate, trichloroethanol and salicylamide is impaired (Axelrod, Schmid & Hammaker, 1957; Peterson & Schmid, 1975; Childs *et al.*, 1959). Thus, multiple forms of UDP glucuronyl transferase probably exist with overlapping substrate specificities, and the form absent in Crigler-Najjar syndrome is specific for bilirubin. There is strong evidence from animal studies that multiple forms of the transferase do exist (Del Villar *et al.*, 1975). Phenobarbitone is without effect in homozygotes for the disorder, as would be expected (Arias *et al.*, 1969).

A second, less severe, condition in which there is still unconjugated hyperbilirubinaemia and jaundice has been described (Jervis, 1959). This disorder differs from Crigler-Najjar syndrome in that, although low, bilirubin conjugating activity is present (Schmid, 1972). Conjugation of salicylamide and menthol is impaired *in vivo* (Arias *et al.*, 1969) and of *o*-aminophenol, 4-methylumbelliferone as well as of *p*-nitrophenol *in vitro* (Arias, 1962; Arias *et al.*, 1969). Bilirubin conjugation is not detectable *in vitro* (Arias *et al.*, 1969). The condition is dramatically improved by treatment with phenobarbitone (Yaffe *et al.*, 1966) and conjugation of menthol and salicylamide is also increased (Arias *et al.*, 1969). Inheritance may be autosomal dominant, but evidence indicates that there is incomplete penetrance with varied expressivity (Arias *et al.*, 1969).

Finally, there is a mild disorder of bilirubin conjugation known as Gilbert's syndrome (Gilbert, Lereboullet & Herscher, 1907). There is mild, chronic elevation of serum unconjugated bilirubin which may go unnoticed

(Foulk *et al.*, 1959). Inheritance is probably autosomal dominant (Powell *et al.*, 1967). Conjugations of bilirubin, *o*-aminophenol and 4-methylumbelliferone *in vitro* have variously been reported as normal (Arias, 1962) and impaired (Metge *et al.*, 1964). However the lowest activity reported is still ten times higher than necessary to eliminate all the bilirubin normally produced. The defect may thus be in the transport mechanism of bilirubin into liver cells (Schmid & Hammaker, 1959).

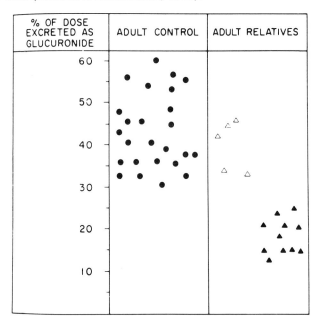

△ homozygous normal

▲ heterozygous

Fig. 3.7. Menthol glucuronidation in relatives of patients with Crigler-Najjar syndrome. Values represent % of 2 g dose of menthol excreted as the glucuronide over 5 h. (From Szabó & Ebrey (1963). By permission of the Publishing House of Hungarian Academy of Sciences.)

In the three conditions described above there is a range of functional impairment of the conjugation of some drugs. Although reports are lacking, it seems likely that subjects suffering from such disorders will be more susceptible to toxic side effects of drugs normally dependent on glucuronide conjugation for their elimination.

Catalase. Acatalasia, or acatalasaemia, is an autosomal recessive disorder in which catalase production is deficient or absent (Figure 3.8) (Takahara, 1952). Numerous variants of the disorder with different modes of inheritance are now known (Table 3.4). The subject has been reviewed in detail by Aebi & Wyss (1978). Symptoms associated with the disorder include oral ulceration and loss of teeth, probably due to the inability to inactivate hydrogen peroxide produced by oral bacteria. The only known drug toxicity caused by this disorder is due to an inability to metabolize topical hydrogen peroxide. The gene frequency varies among different groups from 0.05 to 1.4%. Three forms of the disorder in Japan have been described, mild, moderate and severe (Takahara *et al.*, 1960). However symptoms are not always present, even in the homozygote. Residual catalase in these subjects is without activity and may represent the presence of a sub-unit, the defect perhaps being in an inability to assemble the active enzyme (Shibata *et al.*, 1967). In the Swiss form of the disorder (Aebi *et al.*, 1961) dental defects are absent, probably because of residual catalase activity. This disorder is probably due to a structural gene defect (Aebi, 1967).

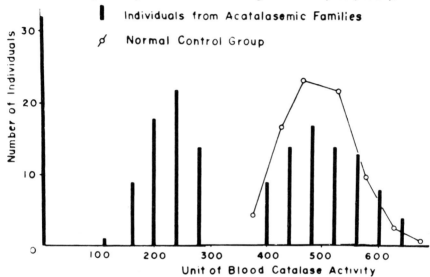

Fig. 3.8. Catalase activity in red blood cells of subjects in Type 1 acatalasaemic families. Catalase activity is distributed trimodally, with a group of subjects with no detectable catalase activity (extreme left), a group with intermediate activity and a group with normal activity (right). (From Takahara (1968). By permission of Grune & Stratton Inc.).

From the foregoing it is apparent that many more examples of genetically determined defects in Phase II reactions, such as acetylation and glucuronidation, are known than in cytochrome P-450 mediated drug oxidations. In fact, there is no example of a defect in drug oxidation that can be positively attributed to some abnormality of a specific form of cytochrome P-450.

Altered excretion of drugs

Dubin-Johnson's syndrome

Very few genetically determined drug side-effects can be attributed to abnormalities of excretion. One example is known in Dubin-Johnson's syndrome, in which bilirubin glucuronide transport into bile is impaired, resulting in conjugated hyperbilirubinaemia (Dubin & Johnson, 1954; Sprinz & Nelson, 1954). Conjugated bilirubin is also present in urine (Dubin, 1958). Transmission is as an autosomal recessive trait. Although there is pigmentation of the liver cells and chronic icterus, the condition is frequently asymptomatic (Dubin, 1958). Early studies with the dye brom-sulphthalein (BSP) revealed that hepatic extraction and storage were normal but BSP excretion into bile was delayed, with appearance of conjugate in plasma and urine (Mandema *et al.*, 1960). However, glucuronide conjugation

Table 3.4.   Variants of acatalasia.

Type of disorder and origin		Families studied		Activity as % normal		Mode of inheritance and other remarks
		Homo-zygotes	Hetero-zygotes	Homo-zygotes	Hetero-zygotes	
I	Japan & Korea	79 79	161	0-0.2	37-56	Incomplete autosomal recessive; homogeneous distribution of residual catalase
II	Japan	1 1	0	0	100	Autosomal recessive
IIIa	Japan	1		0	>50	Overlap between heterozygotes and normals
IIIb	Japan	1 1	?	4	?	
IIIc	Switzerland	3 11	>30	0.1-2	60-85	Unstable catalase variant. May be hybrid enzyme in heterozygote
IV	Israel & USA	2 1	16	8	49-67	Occurs in combination with G6PD deficiency. Homogeneous distribution of residual catalase
V	USA	1 0	6	?	100	Allocatalasia. Variant with increased electrophoretic mobility but otherwise normal

Modified from Aebi & Wyss (1978). By permission of McGraw-Hill Book Corp.

was normal both *in vivo* (Schoenfield *et al.*, 1963) and *in vitro* (Arias, 1961). These observations led to the conclusion that the transport of the conjugate into bile was defective. In addition to bilirubin and BSP glucuronide excretion being impaired, the excretion of rose bengal, indocyanine green and cholecystography contrast media is affected. The excretion of organic cations, bile salts and procainamide ethobromide is unaffected, since they utilize a different transport system. In patients with asymptomatic Dubin-Johnson's syndrome, contraceptive steroids can precipitate jaundice (Cohen, Lewis & Arias, 1972), perhaps because of competition by steroid glucuronides for the bilirubin glucuronide transport system.

Abnormalities in drug response

Increased sensitivity to drugs

Bone marrow depression. There is considerable evidence that chloramphenicol can cause a dose-dependent reversible suppression of bone marrow in all subjects, probably due to mitochondrial injury resulting from inhibition of protein synthesis (Yunis, 1973). However, it can also cause a much rarer idiosyncratic, often irreversible, aplasia of bone marrow that may be a consequence of inhibition of DNA synthesis (Yunis, 1973). Evidence of a genetic contribution to this aplasia is found in a report that a pair of identical twins both developed aplastic anaemia from chloramphenicol within a short time of each other (Nagao & Mauer, 1969). Further, in bone marrow cultures, total gross DNA and RNA synthesis were much more susceptible to inhibition by chloramphenicol in subjects who had recovered from chloramphenicol-induced aplastic anaemia (Figure 3.9) (Yunis & Harrington, 1960). In cultures of bone marrow from the parents

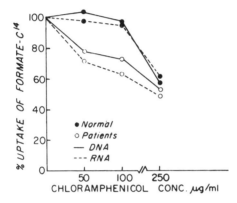

Fig. 3.9.　Effect of chloramphenicol on gross DNA synthesis (——) and gross RNA synthesis (----) in bone marrow cultures from normal subjects (•) and from those who had recovered from chloramphenicol-induced aplastic anaemia (o). Nucleic acid synthesis is expressed as percentage of [14C]formate incorporation into acid-precipitable material, compared with control cultures receiving no chloramphenicol. (Data from Yunis & Harrington (1960). From Atlas & Nebert (1977), by permission of the authors and Taylor & Francis Ltd).

of two of the affected individuals, DNA synthesis was inhibited at intermediate doses of chloramphenicol (Yunis, 1973). Recent studies support the concept that it is the nitrobenzene moiety of chloramphenicol that is responsible for its ability to produce aplastic anaemia (Man-Yan, Arimura & Yunis, 1975).

In studies on bone marrow cultures from normal subjects and those who had recovered from phenylbutazone-induced agranulocytosis, the cells from the affected subjects were much more sensitive to the cytotoxic effects of phenylbutazone and its metabolites, oxyphenbutazone and γ-hydroxyphenylbutazone (Smith, Chinn & Watts, 1977). This has similarly been shown with quinine in subjects who had recovered from quinine-induced agranulocytosis (Sutherland *et al.*, 1977). The optical isomer of quinine, quinidine, was without effect. It would be of obvious interest to determine if there is any degree of overlap in sensitivity to the three drugs in susceptible individuals.

Drug side effects associated with blood group. One interesting outcome of a survey into possible correlations between certain adverse drug reactions and genetic factors was the observation that young women with blood group A or AB have a greater risk of developing venous thromboemboli from the oral contraceptive than those with blood group O (Jick *et al.*, 1969; Lewis *et al.*, 1971). The reason for this is not known.

There has also been a report of increased incidence of cardiac arrhythmias after digoxin in subjects with blood groups other than O. Again the cause is completely unknown (Jick *et al.*, 1972).

Atropine. Subjects with Down's syndrome, a congenital chromosomal abnormality, are abnormally sensitive to the mydriatic and cardioaccelerator effects of atropine but not to the vagotonic effects (Harris & Goodman, 1968). The effect may thus be due to either increased β-receptor sensitivity or increased sympathetic activity.

Ethanol. Increased sensitivity to the effects of ethanol due to decreased metabolism in Eskimoes and Canadian Indians has been described earlier in this chapter. Increased sensitivity to ethanol has also been described in certain oriental groups, particularly Japanese, Taiwanese and Korean, but in these groups ethanol metabolism is normal (Wolff, 1972). These subjects experience marked facial flushing and mild to moderate intoxication on doses of ethanol without effect in Caucasians. Susceptibility may be due to increased autonomic sensitivity to ethanol.

Decreased sensitivity to drugs

Coumarin anticoagulants. Two large pedigrees have been reported in which there is autosomal dominant transmission of resistance to the oral anticoagulant warfarin (O'Reilly *et al.*, 1964; O'Reilly, 1970). Affected subjects are also resistant to dicumarol and phenindione but not to heparin, which has a different mode of action. The dose of warfarin required for normal anticoagulant response in affected individuals is 5-20 times that required in normal subjects (Figure 3.10). Absorption, distribution, metabolism, excretion and protein binding of warfarin were all normal in affected subjects (O'Reilly, Pool and Aggeler, 1968). Warfarin-resistant patients have increased sensitivity to vitamin K when on high doses of anticoagulant, whereas after vitamin K deprivation they are relatively insensitive to vitamin K (O'Reilly *et al.*, 1968). Vitamin K is essential for prothrombin synthesis, being converted to its epoxide in the process. This epoxide is inactive and is converted back to vitamin K in the liver by vitamin K epoxide reductase. Oral anticoagulants are thought to work by inhibiting this conversion. In warfarin-resistant subjects, vitamin K epoxide reductase may have a decreased affinity for both vitamin K and oral anticoagulants, the affinity for the anticoagulants being even less than for vitamin K (O'Reilly, 1970).

Mydriatics. Marked racial differences in response to mydriatics have been reported (Chen & Poth, 1929). Whereas Caucasians respond to ephedrine and related drugs applied to the conjunctival sac with papillary dilation Negroes are virtually insensitive to the mydriatic effects of these compounds (Chen & Poth, 1929). A similar racial difference in sensitivity to atropine mydriasis has been reported (Scott, 1945). Since mydriasis by these compounds is thought to be ultimately mediated through β-receptors it seems possible that in Negro subjects the β-receptor controlling the iris has decreased sensitivity to β-agonists. Whether such a change in sensitivity is reflected other than in the eye remains to be established.

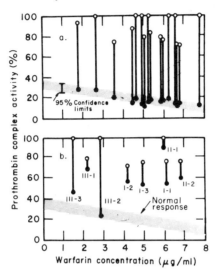

Fig. 3.10. Effect of warfarin on prothrombin complex activity in normal subjects and subjects with warfarin resistance. A single dose of warfarin (1.5 mg/kg) was administered to (*a*) 16 normal subjects and (*b*) 8 subjects related to a warfarin-resistant patient, and plasma concentration of warfarin and prothrombin complex activity measured 48 h later. Initial levels of prothrombin complex activity (o) and levels after warfarin (•), the shaded area shows 95% confidence limits for the normal levels. Roman numerals in (*b*) refer to the generation of the subjects. (From O'Reilly *et al.* (1964). By permission of Massachusetts Medical Society.)

Atypical response to drugs

The following section describes a variety of drug side-effects for which there is evidence of a genetic component and for some of which there is good evidence that the drugs are causing a novel response.

Porphyria. The porphyrias are a group of related disorders involving abnormalities of haem synthesis with the excretion of large amounts of haem precursors. The pathway of haem synthesis is shown in Figure 3.11. δ-Aminolaevulinic acid synthetase (ALAS), the first step in the pathway, is rate-limiting and is repressed at both transcriptional and translational levels by haem. There are six different forms of porphyria and it is now believed that each form may represent an inborn error of a different enzyme in the haem biosynthetic pathway (Brodie, Moore & Goldberg, 1977). In all of the porphyrias, ALAS activity is elevated in liver and leucocytes, presumably

Drug toxicity

due to derepression of ALAS by decreased haem synthesis (Brodie *et al.*, 1977). In subjects with latent porphyria, a variety of drugs, many of them inducers of mixed-function oxidase activity, can precipitate a porphyric attack which may be fatal. Drugs contraindicated are listed in Table 3.5 (Brodie, 1977). Allyl-containing compounds such as allylbarbiturates

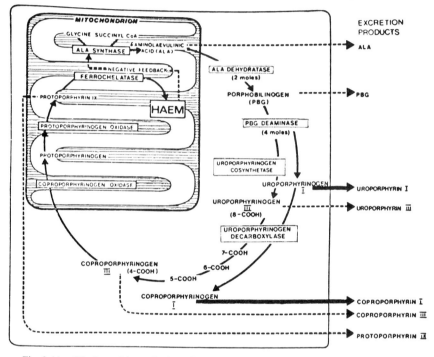

Fig. 3.11.   The haem biosynthetic pathway. (From Brodie *et al.* (1977). By permission of the authors and *The Lancet*.)

(e.g. secobarbital) and allylisopropylacetamide are particularly potent at provoking acute attacks (Eales & Linder, 1962; Granick, 1965). Many, if not all, of these compounds stimulate de novo synthesis of ALAS (Granick & Urata, 1963; Granick, 1966) whilst ALAS degradation is unaffected (Granick, 1966; Strand, Manning & Marver, 1972). There are thus three possible mechanisms for such stimulation. Cytochrome P-450 apoproteins synthesized de novo in response to inducers (Haugen, Coon & Nebert, 1976), are believed to act as positive regulators of ALAS at a translational level and thus their induction will lead to increased synthesis of ALAS (Rajamanickam, Satyanarayana Rao & Padmanaban, 1975). Secondly, removal of haem from the haem pool by incorporation into the apoprotein will derepress ALAS and thus stimulate its formation (Jacob & Monod, 1961). A third possibility is that these inducing compounds can stimulate ALAS synthesis directly (De Matteis & Gibbs, 1972). It may be that a combination of these factors plays a role. The allyl-containing compounds are converted to metabolites that destroy cytochrome P-450, thereby depleting the haem pool and derepressing ALAS (De Matteis, 1971). A third class of ALAS inducers are metabolites of steroids, such as 11β-hydroxy-Δ^4-androstenedione, which are normally converted to 5α-derivatives in the liver by steroid-Δ^4-5α-reductase. In some patients with acute intermittent porphyria, levels of this enzyme are reduced (Kappas *et al.*, 1972), leading to increased amounts of 5β-11 (A-B *cis*) derivatives in which the Δ^4 double bond is not reduced. These 5β metabolites are potent inducers of ALAS. Thus all of these compounds, although acting by different mechanisms, cause increased ALAS activity. Where there is a defect in one of the enzymes of haem synthesis, this increase in ALAS activity will result in accumulation of haem precursors proximal to the defect. This is the basis of

Table 3.5. Drugs believed to precipitate porphyria.

Althesin	Imipramine
Barbiturates	Meprobomate
Bemegride	Methyldopa
Carbromal	Nikethamide
Chloramphenicol	Pentazocine
Chlordiazepoxide	Phenytoin and other hydantoins
Chlorpropamide	Pyrazinamide
Chloroquine	Oestrogens
Dichloralphenazone	Oral contraceptives
Ergot preparations	Sulphonamides
Ethanol	Theophylline derivatives
Glutethimide	Tolbutamide
Griseofulvin	Troxidone

a porphyric attack. The type of porphyria precipitated will depend on which enzyme is defective. Drug-induced attacks have been shown to occur in acute intermittent porphyria, variegate porphyria, hereditary coproporphyria and cutaneous hepatic porphyria (Goldberg, Brodie & Moore, in the press). Certain inducers such as tetrachlorodibenzo-*p*-dioxin and hexachlorobenzene, can cause porphyria in the absence of any defect in the enzymes of the haem biosynthetic pathway (Poland & Glover, 1973).

Pentosuria. Pentosuria is a benign disorder of carbohydrate metabolism in which there is excess urinary excretion of *L*-xylulose, a pentose sugar (Hiller, 1917). The disorder, which is due to a defect in NADP-xylitol dehydrogenase (Wang & van Eys, 1970) which converts *L*-xylulose to xylitol, is inherited as an autosomal recessive trait. It occurs almost entirely in Jews, in whom there is a 1 in 2000 to 1 in 5000 incidence (Wright, 1961). *L*-xylulose can arise from metabolism of *D*-glucuronic acid, produced from uridine diphosphoglucuronic acid, by the so-called glucuronic acid oxidation pathway. Normally the *L*-xylulose thus produced is further metabolized by xylitol dehydrogenase and then enters the pentose phosphate pathway. The absence of symptoms in subjects with pentosuria seems to indicate that the glucuronic acid oxidation pathway does not serve an essential function in man. Administration of glucuronic acid to affected subjects causes increased *L*-xylulose excretion, as would be expected (Enklewitz &

Lasker, 1935). Aminopyrine also causes increased *L*-xylulose production in affected individuals (Margolis, 1929). Aminopyrine, together with chloretone and barbital, has been shown to stimulate glucuronic acid production in animals (Burns *et al.*, 1957). Thus these compounds probably induce one of the enzymes of the glucuronic acid oxidation pathway proximal to xylitol dehydrogenase which will lead to accumulation and excretion of *L*-xylulose in pentosuria.

Anaesthetics. A rare complication of general anaesthesia is malignant hyperthermia in which there is a rapid rise in core temperature, in some cases reaching 112°, generalized muscular rigidity and severe metabolic acidosis. This condition has been observed after anaesthesia with nitrous oxide, methoxyflurane, halothane, ether, cyclopropane and combinations of these. The condition is more common when succinylcholine is used as a premedication. It is often fatal (Kalow, 1972). Inheritance is autosomal dominant and the frequency of the phenotype is about 1 in 20 000. Intravenous procaine can alleviate the symptoms in some cases but curare is without effect (Kalow, 1972). Recent evidence (Moulds & Denborough, 1974) from experiments on muscle biopsy samples has shown that tissue from affected subjects responds to halothane, caffeine, succinylcholine, potassium chloride and increasing the temperature from 25° to 37° with a contracture whereas normal tissue does not. The contracture was blocked by procaine. Thus the defect is probably in the Ca^{2+} storing membranes of the sarcolemma and sarcoplasmic reticulum such that a variety of stimuli produce abnormal release of Ca^{2+}.

Steroid-induced glaucoma. Armaly (1968) has reported that increases in ocular pressure in response to 0.1% dexamethasone 21-phosphate show a trimodal distribution. The tendency to develop high pressures is inherited as an autosomal recessive trait, and is strongly associated with the development of open-angle hypertensive glaucoma and low-tension glaucoma. It has also been shown that chamber angles and depths are, to a large extent, genetically determined (Kellerman & Posner, 1955). Subjects with narrow chambers are thus genetically susceptible to precipitation of narrow angle glaucoma by adrenergic mydriatic agents (Grant, 1955).

Allopurinol. In some patients with gout there is a reduction of HGPRT activity to 1% of normal. (Total lack of HGPRT leads to Lesch-Nyhan syndrome, which has been described above.) The HGPRT deficient form of gout is inherited as an X-linked recessive trait (Kelley *et al.*, 1969). HGPRT normally plays an important role in the purine salvage pathway, catalysing the conversion of guanine and hypoxanthine to GMP and IMP respectively which act as feedback inhibitors of the rate-limiting step in de novo purine biosynthesis. Hypoxanthine may also be converted to xanthine and then uric acid by xanthine oxidase. When HGPRT is deficient, there is decreased conversion of guanine and hypoxanthine to their nucleotides, which results in unregulated purine synthesis due to derepression. The excess purines are metabolized by xanthine oxidase resulting in hyperuricaemia (Kelley *et al.*, 1969). In gout with normal HGPRT levels, allopurinol acts by inhibiting xanthine oxidase thus causing increased IMP levels due to HGPRT activity and hence repression of purine synthesis.

In addition, allopurinol serves as a substrate for HGPRT, and the ribonucleotide thus formed can also repress purine synthesis (Caskey, Ashton & Wyngaarden, 1964). Thus, in HGPRT-deficient gout, although allopurinol decreases uric acid production by inhibition of xanthine oxidase and hence prevents urinary calculi formation, hypoxanthine accumulates without being converted to IMP, nor is allopurinol converted to its ribonucleotide. These two factors result in normal or increased urinary excretion of purines, mainly oxypurines, hypoxanthine and xanthine (Figure 3.12) (Kelley *et al.*, 1969) with possible development of xanthine stones (Sorensen, 1968).

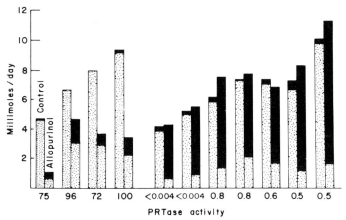

Fig. 3.12. Effect of allopurinol on purine excretion in HGPRT deficiency. Each pair of columns represents daily urinary excretion of uric acid (stippled bar) and other oxypurines (solid bar) before (left column) and after (right column) treatment with allopurinol in individual subjects. HGPRT activity is expressed in nmol/mg protein/h. Four values at left represent normal subjects, two in centre subjects with Lesch-Nyhan syndrome and five at right, subjects with HGPRT deficient gout. (From Kelley *et al.* (1969). By permission of American College of Physicians.)

Glucose-6-phosphate dehydrogenase deficiency. Within a year of its introduction to treat malaria (Mühlens, 1926), pamaquine was reported as causing haemolytic anaemia (Cordes, 1926) in which Heinz bodies were observed in the red cells (Palma, 1928). The familial nature of the sensitivity, racial differences in susceptibility (Dimson & McMartin, 1946) and the similarity of the response to favism (acute haemolytic anaemia on ingestion of fava beans) (Turchetti, 1948) were all noted but the nature of the defect remained unknown. However, soon after the introduction of the structurally similar drug, primaquine, in 1950, it was realized that the defect leading to haemolysis lay in the red cell (Dern *et al.*, 1954), which was found to have diminished levels of reduced glutathione (GSH) in sensitive subjects (Beutler, Dern & Alving, 1955), probably due to defective glucose-6-phosphate dehydrogenase (G6PD) (Carson *et al.*, 1956). G6PD deficiency is the most common genetically determined enzyme abnormality in man. Approximately 100 million people are affected (Vesell, 1972) and the frequency can vary from as high as 53% in male Kurdic Ashkenazi Jews to nil in Eskimoes. Transmission is X-linked incomplete dominant. There are over 80 discrete variants of G6PD each with a slightly different clinical picture (Motulsky, Yoshida & Stomatoyannopoulos, 1971), and varying in a variety of properties such as total red cell activity, electrophoretic mobility, K_m for NADP and G6P, V_{max} for substrate analogues and heat stability. The commonest types are A[-] and A[+], found predominantly in Negroes, Mediterranean, observed in people with Mediterranean ancestry, and Canton, found in South Chinese.

Mature red cells can synthesize glutathione and other cofactors using glucose as an energy source. This is converted to G6P which then provides the necessary energy through anaerobic glycolysis. A small proportion of G6P is metabolized by direct oxidation, a process stimulated by drugs such as primaquine and certain other compounds, for example, cysteine and pyruvate. The first step in this oxidation is catalysed by G6PD and the overall process leads to a net production of 2 moles of NADPH, which is essential for the reduction of oxidized glutathione (GSSG) to GSH and for the activity of methaemoglobin reductase. GSH is rapidly oxidized to GSSG in the red cell under a variety of conditions, whereas reduction of GSSG requires NADPH and glutathione reductase. However, the activity of this enzyme is such that normally less than 0.25% of glutathione in the red cell is oxidized (Srivastava & Beutler, 1968). GSH is thought to play a vital role in maintaining protein sulphydryl groups in the reduced state, thus preventing enzyme or haemoglobin denaturation, i.e. Heinz body formation, and perhaps in maintaining the integrity of the erythrocyte membrane (Barron & Singer, 1943). G6PD, by generating NADPH, is thus essential in maintaining GSH in the reduced state. As red cells age, the level of G6PD decreases. This is particularly marked in G6PD deficiency. However, even in affected subjects, younger cells have sufficient G6PD to protect them against haemolytic drugs (Marks & Gross, 1959). This explains why haemolytic attacks become self-limiting after about one week (Dern, Beutler & Alving, 1954) (Figure 3.13).

Many haemolytic drugs (Table 3.6) are substrates for enzymes of drug metabolism which convert them to reactive intermediates (Fouts & Brodie, 1957; Kiese, 1966; Bickel, 1969). Inter-individual differences in the capacity to activate haemolytic drugs may thus play an extra-erythrocytic role in determining susceptibility in G6PD deficient subjects (Dern, Beutler & Alving, 1955). A variety of mechanisms operate to cause haemolysis in G6PD deficiency. These are all directly or indirectly related to low GSH levels. GSH may be further diminished by oxidation. (Flohé & Günzler, 1974) or conjugation (Habig, Pabst & Jakoby, 1974; Habig, Keen & Jakoby, 1975). In addition, reactive intermediates of the drug may interact directly with protein sulphydryl groups, which would no longer be protected against oxidative attack in G6PD deficiency because of the low levels of GSH. All such reactions can lead to denaturation of haemoglobin, possibly due to oxidation of the cysteine residue at position 93 of the β chain, causing breakdown of the tertiary structure and oxidation of more sulphydryl groups thus revealed (Jacob *et al.*, 1968). Such denatured haemoglobin forms Heinz bodies and these may bind to the cell membrane by sulphydryl

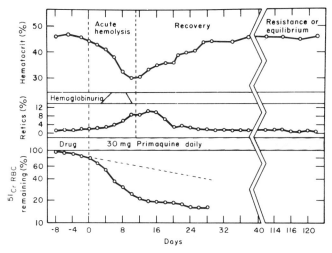

Fig. 3.13. Time course of primaquine-induced haemolytic anaemia. Composite data from 3 Negro male subjects with A⁻ G6PD deficiency. At -8 days each subject was injected with a sample of his own erythrocytes tagged with ^{51}Cr. Primaquine (80 mg daily) was started at day 0. Haematocrit as percent (upper), reticulocytes (centre) and % ^{51}Cr red cells remaining (lower). Broken line represents normal curve for erythrocyte destruction. Note haemoglobinuria during acute phase of haemolysis. (From Kellermeyer *et al.* (1961). By permission of the authors and C. V. Mosby Corp.)

bridges causing changes in shape or plasticity of the cells. Such damage, together with the presence of Heinz bodies within the cells, interferes with cell progress through splenic sinusoids where they are then destroyed by reticuloendothelial cells (Beutler, 1972). Deficiency of G6PD, which has a high incidence in areas where malaria is prevalent, was found to protect red cells from parasite infestation, thereby conferring an evolutionary advan-

Table 3.6. Drugs and other agents that can cause haemolytic anaemia in subjects with G6PD deficiency. (From Marks & Banks (1965). By permission of the authors, John Wiley & Sons Inc. and the New York Academy of Sciences.

Primaquine	Quinine
Pamaquine	Quinidine
Pentaquine	*p*-Aminosalicylic acid
Quinocide	Antipyrine
Sulphanilamide	Probenecid
Sulphapyridine	Acetanilide
Sulphisoxazole	Phenylhydrazine
Sulphacetamide	Acetophenetidin
Sulphamethoxypyridazine	Pyramidone
Salicylazosulphapyridine	Chloroquine
Sulphones (sulphoxone)	Chloramphenicol
Naphthalene	Fava bean
Methylene blue	Viral respiratory infections
Vitamin K	Infectious hepatitis
Acetylsalicylic acid	Infectious mononucleosis
Nitrofurantoin	Bacterial pneumonias and septicaemias (e.g. typhoid)
Furazoladone	Diabetic acidosis
	Uremia

tage on the heterozygous female carrier (Luzzatto, Usanga & Reddy, 1969).

Other defects associated with the erythrocyte glutathione system. In addition to the 80 or so variants of G6PD that may lead to haemolysis, several defects in some of the other enzymes of GSH metabolism have been observed. Two cases of defective γ-glutamylcysteine synthetase, which is involved in glutathione synthesis, both associated with haemolysis have been reported (Boivin, Galand & Bernard, 1973). Autosomal recessive inheritance of a defect in glutathione synthetase, also associated with haemolysis, has been reported (Konrad *et al.*, 1972). Deficiency of either of these enzymes may also reduce transport of glutathione amino acid precursors into the red cell (Meister, 1974). Deficiency of glutathione reductase, which has been associated with haemolysis, is inherited as an autosomal dominant trait, the defect being in a reduced affinity for flavine adenine dinucleotide (Löhr *et al.*, 1974). Deficient glutathione peroxidase also associated with haemolysis has been observed. This is an autosomal autonomous trait (Necheles, 1974). Finally, defects in 6-phosphogluconate dehydrogenase, which, together with G6PD, is responsible for NADPH production in the erythrocyte, have been reported. The defect is inherited by autosomal autonomous transmission, but does not appear to increase the sensitivity of affected subjects to haemolytic drugs (Beutler, 1969).

Haemoglobin M. Over 100 variants of human haemoglobin (Hb) are known and some of these are unstable or prone to methaemoglobin (metHb) formation. A variety of drugs, some directly and some after metabolic activation (Table 3.7), can convert Hb to metHb in normal red cells (Prankerd, 1961; Kiese, 1966). This is rapidly metabolized back to Hb by metHb reductase. However, some variants of Hb, designated HbM,

Table 3.7.   Drugs that can cause methaemoglobinaemia.

Direct-acting	Requiring metabolic activation
Nitrites	Nitrates
Chlorates	Aromatic amino and nitro compounds
Quinones	Anilines
Methylene blue	Acetanilide
	Phenacetin
	Nitrobenzenes
	Nitrotoluenes
	Sulphonamides

Modified from Prankerd (1961). By permission of Blackwell Scientific Publications Ltd.

after conversion to metHb are resistant to metabolism by metHb reductase. This is due to amino acid substitution in the haem pocket such that any metHb produced is stabilized in this form (Singer, 1955). Subjects with any of the forms of HbM, inherited as autosomal dominant traits, will thus have increased sensitivity to the drugs listed in Table 3.7 that produce metHb, and since metHb cannot give up oxygen, such subjects will become cyanosed on exposure to these drugs.

Drug-sensitive haemoglobins. In addition to the drug-sensitive forms of HbM, several other Hb variants are sensitive to drugs, particularly sulphonamides and primaquine (Frick, Hitzig & Betke, 1962). These forms of Hb, such as Hb$_{Zürich}$ (Muller & Kingma, 1961), Hb$_{Köln}$ (Carrell, Lehmann & Hutchinson, 1966) and Hb$_{Hammersmith}$ (Dacie *et al.*, 1967) have amino acid substitutions in the haem pocket such that the haem easily dissociates on exposure to certain drugs. The globin then forms Heinz bodies, which leads to severe haemolysis by a mechanism similar to that in G6PD deficiency (Jacob *et al.*, 1968). Another unstable form of Hb, inherited as an autosomal recessive trait is HbH, a β-chain tetramer and thus a form of α-thalassaemia (Baglioni, 1963). HbH is sensitive to the drugs listed in Table 6 under G6PD deficiency which tend to cause accumulation of metHb in older cells with a consequent reduction in red cell life span. In Thailand 1 person in 300 is affected and levels of HbH can vary from 5 to 30% in individuals.

NADH-methaemoglobin reductase deficiency. Normally red cells have less than 1% metHb because of its continual reduction back to Hb (Harris, 1970) primarily by NADH-metHb reductase (Keitt, 1972). NADH production, by glyceraldehyde-3-phosphate dehydrogenase, is rate-limiting. In hereditary methaemoglobinaemia, an autosomal recessive disorder, NADH-metHb reductase is absent. Although other mechanisms exist that can reduce metHb to Hb, deficiency of this enzyme leads to accumulation of metHb on exposure to a variety of drugs including nitrates, chlorates, dapsone and primaquine (Table 3.7), which may lead to cyanosis. Although younger red cells have reduced levels of NADH-metHb reductase in this disorder, there is sufficient present to protect them (Keitt, Smith & Jandl, 1966) and only older cells accumulate metHb, thus accounting for the self-limiting nature of cyanotic attacks during exposure to drugs. At least six different variants of defective NADH-metHb reductase are now known (Hsieh & Jaffé, 1971).

Other drug side effects that may have a genetic basis

It is becoming increasingly apparent that the first step in a wide variety of drug toxicities is metabolic activation of the drug. The mechanisms involved have already been considered in Chapter 1. The reader is also referred to the article by Mitchell *et al.* (1975). These mechanisms will therefore not be considered here. For any drug there may be a multiplicity of possible routes of metabolism (Figure 3.5), some leading to activation, some to inactivation of any intermediate thus formed, and some to products less toxic than the parent compound. The synthesis of each individual enzyme involved will be regulated by one or a small number of structural genes which may be controlled by one or more regulatory genes. Mutation of any such gene may alter drug toxicity by alteration in the activity of the routes of activation and deactivation. An example of this is phenacetin-induced methaemoglobinaemia due to decreased *O*-deethylase activity (Shahidi, 1968). Thus the defect may result in a relatively specific abnormality in detoxication, but it can also result in a more generalized abnormality with the metabolism of many drugs affected such as in Crigler-Najjar syndrome. There are many mechanisms whereby such intermediates may be toxic, such as direct covalent interaction with essential proteins and peroxidative damage of the cell membrane. Other mechanisms may include direct interaction with specific cell receptor sites and interference with intermediary metabolism through competition for or destruction of endogenous cofactors. In each of these systems there is multifactorial regulation, so that differences in single genes at any one of many sites could influence drug toxicity. Thus genetic differences in the pathways of metabolism or in the systems affected by the drugs, or their metabolites, may affect toxicity. These differences may be so subtle that they have avoided detection to date, so it is probable that many drug idiosyncracies, the causes of which are at present unknown, will be attributable, at least in part, to genetic factors.

Chemical carcinogens

It is outside the scope of this article to discuss mechanisms of drug-induced cancer (aspects of which are covered in Chapters 4 and 9), chemical terato-genesis (see Chapter 10) or allergic reactions to drugs (see Chapters 11 and 14). However, there could be genetic involvement in such effects. The possible role of acetylation polymorphism in protection against bladder cancer from aromatic amines has already been considered. There is con-siderable evidence that many forms of human cancer are caused by drugs and other exogenous compounds, the majority of which require metabolic activation to the ultimate carcinogenic species (Heidelberger, 1975). Genetic differences in the metabolism of such compounds may well influence susceptibility to cancer. Ample evidence exists for this in experimental animals (Thorgeirsson & Nebert, 1977) and there is some evidence that this may also be so in man (see Nebert & Atlas, 1977). In addition, genetic differences in DNA repair mechanisms or immune surveillance may play a role in determining susceptibility to chemical carcinogens.

Chemical teratogens

There is increasing evidence that genetic factors play a role in chemical teratogenesis. For example, Biddle (1974) has shown strain differences to susceptibility to teratogenesis by acetazolamide in inbred mice. There is also a single gene difference among certain strains of mice in their responsive-ness to induction by polycyclic hydrocarbons and this is positively associ-ated with susceptibility of responsive strains to stillborns, foetal malforma-tions and resorptions caused by polycyclic hydrocarbons (Shum, Lambert & Nebert, 1977). There is evidence that phenytoin teratogenesis, in experi-mental animals at least, is due to the formation of an epoxide intermediate (Martz, Failinger & Blake, 1977). Genetically determined differences in the rate of formation of this metabolite, or in the rate of its inactivation, could conceivably lead to differences in susceptibility to phenytoin tera-togenesis in man. The extent to which genetic factors influence terato-genesis in man is an important, but as yet unanswered, question.

Drug allergy and sensitivity

Many drugs produce allergic reactions in man and there is considerable evidence that these reactions can be modified by genetic factors. The role of the genetic polymorphism for acetylation in the formation of drug-induced antinuclear antibodies and the development of SLE has already been considered. Hereditary defects in both the complement system and the synthesis of immunoglobulins have been described (Ruddy & Austen, 1972; Rosen & Merler, 1972). The role of such abnormalities in drug-induced allergic reactions remains to be elucidated. Genetic differences in susceptibility to a variety of allergic conditions, including asthma, rhinitis and dermatitis have been observed (Holst & Möller, 1975) and there has been a report of a high degree of concordance in identical twins for contact sensitivity to benzalkonium chloride and potash soap (Max Kjellman, 1977). Genetic factors may influence allergic reactions through differences in formation of metabolites that can act as haptens or through differences in the immune system itself.

Drug dependence

The extent to which genetic factors play a role in drug dependence is not known. Genetic differences among inbred rat strains in ethanol preference that may depend on differences in ethanol disposition have been described (Koivula, Koivusalo & Lindros, 1975). There is also evidence that in man there is a genetic predisposition in coffee drinking and cigarette smoking (Conterio & Chiarelli, 1962). It is possible that genetic differences also exist in the sensitivity or response to the opiate receptor (Kosterlitz & Hughes, 1975) thus affecting susceptibility to opiate dependence. This may prove to be one of the most exciting areas of pharmacogenetic research over the next few years.

Genetic factors in response to environmental stimuli

Finally, one aspect of the effects of genetic factors in drug toxicity not yet considered is the role of genetic susceptibility to environmental factors that affect drug metabolism. Genetic differences in the inducibility of aryl hydrocarbon hydroxylase by polycyclic hydrocarbons in inbred strains of mice have been described (Nebert *et al.*, 1975). Differences in inducibility by barbiturates and related compounds in inbred rat strains have been reported (Jori, Pugliatti & Santini, 1972). There is also evidence for genetic differences in aryl hydrocarbon hydroxylase inducibility in man (see Nebert & Atlas, 1977). Induction is thought to be a receptor phenomenon in which the inducing compound interacts with a cytosolic receptor (Poland & Glover, 1975; Poland, Glover & Kende, 1976). There is probably a specific receptor for each type of inducer, each one being the product of a single structural gene. Differences in these genes would account for inducibility polymorphisms. Thus, even for those drug side-effects not affected by polymorphic drug metabolism, genetic differences in the inducibility of those enzymes could still result in polymorphic toxicity.

References

Aebi, H.E. (1967). In *Proceedings of the Third International Congress on Human Genetics, Chicago*, 1966, Editors: Crow, J.F. and Neel, J.V. p. 189. Baltimore: Johns Hopkins University Press.

Aebi, H.E. Heiniger, J.P. Bütler, R. and Hässig, A. (1961). *Experentia*, 17, 466.

Aebi, H.E. and Wyss, S.R. (1978). In *The Metabolic Basis of Inherited Disease*, 4th Ed., Editors: Stanbury, J.B., Wyngaarden, J.B. and Frederickson, D.S., p. 1792. New York: McGraw-Hill.

Alarćon-Segovia, D., Fishbein, E. and Alcala, H. (1971). *Arthritis Rheum.*, 14, 748.

Angelo, M.M. Dring, L.G., Idle, J.R., Lancaster, R., Mahgoub, A. and Smith, R.L. (1977). *Br. J. clin. Pharmac.*, 4, 725P.

Arias, I.M. (1961). *Am. J. Med.*, 31, 510.

Arias, I.M. (1962). *J. clin. Invest.*, 41, 2233.

Arias, I.M., Gartner, L.M., Cohen, M., BenEzzer, J. and Levi, A.J. (1969). *Am. J. Med.*, 47, 395.

Armaly, M.F. (1968). *Ann. N.Y. Acad. Sci.*, 151, 861.

Atlas, S.A. and Nebert, D.W. (1977). In *Drug Metabolism — from Microbe to Man*, Editors: Parke, D.V. and Smith, R.L., p. 293. London: Taylor & Francis.

Axelrod, J., Schmid, R. and Hammaker, L. (1957). *Nature, Lond.*, 180, 1426.

Baglioni, C. (1963). In *Molecular Genetics*, Editor: Taylor, J.H. New York: Academic Press.

Barron, E.S.G. and Singer, T.P. (1943). *Science, N.Y.*, 97, 356.

Bearn, A.G. (1953). *Am. J. Med.*, 15, 442.

Beierwaetes, W.H., Carr, E.A. and Hunter, R.L. (1961). *Trans. Ass. Am. Physicians*, 74, 170.

Beierwaetes, W.H. and Robbins, J. (1959). *J. clin. Invest.*, 38, 1683.

Beutler, E. (1969). *Pharmac. Rev.*, 21, 73.

Beutler, E. (1972). In *The Metabolic Basis of Inherited Disease*, 3rd Ed., Editors: Stanbury, J.B., Wyngaarden, J.B. and Frederickson, D.S., p. 1358. New York: McGraw-Hill.

Beutler, E., Dern, R.J. and Alving, A.S. (1955). *J. Lab. clin. Med.*, 45, 286.

Bickel, M.H. (1969). *Pharmac. Rev.*, 21, 325.

Biddle, F.G. (1974). *Teratology*, 11, 37.

Biehl, J.P. (1957). In *Transactions of the 16th Conference on the Chemotherapy of Tuberculosis*, p. 108. Washington, D.C.: Veterans Administration: Army: Navy.

Boivin, P., Galand, C. and Bernard, J.F. (1973). In *Glutathione. Proceedings of the 16th Conference of the German Society of Biological Chemistry, Tübingen, March 1973*. Editors: Flohé, L., Benöhr, H.C., Sies, H., Waller, H.D. and Wendel, A., p. 146. New York: Academic Press.

Bönicke, R. and Lisboa, B.P. (1957). *Naturwiss.*, 44, 314.

Brodie, M.J. (1977). MD Thesis, Glasgow.

Brodie, M.J., Moore, M.R. and Goldberg, A. (1977). *Lancet*, 2, 699.

Burns, J.J., Evans, C. Trousof, N. and Kaplan, J. (1957). *Fedn Proc. Fedn Am. Socs exp. Biol.*, 16, 286.

Brown, R.S., Kelley, W.N., Seegmiller, J.E. and Carbone, P.P. (1968). *J. clin. Invest.*, 47, 12a.

Carlson, H.B., Anthony, E.M., Russel, W.F. and Middlebrook, G. (1956). *New Engl. J. Med.*, 255, 118.

Carrell, R.W., Lehmann, H. and Hutchinson, H.E. (1966). *Nature, Lond.*, 210, 915.

Carson, P.E., Flanagan, C.L., Ickes, C.E. and Alving, A.S. (1956). *Science, N.Y.*, 124, 484.

Caskey, C.T., Ashton, D.M. and Wyngaarden, J.B. (1964). *J. biol. Chem.*, 239, 2570.

Cavalieri, R.R. and Searle, G.L. (1966). *J. clin. Invest.*, 45, 939.

Chabner, B.A., Johns, D.G. Coleman, C.N., Drake, J.C. and Evans, W.H. (1974). *J. clin. Invest.*, 53, 922.

Chen, K.K. and Poth, E.J. (1929). *J. Pharmac. exp. Ther.*, 36, 429.

Childs, B., Sidbury, J.B. and Migeon, C.J. (1959). *Pediatrics, Springfield*, 23, 903.

Cohen, L., Lewis, C. and Arias, I.M. (1972). *Gastroenterology*, 62, 1182.

Conolly, M.E., Briant, R.H., George, C.F. and Dollery, C.T. (1972). *Eur. J. clin. Pharmac.*, 4, 222.

Conterio, F. and Chiarelli, B. (1962). *Heredity, Lond.*, 17, 347.

Cordes, W. (1926). In *15th Annual Report of the United Fruit Company* (*Medical Department*), p. 66.

Crigler, J.F., Jr. and Gold, N.I. (1969). *J. clin. Invest.*, 48, 42.

Dacie, J.V., Shinton, N.J., Gaffney, P.J., Carrell, R.W. and Lehmann, H. (1967). *Nature, Lond.*, 216, 663.

Das, K.M., Eastwood, M.A., McManus, J.P.A. and Sircus, W. (1973). *New Engl. J. Med.*, 289, 491.

Davidson, J.D. and Winter, T.S. (1964). *Cancer Res.*, 24, 261.

Davies, R.O., Marton, A.V. and Kalow, W. (1960). *Can. J. Biochem. Physiol.*, 38, 545.

Del Villar, E., Sanchez, E., Autor, A.P. and Tephly, T.R. (1975). *Molec. Pharmac.*, 11, 236.

De Matteis, F. (1971). *Biochem. J.*, 124, 767.

De Matteis, F. and Gibbs, A. (1972). *Biochem. J.*, 126, 1149.

Dern, R.J., Beutler, E. and Alving, A.S. (1954). *J. Lab. clin. Med.*, 44, 171.

Dern, R.J., Beutler, E. and Alving, A.S. (1955). *J. Lab. clin. Med.*, 45, 30.

Dern, R.J., Weinstein, I.M., LeRoy, G.V., Talmage, D.W. and Alving, A.S. (1954). *J. Lab. clin. Med.*, 43, 303.

Devadatta, S., Gangadharam, P.R.J., Andrews, R.H., Fox, W., Ramakrishnan, C.V., Selkon, J.B. and Velu, S. (1960). *Bull. Wld Hlth Org.*, 23, 587.

Dimson, S.B. and McMartin, R.B. (1946). *Q. Jl Med.*, 15, 25.

Dubin, I.N. (1958). *Am. J. Med.*, 24, 268.

Dubin, I.N. and Johnson, F.B. (1954). *Medicine, Baltimore*, 33, 155.

Drayer, D.E. and Reidenberg, M.M. (1977). *Clin. Pharmac. Ther.*, 22, 251.

Eales, L. and Linder, G.C. (1962). *S. Afr. med. J.*, 36, 284.

Ebadi, M.S. and Kugel, R.B. (1970). *Pediat. Res.*, 4, 187.

Ellard, G.A. (1976). *Clin. Pharmac. Ther.*, 19, 610.

Ellard, G.A. and Gammon, P.T. (1977). *Br. J. clin. Pharmac.*, 4, 5.

Endrenyi, L., Inaba, T. and Kalow, W. (1976). *Clin. Pharmac. Ther.*, 20, 701.

Enklewitz, M. and Lasker, M. (1935). *J. biol. Chem.*, 110, 443.

Evans, D.A.P. (1965). *Ann. N.Y. Acad. Sci.*, 123, 178.

Evans, D.A.P. (1977). In *Drug Metabolism — from Microbe to Man*, Editors: Parke, D.V. and Smith, R.L., p. 369. London: Taylor & Francis.

Evans, D.A.P., Davison, K. and Pratt, R.T.C. (1965). *Clin. Pharmac. Ther.*, 6, 430.

Evans, D.A.P., Manley, K. and McKusick, V.A. (1960). *Br. med. J.*, 2, 485.

Evans, D.A.P. and White, T.A. (1964). *J. Lab. clin. Med.*, 63, 394.

Eze, L.C., Tweedie, M.C.K., Bullen, M.F., Wren, P.J.J. and Evans, D.A.P. (1974). *Ann. hum. Genet.*, 37, 333.

Fenna, D., Mix, L., Schaefer, O. and Gilbert, J.A.L. (1971). *Can. med. Ass. J.*, 105, 472.

Flohé, L. and Günzler, W.A. (1974). In *Glutathione. Proceedings of the 16th Conference of the German Society of Biological Chemistry, Tübingen, March 1973*. Editors: Flohé, L., Benöhr, H.C., Sies, H., Woller, H.D. and Wendel, A., p. 132. New York: Academic Press.

Foulk, W.T., Butt, H.R., Owen, C.A., Whitcomb, F.F. and Mason, H.L. (1959). *Medicine, Baltimore*, 38, 25.

Fouts, J.R. and Brodie, B.B. (1957). *J. Pharmac. exp. Ther.*, 119, 197.

Frick, P.G. Hitzig, W.H. and Betke, K. (1962). *Blood*, 20, 261.

Gilbert, A., Lereboullet, P. and Herscher, M. (1907). *Bull. Mém. Soc. méd. Hôp. Paris*, 24, 1203.

Goedde, H.W. and Baitsch, H. (1964). *Br. Med. J.*, 2, 310.

Goldberg, A., Brodie, M.J. and Moore, M.J. (in the press). In *Price's Textbook of Medicine*, 12th Ed. London; Oxford University Press.

Granick, S. (1965). *Ann. N.Y. Acad. Sci.*, 123, 188.

Granick, S. (1966). *J. biol. Chem.*, 241, 1359.

Granick, S. and Urata, G. (1963). *J. biol. Chem.*, 238, 821.

Grant, W.M. (1955). *Pharmac. Rev.*, 7, 143.

Grunberg, E., Leiwant, B., D'Ascensio, I.-L. and Schnitzer, R.J. (1952). *Dis. Chest.*, 21, 369.

Habig, W.H., Keen, J.H. and Jakoby, W.B. (1975). *Biochem. biophys. Res. Commun.*, 64, 501.

Habig, W.H., Pabst, M.J. and Jakoby, W.B. (1974). *J. biol. Chem.*, 249, 7130.

Harris, H., Hopkinson, D.A., Robson, E.B. and Whittaker, M. (1963). *Ann. hum. genet.*, 26, 359.

Harris, H. and Whittaker, M. (1963). *Ann. hum. Genet.*, 27, 53.

Harris, J.W. (1970). In *The Red Cell.* Cambridge: Harvard University Press.

Harris, W.S. and Goodman, R.M. (1968). *New Engl. J. Med.*, 279, 407.

Haugen, D.A., Coon, M.J. and Nebert, D.W. (1976). *J. biol. Chem.*, 251, 1817.

Heidelberger, C. (1975). *A. Rev. Biochem.* 44, 79.

Herbert, V. and Castle, W.B. (1964). *New Engl. J. Med.*, 270, 181.

Hiller, A. (1917). *J. biol. Chem.*, 30, 129.

Holst, R. and Möller, H. (1975). *Br. J. Derm.*, 93, 145.

Hopkinson, D.A., Spencer, N. and Harris, H. (1963). *Nature, Lond.*, 199, 969.

Hsieh, H. and Jaffé, E.R. (1971). *J. clin. Invest.*, 50, 196.

Hughes, H.B. (1953). *J. Pharmac. exp. Ther.*, 109, 444.

Hughes, H.B., Biehl, J.P., Jones, A.P. and Schmidt, L.H. (1954). *Am. Rev. Tuberc. pulm. Dis.*, 70, 266.

Hughes, H.B., Schmidt, L.H. and Biehl, J.P. (1955). In *Transactions of the 14th Conference on the Chemotherapy of Tuberculosis*, p. 217. Washington, D.C.: Veterans Administration: Army: Navy.

Ingbar, S.H. (1961). *J. clin. Invest.*, 40, 2053.

Jacob, F. and Monod, J. (1961). *J. molec. Biol.*, 3, 318.

Jacob, H.S., Brain, M.C., Dacie, J.V., Carrell, R.W. and Lehmann, H. (1968). *Nature, Lond.*, 218, 1214.

Jenne, J.W. (1965). *J. clin. Invest.*, 44, 1992.

Jenne, J.W., McDonald, F.M. and Mendoza, E. (1961). *Am. Rev. resp. Dis.*, 84, 371.

Jervis, G.A. (1959). *A.M.A. Archs Neurol. Psychiatry*, 81, 55.

Jick, H., Slone, D., Shapiro, S., Heinonen, O.P., Lawson, D.H., Lewis, G.P., Jusko, W., Ballingall, D.L.K., Siskind, V., Hartz, S., Gaetano, L.F., MacLaughlin, D.S., Parker, W.J., Wizwer, P., Dinan, B., Baxter, C. and Miettinen, O.S. (1972). *Circulation*, 45, 352.

Jick, H., Slone, D., Westerholm, B., Inman, W.H.W., Vessey, M.P., Shapiro, S., Lewis, G.P. and Worcester, J. (1969). *Lancet*, 1, 539.

Johnstone, E.C. (1976). *Psychopharmacologia*, 46, 289.

Jori, A., Pugliatti, C. and Santini, V. (1972). *Pharmacology*, 7, 296.

Kalow, W. (1962). *Pharmacogenetics: Heredity and the Response to Drugs*, p. 146. Philadelphia: W.B. Saunders.

Kalow, W. (1972). *Fedn Proc. Fedn Am. Socs exp. Biol.*, 31, 1270.

Kalow, W. and Davies, R.O. (1959). *Biochem. Pharmac.*, 1, 183.

Kalow, W. and Genest, K. (1957). *Can. J. Biochem. Physiol.*, 35, 339.

Kalow, W. and Lindsay, H.A. (1955). *Can. J. Biochem. Physiol.*, 33, 568.

Kalow, W., Kadar, D., Inaba, T. and Tang, B.K. (1977). *Clin. Pharmac. Ther.*, 21, 530.

Kappas, A., Bradlow, H.L., Gillette, P.N., Levere, R.D. and Gallagher, T.F. (1972). *Fedn Proc. Fedn Am. Socs exp. Biol.*, 31, 1293.

Katz, M., Lee, S.K. and Cooper, B.A. (1972). *New Engl. J. Med.*, 287, 425.

Keitt, A.S., Smith, T.W. and Jandl, J.H. (1966). *New Engl. J. Med.*, 275, 398.

Keitt, A.S. (1972). In *The Metabolic Basis of Inherited Disease*, 3rd Ed., Editors: Stanbury, J.B., Wyngaarden, J.B. and Frederickson, D.S., p. 1389. New York: McGraw-Hill.

Kellerman, L. and Posner, A. (1955). *Am. J. Ophthal.*, 40, 681.

Kellermeyer, R.W., Tarlov, A.R., Schrier, S.L., Carson, P.E. and Alving, A.S. (1961). *J. Lab. clin. Med.*, 58, 225.

Kelley, W.N., Greene, M.L., Rosenbloom, F.M., Henderson, J.F. and Seegmiller, J.E. (1969). *Ann. intern. Med.*, 70, 155.

Kelley, W.N., Rosenbloom, F.M., Henderson, J.F. and Seegmiller, J.E. (1967). *Proc. natn. Acad. Sci. U.S.A.*, 57, 1735.

Kiese, M. (1966). *Pharmac. Rev.*, 18, 1091.

Knight, R.A., Selin, M.J. and Harris, H.W. (1959). In *Transactions of the 18th Conference on the Chemotherapy of Tuberculosis*, p. 52.

Koivula, T., Koivusalo, M. and Lindros, K.O. (1975). *Biochem. Pharmac.*, 24, 1807.

Konrad, P.N., Richards, F., Valentine, W.N. and Paglia, D.E. (1972). *New Engl. J. Med.*, 286, 557.

Kosterlitz, H.W. and Hughes, J. (1975). *Life Sci.*, 17, 91.

Kutt, H., Winters, W., Kokenge, R. and McDowell, F. (1964a). *Archs Neurol., Chicago*, 11, 642.

Kutt, H., Winters, W. and McDowell, F.H. (1966). *Neurology, Minneap.*, 16, 594.

Kutt, H., Wolk, M., Scherman, R. and McDowell, F. (1964b). *Neurology, Minneap.*, 14, 542.

La Du, B.N. (1972). *Fedn Proc. Fedn Am. Socs exp. Biol.*, 31, 1276.

Lehmann, H. and Liddell, J. (1964). *Progr. med. Genet.*, 3, 75.

Lehmann, H. and Ryan, E. (1956). *Lancet*, 2, 124.

Lewis, G.P., Jick, H., Slone, D. and Shapiro, S. (1971). *Ann. N.Y. Acad. Sci.*, 179, 729.

Löhr, G.W., Blume, K.G., Rüdiger, H.W. and Arnold, H. (1974). In *Glutathione. Proceedings of the 16th Conference of the German Society of Biological Chemistry, Tübingen, March 1973*. Editors: Flohé, L. Benöhr, H.C., Sies, H., Waller, H.D. and Wendel, A., p. 165. New York: Academic Press.

Lubin, A.H., Garry, P.J. and Owen, G.M. (1971). *Science, N.Y.*, 173, 161.

Luzzatto, L., Usanga, E.A. and Reddy, S. (1969). *Science, N.Y.*, 164, 839.

McIntyre, O.R., Sullivan, L.W., Jeffries, G.H. and Silver, R.H. (1965). *New Engl. J. Med.*, 272, 981.

Mahgoub, A., Idle, J.R., Dring, L.G., Lancaster, R. and Smith, R.L. (1977). *Lancet*, 2, 584.

Mandema, E., de Fraiture, W.H., Niewig, H.O. and Arends, A. (1960). *Am. J. Med.*, 28, 42.

Man-Yan, D.R., Arimura, G.K. and Yunis, A.A. (1975). *Molec. Pharmac.*, 11, 520.

Margolis, J.L. (1929). *Am. J. med. Sci.*, 177, 348.

Marks, P.A. and Banks, J. (1965). *Ann. N.Y. Acad. Sci.*, 123, 198.

Marks, P.A. and Gross, R.T. (1959). *J. clin. Invest.*, 38, 2253.

Martz, F., Failinger, C. and Blake, D.A. (1977). *J. Pharmac. exp. Ther.*, 203, 23.

Max Kjellman, N.-I. (1977). *Acta paediat. Scand.*, 66, 465.

Meister, A. (1974). In *Glutathione. Proceedings of the 16th Conference of the German Society of Biological Chemistry, Tübingen, March 1973*. Editors: Flohé, L., Benöhr, H.C., Sies, H., Waller, H.D. and Wendel, A., p. 56. New York: Academic Press.

Metge, W.R., Owen, C.A., Foulk, W.T. and Hoffman, N.H. (1964). *J. Lab. clin. Med.*, 64, 89.

Miller, J.A. (1970). *Cancer Res.*, 30, 559.

Mitchell, J.R., Potter, W.Z., Hinson, J.A., Snodgrass, W.R., Timbrell, J.A. and Gillette, J.R. (1975). In *Concepts in Biochemical Pharmacology. Handbook of Experimental Pharmacology*, Editors: Gillette, J.R. and Mitchell, J.R. Vol. XXVIII: 3, p. 383. Berlin, Heidelberg, New York: Springer-Verlag.

Mitchell, J.R., Thorgeirsson, U.P., Black, M.J., Timbrell, J.A., Snodgrass, W.R., Potter, W.Z., Jollow, D.J. and Keiser, H.R. (1975). *Clin. Pharmac. Ther.*, 18, 70.

Motulsky, A.G. (1957). *J. Am. med. Ass.*, 165, 835.

Motulsky, A.G. (1964). *Prog. med. Genet*, 3, 49.

Motulsky, A.G., Yoshida, A. and Stomatoyannopoulos, G. (1971). *Ann. N.Y. Acad. Sci.*, 179, 636.

Moulds, R.F.W. and Denborough, M.A. (1974). *Br. med. J.*, 2, 241.

Mühlens, P. (1926). *Naturwiss.*, 14, 1162.

Muller, C.J. and Kingma, S. (1961). *Biochim. biophys. Acta.*, 50, 595.

Nagao, T. and Mauer, A.M. (1969). *New Engl. J. Med.*, 281, 7.

Nebert, D.W. and Atlas, S.A. (1977). In *Genetics of Human Cancer*, Editors: Mulvihill, J.J., Miller, R.W. and Fraumeni, J.F., p. 301. New York: Raven Press.

Nebert, D.W., Robinson, J.R., Niwa, A., Kumaki, K. and Poland, A.P. (1975). *J. cell Physiol.*, 83, 393.

Necheles, T.F. (1974). In *Glutathione: Proceedings of the 16th Conference of the German Society of Biological Chemistry, Tübingen, March 1973*, Editors: Flohé, L., Benöhr, H.C., Sies, H., Waller, H.D. and Wendel, A., p. 173. New York: Academic Press.

Neitlich, H.W. (1966). *J. clin. Invest.*, 45, 380.

Nelson, S.D., Snodgrass, W.R. and Mitchell, J.R. (1975). *Fedn Proc. Fedn Am. Socs. exp. Biol.*, 34, 784.

O'Reilly, R.A. (1970). *New Engl. J. Med.*, 282, 1448.

O'Reilly, R.A., Aggeler, P.M., Hoag, M.S., Leong, L.S. and Kropatkin, M. (1964). *New Engl. J. Med.*, 271, 809.

O'Reilly, R.A., Pool, J.G. and Aggeler, P.M. (1968). *Ann. N.Y. Acad. Sci.*, 151, 913.

Palma, M.D. (1928). *Rif. Med.*, 44, 753.

Perry, H.M. (1973). *Am. J. Med.*, 54, 58.
Perry, H.M., Tan, E.M., Carmody, S. and Sakamoto, A. (1970). *J. Lab. clin. Med.*, 76, 114.
Peters, J.H., Miller, K.S. and Brown, P. (1965). *Analyt. Biochem.*, 12, 379.
Peterson, R.E. and Schmid, R. (1957). *J. clin. Endocr. Metab.*, 17, 1485.
Poland, A. and Glover, E. (1973). *Science, N.Y.*, 179, 476.
Poland, A.P., and Glover, E. (1975). *Molec. Pharmac.*, 11, 389.
Poland, A.P., Glover, E. and Kende, A.S. (1976). *J. biol. Chem.*, 251, 4936.
Powell, L.W., Hemingway, E., Billing, B.H. and Sherlock, S. (1967). *New Engl. J. Med.*, 277, 1108.
Prankerd, T.A.J. (1961). *The Red Cell: An Account of its Chemical Physiology and Pathology*. Oxford: Blackwell Scientific Publications Ltd.
Prescott, L.F., Steel, R.F. and Ferrier, W.R. (1970). *Clin. Pharmac. Ther.*, 11, 496.
Rajamanickam, C., Satyanarayana Rao, M.R. and Padmanaban, G. (1975). *J. biol. Chem.*, 250, 2305.
Robitzek, E.H., Selikoff, I.J. and Ornstein, G.G. (1952). *Q. Bull. Sea View Hosp.*, 13, 27.
Robson, J.M. and Sullivan, F.M. (1963). *Pharmac. Rev.*, 15, 169.
Rosen, F.S. and Merler, E. (1972). In *The Metabolic Basis of Inherited Disease*, 3rd Ed., Editors: Stanbury, J.B., Wyngaarden, J.B. and Frederickson, D.S., p. 1633. New York: McGraw-Hill.
Rubinstein, H.M., Dietz, A.A., Hodges, L.K., Lubrano, T. and Czebotar, V. (1970). *J. clin. Invest.*, 49, 479.
Ruddy, S. and Austen, K.F. (1972). In *The Metabolic Basis of Inherited Disease*, 3rd Ed., Editors: Stanbury, J.B., Wyngaarden, J.B. and Frederickson, D.S., p. 1655. New York: McGraw-Hill.
Schmid, R. (1972). In *The Metabolic Basis of Inherited Disease*, 3rd Ed., Editors: Stanbury, J.B., Wyngaarden, J.B. and Frederickson, D.S., p. 1141. New York: McGraw-Hill.
Schmid, R. and Hammaker, L. (1959). *New Engl. J. Med.*, 260, 1310.
Schoenfield, L.J., McGill, D.B., Hunter, D.B., Foulk, W.F. and Butt, H.R. (1963). *Gastroenterology*, 44, 101.
Scott, E.M. (1970). *Biochem. biophys. Res. Commun.*, 38, 902.
Scott, E.M. (1973). *Ann. hum. Genet.*, 37, 139.
Scott, T.G. (1945). *Br. J. Opthal.*, 29, 12.
Seegmiller, J.E., Rosenbloom, F.M. and Kelley, W.N. (1967). *Science, N.Y.*, 155, 1682.
Shahidi, N.T. (1967). *Am. J. Dis. Child.*, 113, 81.
Shahidi, N.T. (1968). *Ann. N.Y. Acad. Sci.*, 151, 822.
Shibata, Y., Higashi, T., Hirai, H. and Hamilton, H.B. (1967). *Archs Biochem. Biophys.*, 118, 200.
Shum, S., Lambert, G.H. and Nebert, D.W. (1977). *Pediat. Res.*, 11, 529.
Singer, K. (1955). *Am. J. Med.*, 18, 633.
Smith, C.S., Chinn, S. and Watts, R.W.E. (1977). *Biochem. Pharmac.*, 26, 847.
Smith, J., Tyrrell, W.F., Gow, A., Allan, G.W. and Lees, A.W. (1972). *Chest.*, 61, 587.
Smith, M., Hopkinson, D.A. and Harris, H. (1973). *Ann. hum. Genet.*, 37, 49.
Smith, R.L., Idle, J.R. Mahgoub, A.A., Sloan, T.P. and Lancaster, R. (1978). *Lancet*, 1, 943.
Solomon, H.M. (1968). *Ann. N.Y. Acad. Sci.*, 151, 932.
Sorensen, L.B. (1968). *Fedn Proc. Fedn Am. Socs exp. Biol.*, 27, 1099.
Sprinz, H. and Nelson, R.S. (1954). *Ann. intern. Med.*, 41, 952.
Srivastava, S.K. and Beutler, E. (1968). *Lancet*, 2, 23.
Strand, L.J., Manning, J. and Marver, H.S. (1972). *J. biol. Chem.*, 247, 2820.
Sutherland, R., Vincent, P.C., Raik, E. and Burgess, K. (1977). *Br. med. J.*, 1, 605.
Szabó, L. and Ebrey, P. (1963). *Acta paediat. hung.*, 4, 153.
Takahara, S. (1952). *Lancet*, 2, 1101.
Takahara, S. (1968). In *Hereditary Disorders of Erythrocyte Metabolism*, Editor: Beutler, E., Vol. 1, p. 21. New York: Grune & Stratton.
Takahara, S., Hamilton, H.B., Neel, J.V., Kobara, T.Y., Ogura, Y. and Nishimura, E.T. (1960). *J. clin. Invest.*, 39, 610.
Teng, Y.-S., Anderson, J.E. and Giblett, E.R. (1975). *Am. J. hum. Genet.*, 27, 492.
Thorgeirsson, S.S. and Nebert, D.W. (1977). *Adv. Cancer Res.*, 25, 149.
Timbrell, J.A., Wright, J.M. and Baillie, T.A. (1977). *Clin. Pharmac. Ther.*, 22, 602.
Tucker, G.T., Silas, J.H., Iyun, A.O., Lennard, M.S. and Smith, A.J. (1977). *Lancet*, 2, 718.

Turchetti, A. (1948). *Rif. Med.*, 62, 325.

Vesell, E.S. (1972). *New Engl. J. Med.*, 287, 904.

Vesell, E.S., Page, J.G. and Passananti, G.T. (1971). *Clin. Pharmac. Ther.*, 12, 192.

Wang, Y.M. and van Eys, J. (1970). *New Engl. J. Med.*, 282, 892.

von Wartburg, J.P. and Schürch, P.M. (1968). *Ann. N.Y. Acad. Sci.*, 151, 936.

Weber, W.W. (1971). In *Concepts in Biochemical Pharmacology. Handbook of Experimental Pharmacology.* Editors: Brodie, B.B. and Gillette, J.R., Vol. XXVIII: 2, p. 564. Berlin, Heidelberg, New York: Springer-Verlag.

Weber, W.W., Cohen, S.N. and Steinberg, M.S. (1968). *Ann. N.Y. Acad. Sci.*, 151, 734.

Wolff, P.H. (1972). *Science, N.Y.*, 175, 449.

Woosley, R.L., Nies, A.S., Drayer, D., Reidenberg, M. and Oates, J.A. (1977). *Clin. Res.*, 25, 379A.

Wright, W.T. (1961). *New Engl. J. Med.*, 265, 1154.

Yaffe, S.J., Levy, G., Matsuzawa, T. and Baliah, T. (1966). *New Engl. J. Med.*, 275, 1461.

Yoshida, A. and Motulsky, A.G. (1969). *Am. J. hum. Genet.*, 21, 486.

Yunis, A.A. (1973). *Semin. Hematol.*, 10, 225.

Yunis, A.A. and Harrington, W.J. (1960). *J. Lab. clin. Med.*, 56, 831.

Zacest, R. and Koch-Weser, J. (1972). *Clin. Pharmac. Ther.*, 13, 420.

Zingale, S.B., Minzer, L., Rosenberg, B. and Lee, S.L. (1963). *Ann. intern. Med.*, 112, 63.

4. The effect of diet on the toxicity of drugs

M. Angeli-Greaves and A. E. M. McLean

Introduction

The chemical environment of man, that is all the molecules that impinge upon him, can be thought of as falling into five categories:
1. Air, and inhaled substances, such as smoke and dust;
2. Water;
3. Food and drink;
4. Substances ingested for social or therapeutic purposes, or for pleasure (medications, herbs, drugs, betel chewing);
5. Substances applied to the skin — cosmetics, soaps, oils, etc., applied either by individual choice or through industrial exposure.

However, from the point of view of, say, a liver cell, it does not matter whether a molecule arrives via an anal suppository, an industrial smoke, or a food colourant.

The bulk of the molecules that come into contact with cells come as food. We eat 1-3 kilograms of food per day, and food is inextricably a part of man's culture. It has great symbolic significance, and food habits merge gradually into social customs, such as dancing, drinking, the use of herbs and spices, washing or cosmetics, making it difficult to isolate single factors in food.

The components of the diet can be looked at from three points of view:
1. General nutritional adequacy;
2. Contamination with toxic substances;
3. Factors in the food that alter metabolic networks, and so alter response to toxic substances.

The role of diet on drug toxicity is complex, and few generalizations are possible, but there are a number of suggested relationships between diet and toxicity for which the evidence is strong. The view that diet may alter response to toxic materials has emerged as the result of two lines of investigation: firstly, animal experiments in which diet is a variable that affects an experimental toxicity model; and secondly, epidemiological studies followed by formulation of hypotheses to explain a possible correlation found between dietary habits in a community or group of patients and a particular pattern of disease.

Pharmacokinetic considerations

A drug follows a route of absorption, distribution, metabolism and excretion which depends on a number of systems that can be influenced and modified through changes in the diet. There is little information about drug absorption in malnourished states.

Orally administered drugs are generally absorbed through the digestive tract mucosa and especially through the small intestine epithelium. In long-term protein deficiency, severe mucosal atrophy is found (Trowell, Davies & Dean, 1954).

The pharmacokinetics of a compound can be of importance in the process of acute toxicity (Mitchell, 1975) as peak plasma levels of a drug may cause such high tissue levels in the liver that normally safe metabolic pathways are saturated. When this happens, minor pathways may become significant and a higher proportion of these alternative metabolites produced, which may be toxic (see Chapter 1). Conversely, if absorption of the drug is retarded, the safe pathway will not be saturated as high peak plasma levels will not be reached and toxic metabolites will not be produced in appreciable amounts.

Once absorbed, drugs are transported in the bloodstream to their active sites and places of metabolism and excretion. Many drugs are transported in an albumin-bound form. In low protein states such as kwashiorkor, one of the earliest and most striking changes is the decrease in the levels of plasma albumin. When this occurs, saturation of drug binding sites in the albumin fraction will take place at lower plasma levels than normal and probably at lower doses than normal. This could be an important factor in the toxicity of some drugs. For example, the diuretic frusemide has been shown experimentally to produce kidney damage as a consequence of overdose. Toxicity seems to develop on saturation of the plasma albumin frusemide carrier. Excess frusemide then stays unbound in the plasma, the levels of free drug reaching the kidney increase and toxic effects are seen (Mitchell, 1975).

Frusemide metabolism and plasma protein binding in malnourished states has not been studied and might offer some interesting information, as would studies of diphenylhydantoin kinetics in the malnourished, as a similar mechanism has been described for this drug.

A great deal of evidence exists, both experimentally and in human studies, correlating protein-calorie deficiencies with alterations in the kidney function (Klahr & Alleyne, 1973). The observed fall in glomerular filtration and renal plasma flow would be expected to change the elimination kinetics of many drugs.

Metabolic considerations

Perhaps the best studied aspect of the influence of nutrition on the fate of drugs is the change in drug-metabolizing enzymes in the liver.

The level of cytochrome P-450 in the liver of an experimental animal depends on its nutritional and hormonal state (Marshall & McLean, 1969). This level can easily be increased, and the activity of the system induced by giving any of a series of compounds such as DDT, polycyclic hydrocarbons or phenobarbitone (Conney & Burns, 1962) or decreased by compounds such as cobalt chloride. By altering the diet one can change the basal levels of cytochrome P-450 and also the response to inducing agents (Sachan, 1975; Wade & Norred, 1976; Campbell & Hayes, 1974; Marshall & McLean, 1971a and b).

The level of enzyme induction depends on both protein and fat intakes (Table 4.1). What matters is not only the total amount of fat (Table 4.2) but also the type of fat fed to the experimental animal (Table 4.3).

Table 4.1. Interaction of dietary protein and polyunsaturated fat (herring oil) on concentration of cytochrome P-450 in the liver of rats. Male rats (initial body weight 110-130g) were fed on the diets for 10 days, four rats to each group.

Diet	Microsomal cytochrome P-450 (nmol/g liver)	
	Water	Phenobarbitone
No protein, no fat	8 ± 1	24 ± 6
No protein, 15% herring oil	13 ± 1	53 ± 17
20% casein, no fat	18 ± 3	60 ± 7
20% casein, 15% herring oil	24 ± 7	123 ± 19
Stock pellets (41B diet)	30 ± 3	124 ± 7

Modified from Marshall & McLean (1971a).

Table 4.2. The permissive effect of dietary cod liver oil on the induction of hepatic microsomal cytochrome P-450 by phenobarbitone in rats fed 3% and 20% casein diets.

Concentration of oil in diet	Liver cytochrome P-450 (nmol/g liver)	
	3% Casein	20% Casein
0%	33 ± 9 (12)	45 ± 8 (28)
1%		57 ± 13 (4)
2.5%	50 ± 5 (4)	92 ± 14 (4)
5%	57 ± 3 (4)	92 ± 17 (8)
7.5%	70 ± 18 (4)	107 ± 19 (4)
10%	56 ± 11 (4)	111 ± 18 (8)

From Marshall & McLean, unpublished data.

Table 4.3. The effect of dietary fats on the induction of cytochrome P-450 by phenobarbitone in the liver of rats.

Diet	Cytochrome P-450 (nmol/g liver)
20% casein, no fat	45 ± 8
10% coconut oil	58 ± 17
10% olive oil	66 ± 9
10% maize oil	81 ± 12
10% herring oil	111 ± 9
10% cod liver oil	120 ± 13
Pellets (41B diet)	120 ± 21

Modified from Marshall & McLean (1971b).

Cytochrome P-450 is not a single protein but rather a group of enzymes which exist as part of the endoplasmic reticulum membrane and depend on it for their function. When the lipid content of the diet is altered, fatty acid composition of cell lipids is also altered and this might influence the activity of the system (Coniglio, Buck & Grogan, 1976; Kyriakides *et al.*, 1976; Wade & Norred, 1976).

Vesell & Page (1969), in a pioneering series of experiments in humans, showed that the clearance of such drugs as antipyrine and phenylbutazone could be used as a measure of drug-metabolizing activity. The latter was shown to be subject to genetic factors. In further studies in twins, Vesell pointed out environmental influences over the metabolism of drugs.

Recent experiments by Kappas *et al.* (1976) have related protein and carbohydrate intake to drug metabolism.

Dietary influences over cytochrome P-450 activity include not only protein fat and caloric content but also the presence of inducing agents in the diet. Fraser *et al.* (1977) studied a population group in Gambia and found that despite their low protein intake their antipyrine half-life did not differ significantly from British or American populations. They attributed this to the presence of inducing agents in their diet. On the other hand, between two groups of subjects in Britain, one vegetarian and the other non-vegetarian, there were significant differences in their antipyrine half-lives. This study, however, did not rule out the possibility of a genetic variable, as the vast majority of the vegetarians were Asian and the non-vegetarians were Caucasian. Metabolism of antipyrine in healthy Caucasian volunteers from Washington, Dundee, Hanover and Stockholm has not shown any significant differences (Table 4.4).

Table 4.4.   Metabolism of antipyrine in healthy volunteers.

Population	Reference	Antipyrine half-life (h, mean ± SD)	Number of subjects studied
Washington	Vesell & Page (1969)	10.9 ± 3.0	36
Dundee	O'Malley *et al.* (1973)	12.0 ± 3.5	61
Hanover	May *et al.* (1974)	11.9 ± 2.2	21
Stockholm	Kolmodin *et al.* (1969)	13.1 ± 7.5	33

These nutritional-pharmacological interactions may have considerable importance in cases such as debilitated or chronically ill patients. Nowadays, a significant segment of the population manipulate their diets in order to reduce weight. Others use diets as part of a therapy programme, as in the case of diabetic or hypertensive patients, while post-operative and unconscious patients fed intravenously usually ingest very little protein during these periods.

Nutrition and toxicity

Carbon tetrachloride

Carbon tetrachloride is eliminated mainly unchanged in the expired air, but a small fraction of the dose may be metabolized by cytochrome P-450 in the liver.

The resultant metabolite is a highly reactive compound, believed to be a trichloromethyl ($\cdot CCl_3$) free radical that can react with and bind to proteins in the cell. This has been suggested as the molecular basis of carbon tetrachloride toxicity by Slater (see Chapter 6) and also by Castro (1974).

Lipid peroxidation has also been proposed as the mechanism of carbon tetrachloride toxicity by Recknagel (1967), but the failure of vitamin E to protect against the hepatotoxic effects suggests that autocatalytic peroxidation is probably not one of the major reactions relevant to cell injury. Chloroform, which is a hepatotoxin chemically closely related to carbon tetrachloride, fails to induce autocatalytic peroxidation (Klaasen & Plaa, 1969; McLean & McLean, 1969).

Induction of cytochrome P-450 increases the susceptibility of the liver to carbon tetrachloride, and the decrease in LD_{50} correlates well with the level of activity of cytochrome P-450, as shown in Table 4.5.

Table 4.5. The effect of diet and enzyme induction on the toxicity of carbon tetrachloride.

Diet	Pretoxin	Pretoxin in dose LD_{50} (mg/kg)	Total amount metabolized	
			% of dose	mg/kg
Protein-free	CCl_4	24 000	0.1	24
Stock	CCl_4	6 000	0.3	18
Stock + phenobarbital	CCl_4	800	3.0	24

Modified from McLean (1974).

Conversely, decreasing the protein content of the diet, which reduces cytochrome P-450 levels in the liver to about one third of that of control animals, protects against damage by carbon tetrachloride, making the animals unusually resistant to its toxic effects. Measurement of the pulmonary elimination of unchanged $^{14}CCl_4$ showed that this route is not altered when the protein content of the diet is decreased, but the total amount of labelled carbon dioxide, an indicator of $^{14}CCl_4$ metabolism by cytochrome P-450 in the liver, is drastically different, as shown in Figure 4.1 (McLean, 1975).

It seems likely then, that carbon tetrachloride combines with cytochrome P-450 and is there converted into a highly reactive trichloromethyl radical. This in turn attacks numerous cell sites; this explains why toxicity occurs only in cells possessing the cytochrome P-450 system, and the protection conferred by low protein diets. This is an example in which malnutrition

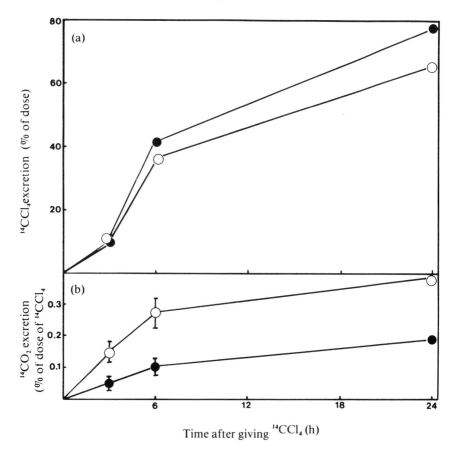

Fig. 4.1. Expiration of $^{14}CCl_4$ (*a*) and $^{14}CO_2$ (*b*) after rats given stock (open circles) or protein-free (closed circles) diets had been given $^{14}CCl_4$ (2.5 ml/kg). Each point marks the mean and range of measurements made on at least 3 rats.

From Seawright & McLean (1967).

proves to be an advantage to the rat, at least in the toxicology laboratory!

When mechanisms of toxicity are being investigated, other factors must be taken into account. The liver has built-in defence mechanisms to cope with highly reactive metabolites. Glutathione, a tripeptide, reacts with some toxic metabolites and renders them harmless by binding via its thiol group, and so prevents the toxic metabolite from reacting with the cell's proteins, enzymes and nucleic acids.

Carbon tetrachloride toxicity does not depend at all on glutathione levels, perhaps because, being a very lipid-soluble substance, the reactive metabolite never leaves the membrane, so that the water-soluble glutathione cannot reach it. However, liver glutathione levels have been shown to be of importance in the case of paracetamol.

Paracetamol

The role of glutathione in paracetamol toxicity has been described by Mitchell *et al.* (1973a) and the possibility of preventing toxic effects of paracetamol overdoses by dietary means by McLean & Day (1975).

Paracetamol is metabolized in the liver mainly to the glucuronide and sulphate conjugates, but a small amount goes through the cytochrome P-450 system and is converted into a toxic metabolite (Mitchell *et al.*, 1974).

Dietary protein levels do not affect glucuronide or sulphate conjugation but do change cytochrome P-450 levels and therefore modify the rate of formation of the toxic metabolite.

On the basis of experience with carbon tetrachloride, it would have been logical to expect that low protein diets would protect against paracetamol liver damage, but in fact the opposite takes place. Low casein diets or 25% yeast diets make rats highly susceptible to the liver necrosis of paracetamol overdosage. A likely explanation is that both the low protein diet and the yeast diet lower glutathione levels in the liver and thus make it more vulnerable to the small amount of toxic metabolite that the reduced amount of cytochrome P-450 is capable of producing. Addition of methionine almost completely prevents the liver necrosis (McLean & Day, 1975).

Evidence supporting this theory shows that liver slices incubated with paracetamol *in vitro* for two hours and then placed in fresh Ringer solution for another four hours leak potassium at a significantly higher rate than control slices incubated without paracetamol (McLean & Nuttall, 1978), as shown in Figure 4.2. Glutathione becomes depleted in the slices, and addition of methionine to the incubation medium of liver slices exposed to paracetamol accelerates repletion of glutathione in the slice, as shown in Figure 4.3. Glutathione repletion, however, does not prevent potassium leakage from the slice, indicating that, whatever damage takes place, it is not reversed by increasing the levels of glutathione. This reinforces the theory that glutathione acts in preventing the biochemical lesion from taking place, but once this has occurred, is powerless to reverse it (McLean & Nuttall, personal communication).

Cancer and nutrition

There is massive evidence linking dietary habits with cancer incidence. Information is mainly epidemiological, although experimental data exist to confirm several of these findings. Human data on an international basis have been compiled by Armstrong & Doll (1975). There is also a series of studies on migrant families of Japanese origin who settled in California and Hawaii, in which a correlation is found between the change in dietary habits as the families adapt to the new country and the change in incidence of specific cancers (Dunn, 1975; Hankin, Nomura & Rhoads, 1975).

There have also been case control studies that have attempted to determine, with hindsight, the probable role of diet on specific cases or patients. These studies are at the very least difficult to control and interpret, and can be misleading.

Drug toxicity

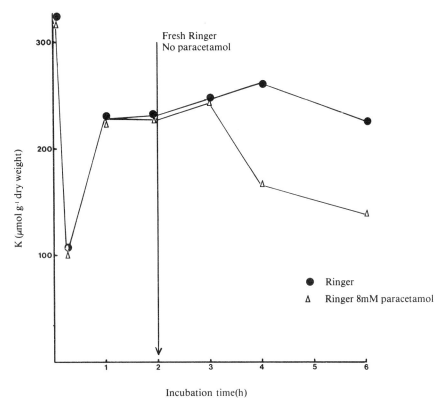

Fig. 4.2. Effect of 2h incubation with 8mM paracetamol on potassium content during 4h subsequent incubation in Ringer albumin solution in liver slices from phenobarbital-treated rats.

Liver slices from two rats were incubated with Ringer, with and without 8mM paracetamol for 2h. The slices were then incubated in fresh Ringer albumin solution without paracetamol for a further 4h.

Potassium content of the slices were measured as described by McLean (1963) *Biochem. J., 87*, 161. Each value represents the mean ± SD of at least 4 separate slices.

Animal data have been obtained from two main types of experiment, using either strains that develop spontaneous carcinomas, or conventional experimental animals which are exposed to a carcinogen. In both cases, diet is used to manipulate the incidence of cancer. These experiments have the inherent problem of being unrelated to the situation in humans, unless the model is shown to behave identically to human cancers on a number of criteria (Hill, 1978).

Experiments relating caloric intake and longevity have shown that under-fed rats have a longer lifespan than rats fed *ad libitum* (Ross & Bras, 1971). Epidemiological data from human beings show a correlation between fat content of the diet and incidence of colorrectal cancers. Hormone and tobacco-related cancers also show a positive correlation with fat intake (Armstrong & Doll, 1975).

Should this be extrapolated to the whole human population? Perhaps we ought to consider the possibility of overnutrition in the western world being involved in the causation of cancer.

Malnutrition, on the other hand, has been blamed for a series of cancers but it seems clear now that cancers related to malnutrition can be attributed to specific dietary contaminants. For example, a good correlation has been found between aflatoxin intake in the diet and liver cancer incidence in countries where contamination of foodstuffs by this mycotoxin is common (Lopez & Crawford, 1967; Peers & Linsell, 1973).

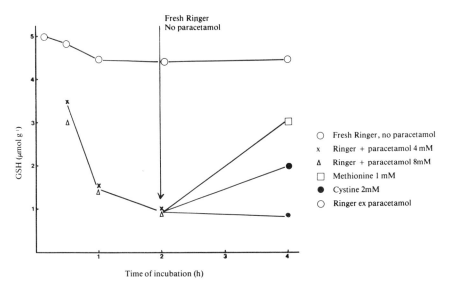

Fig. 4.3. Glutathione content (μmol/g wet weight of slice) of liver slices incubated with and without paracetamol (4 and 8mM) for 2h (phenobarbital-treated rat). Subsequent incubation in Ringer solution with and without addition of methionine and cystine. Each point represents the mean value of two slices and the graph is representative of several similar experiments.

To conclude, let us consider our diet and our grandparents' diet: our generation consumes a great deal more man-made chemicals than did previous generations (Sanders, 1966). Environmental pollutants, food preservatives, colourings and taste enhancers find their way into what we eat. On the other hand, some of these food additives ensure that the risk of fungal contamination and spoilage of foodstuffs is minimal, compared with the pre-additives era. It is likely that this will result in different patterns of disease.

The evidence we have suggests that different dietary habits may account for differences in drug metabolism and toxicity. This should be borne in mind when planning the testing and marketing of drugs on a world-wide scale: a drug tested in a third-world population might show unexpected patterns of toxicity when used on North American or European populations.

References

Armstrong, B. and Doll, R. (1975). *Int. J. Cancer,* 15, 617.

Campbell, T.C. and Hayes, J.R. (1974). *Pharmac. Rev.,* 26, 171.

Castro, J.A. (1974). *Biochem. Pharmac.,* 23, 295.

Coniglio, J.G., Buch, D. and Grogan, W.M. (1976). *Lipids,* 11, 143.

Conney, A.H. and Burns, J.J. (1962). *Adv. Pharmac.,* 1, 31.

Crawford, M.D., Gardner, M.J. and Morris, J.M. (1971). *Lancet,* iii, 327.

Dunn, J.E. (1975). *Cancer Res.,* 35, 3240.

Fraser, H.S., Mucklow, J.C., Bulpitt, C.F., Khan, C., Mould, G. and Dollery, C.T. (1977). *Clin. Pharmac. Ther.,* 22, 799.

Hankin, J.H., Nomura, A. and Rhoads, G.C. (1975). *Cancer Res.,* 35, 3259.

Hill, M. (1978). *Br. Nutr. Food Bull.* (in the press).

Kappas, A., Anderson, K.E., Conney, A.H. and Alveres, A.P. (1976). *Clin. Pharmac. Ther.,* 20, 643.

Klaasen, D.C. and Plaa, G.L. (1969). *Biochem. Pharmac.,* 18, 2019.

Klahr, S. and Alleyne, G.A.O. (1973). *Kidney International,* 3, 129.

Kolmodin, B., Azarnoff, D.L. and Sjoqvist, F. (1969). *Clin. Pharmac. Ther.,* 10, 638.

Kyriakides, E.C., Beeler, D.A., Edmonds, R.H. and Balint, J.A. (1976). *Biochim. Biophys. Acta,* 431, 399.

Lopez, A. and Crawford, M.A. (1967). *Lancet,* ii, 1351.

McLean, A.E.M. (1974). *Israel J. Med. Sci.,* 10, 431.

McLean, A.E.M. (1975). In *Drugs and the Liver,* IIIrd International Symposium, Editors: Gerok, W. and Sickinger, K., p. 143.

McLean, A.E.M. and Day, P. (1975). *Biochem. Pharmac.,* 24, 37.

McLean, A.E.M. and McLean, E.K. (1969). *Br. med. Bull.,* 25, 278.

McLean, A.E.M. and Nuttall, L. (1978). *Biochem. Pharmac.,* 27, 425.

Marshall, W.J. (1970). University of London Ph.D. Thesis, p. 73.

Marshall, W.J. and McLean, A.E.M. (1969). *Biochem. J.,* 115, 27.

Marshall, W.J. and McLean, A.E.M. (1971a). *Biochem. J.,* 122, 569.

Marshall, W.J. and McLean, A.E.M. (1971b). *Proc. Nutr. Soc.,* 30, 66A.

May, B., Helmstaedt, D., Büstgens, L. and McLean, A.E.M. (1974). *Clin. Sci.,* 46, 11.

Mitchell, J.R. (1975). *Proceedings of the Fifth International Congress on Pharmacology* (Helsinki).

Mitchell, J.R., Jollow, D.J., Potter, W.Z., Gillette, J.R. and Brodie, B.B. (1973). *J. Pharmac. exp. Ther.,* 187, 211.

Mitchell, J.R., Thorgeirsson, S., Potter, W.Z., Jollow, D.J. and Keisler, H. (1974). *Clin. Pharmac. Ther.,* 16, 676.

O'Malley, K.O., Browning, M., Stevenson, I. and Turnbull, M.J. (1973). *Eur. J. clin. Pharmac.,* 6, 102.

Peers, F.G. and Linsell, C.A. (1973). *Br. J. Cancer,* 27, 473.

Recknagel, R.O. (1967). *Pharmac. Rev.,* 19, 145.

Ross, M.H. and Bras, G. (1971). *J. Natl. Cancer Inst.,* 47, 1095.

Sachan, D.S. (1975). *J. Nutr.,* 105, 1631.

Sanders, H.J. (1966). *Chem. Eng. News.* Food Additives, part I, p. 100.

Seawright, A.A. and McLean, A.E.M. (1967). *Biochem. J.,* 105, 1055.

Smith, D.A. and Woodruff, M.F.A. (1951). Medical Research Council Special Report No. 274.

Trowell, H.C., Davies, J.N.P. and Dean, R.F.A. (1954). *Kwashiorkor.* Arnold, London.

Vesell, E.S. and Page, J.G. (1969). *J. clin. Invest.,* 48, 2202.

Wade, A.E. and Norred, W.P. (1976). *Fedn Proc.,* 35, 2475.

5. Side effects caused by differences in formulation of drugs

M. J. Groves

Introduction

In the 'Preface' to the First United States Pharmacopoeia published in 1820 there is the statement that 'It is the object of the Pharmacopoeia to select from among substances which possess medical power, those, the utility of which is most fully established and best understood; and to form from them preparations and compositions, in which their powers may be exerted to the greatest advantage'. This suggests that the influence that formulation and preparation may have on the biological activity of a drug has been appreciated for a considerable time. However, it is only relatively recently that the subject has become a branch of scientific activity in its own right. In the early nineteenth century there were few really potent drugs as we understand them, since most appear to have been laxatives of vegetable origin in one form or another. With the advent of the more potent isolated active ingredients, followed by the synthetic drugs of today, the influence of formulation upon activity and, by implication, toxicity and side effects, has become of considerable interest.

The drug is unlikely to be absorbed or excreted unless it is first released from its formulation. It is this stage of the process which is the first and most critical step for the activity of many drugs. If the formulation does not release the drug, the rest of the process becomes somewhat pointless.

Over the past decade or so there have been a number of reviews of the influence that formulation may have on activity (e.g. Levi, 1963a; Groves, 1966; Gibaldi, 1976; Wagner, 1971) and it is reasonably well established that, in some situations, the clinical effectiveness and toxicity of a drug, especially if it is pharmacologically potent (i.e. has a high effect-to-dose ratio), may be influenced by the manipulative processes involved in getting a chemical compound from the producer to the patient. Indeed, the scientific study of this phenomenon has entered the political arena. This has mainly come about because of enormous political pressure to reduce the cost of drug therapy and the encouragement to non-innovative producers to make generic copies of drugs which are the products of innovative research. The realization that the generic drugs did not always have exactly the same clinical effects as those produced by the original drug has resulted in considerable effort being placed on the study of biopharmaceutics. In fairness, the number of examples that can now be cited with confidence where toxicity has been influenced by deliberate or inadvertent interference with the release rate is relatively small. This may be simply because most drugs have a benefit-to-risk ratio sufficiently high so as to minimize any danger of toxicity due to slight changes of release rates. However, if we look at another aspect of the same problem and consider possible clinical failure because the formulation is variable this may be another matter entirely. Even the same formulation containing the same drug and formulation adjuvants may be strongly influenced by the compression to which it is subjected during a tabletting or capsulation process.

It might be argued that the simplest way around the problem would be to administer any drug as a solution in water thereby avoiding the difficulties altogether. However, since small accurately measured doses of a drug are required repeatedly, reproducible dilutions must be used. Further, the water itself is to be regarded as the formulation vehicle, and the drug substance must be water-soluble and stable in solution, which many are not. If we take into account the need for accuracy, stability and optimum performance *in vivo*, the problem can become complex. To take as an example the formulation of a simple single drug substance in a film-coated tablet, the number and chemical variety of the formulation adjuvants which are necessary to achieve the required aim becomes very formidable. (Figure 5.1).

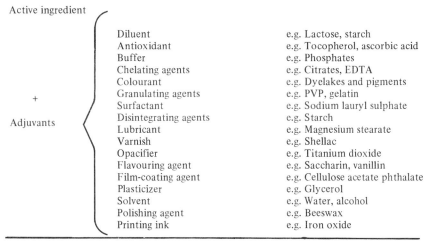

Fig. 5.1. A typical drug formulation (a film-coated tablet).

The difficulties of choosing the appropriate excipients have recently been reviewed by Hess (1977) and attention also drawn to the problems of international acceptability and commercial availability.

Direct toxicity of formulation adjuvants

Direct attribution of toxicity to the formulation adjuvants is not common and, it is usually assumed that the diluents and other ingredients are totally innocuous. That this may not always be so may be seen in the case of the ubiquitous lactose or milk sugar which is often included in tablets, capsules and some injectable products. In general it is well tolerated, but there are some individuals, such as some inhabitants of the Indian sub-continent who may be genetically incapable of tolerating lactose (see Chapter 3). Care is therefore required when selecting formulations for export into the parts of the world affected by this idiosyncrasy. In fact, in the modern world with ready transport and considerable immigration and integration between groups, this type of interaction may be more common than we realize.

An object lesson in the selection of a vehicle for a new drug was encountered in the late 1930s when attempts were made to formulate the new drug sulphanilamide. This drug is not very soluble in water, and a firm called Massengill in the United States produced a syrupy clear elixir formulation which was easy to take. The figures illustrate how easy it is to be misled. The drug is not very soluble in glycerol, which has an LD_{50} in mice of 31.5 g/kg, but there are other glycols which have the characteristic sweet taste and a much higher solvent capacity. Ethylene glycol has an LD_{50} of 13.7 g/kg to mice and 8.5 g/kg to rats, so it is slightly more toxic than diethylene glycol, which has an LD_{50} to rats of 20.8 g/kg, similar to that for glycerol (*Merck Index*, 9th Edt.). The drug, which is itself inherently toxic, was marketed in a 75% aqueous diethylene glycol flavoured elixir. Early in 1937 came the first reports of deaths, and the situation remained obscure for about six months until it became clear that the toxic ingredient in the elixir was the diethylene glycol. Even as early as March 1937, Haag & Ambrose were reporting that the glycol was excreted substantially unchanged in dogs, suggesting it was likely to be safe. Within a few weeks Holick (1937) confirmed that a low concentration of diethylene glycol in drinking water was fatal to a number of species. Hagenbusch (1937) found that necropsies on patients who had been taking 60-70 ml of the solvent per day had similar pictures to rats, rabbits and dogs taking the same dose with or without the drug. This clearly implicated the solvent, although some authors considered that it was simply potentiating the toxicity of the drug. Some idea of the magnitude of this disaster may be found in the paper of Calvary & Klumpp (1939), who reported data on 105 deaths and a further 260 survivors who were affected to different degrees, usually with progressive failure of the renal system. It is easy to be wise after the event, but the formulator fell into a classical trap in that the difference between acute and chronic toxicity had not been adequately considered. In passing, the widespread use of ethylene glycol itself as an antifreeze has led to a number of accidental deaths which suggest that the lethal dose in man is around 1.4 ml/kg, or a volume of about 100 ml.

It is unlikely that a modern formulator would fall into the same trap, but the problem of long-term toxicity of adjuvants is still with us, in particular the possibility of some materials having carcinogenic activity. Almost every country has a list of permitted colourants and food additives. Artificial colours may contain traces of toxic heavy metals or may themselves be directly toxic, but evidence on which a particular material is banned may sometimes be queried, at least in private. The quantity of a colourant, for example, ingested in the course of treatment with the average pharmaceutical product must be considerably less than that taken with foodstuffs. The situation has come to a head over sweeteners with talk of banning saccharin. The problems encountered in pharmaceutical industry when cyclamates were banned were considerable although this material may be allowed back in limited applications. The formulator of products both for export and home consumption does have problems in selecting the appropriate colourants and sweeteners for particular markets.

Contamination

While considering the problems of the toxicity of materials deliberately added to formulations, some comments on the problems of materials inadvertently contaminating products should also be made. This has recently been discussed by Flaum (1978), working in the US Food and Drug Administration. In recent years the contamination of pharmaceutical products with penicillin handled in the same plant has been a source of some concern because of its potential allergenic activity. Flaum also cites the classical case of contamination of isoniazid tablets with diethylstilboestrol by cross-flow of dust in a manufacturing unit. Microbial contamination may be a major source of difficulty as was shown by the outbreak of salmonellosis in Sweden in 1966, which was traced to contaminated defatted thyroid extract. As a consequence of this incident, attention has been turned to bacterial contamination of other pharmaceutical products, and controls are being imposed to ensure that hygienic conditions are maintained during production and storage. The microbial hazard of infusion solution therapy is well recognized as a contamination problem (Phillips, Meers & D'Arcy, 1976).

Contamination can occur in parenteral products, especially the large volume solutions which may introduce substantial quantities of unwanted and, in some cases, undesirable materials directly into the blood stream so that the front-line defences of the body are by-passed. Whilst there is little objective evidence to suggest that patients have actually died, patients who were already seriously ill may have been made worse because of complications produced by particles (Garvan & Gunner, 1964; Winding, 1978). Winding has also demonstrated (1977) that even diagnostic angiographic contrast media are heavily contaminated with particulate material, which should not be present. The main hazards are likely to be due to foreign body reactions produced by materials such as cellulose or talc and in some cases physical blockage of essential tissues and organs (Groves, 1973b; Groves & de Malka, 1976). Winding (1978) has demonstrated the blockage of areas of kidney *in vivo* by particles in the size range 10-15 μm. Although the contamination can be substantially removed by modern manufacturing methods, there is an increasing belief that much detritus is also introduced at the stage of administration by medical and nursing staff (Groves, 1977). This is hardly a formulation problem, but it does make the point that there may be a need to protect the patient from side effects which come about from incorrect use of drugs rather than the relatively minor effects which result from formulation effects. To illustrate the types of foreign materials found in intravenous products, Figure 5.2 classifies detritus into intrinsic and extrinsic sources, although these may not be hard and fast groupings.

Intrinsic	Extrinsic
Glass	Insect parts
Metal	Cellulose fibres
Bacteria	Trichomes
Fungi	Talc
Spores and fragments	Asbestos fibrils
	Glass fibres
	Carbon flakes
	Rubber and associated fillers
	Plastic particles

Fig. 5.2. Contaminants reported in intravenous fluid.

The sequence of events in drug absorption

The initial stage of drug release from the formulation, both in terms of the amount and the rate of release may exercise considerable influence at the clinical response level. A close study of the formulation parameters of any drug is therefore essential during the development of any new drug and, indeed, there are examples where formulations of established drugs also appear to require additional investigation.

A product of the type illustrated in Figure 5.1 may not always release its active component at a reproducible rate *in vivo*. Additives may have various influences on the release of a drug from its formulation. The degree to which formulation variables will influence the absorption characteristics, and result in detrimental or beneficial effects on the patient, depends on the changes in each of the subsequent series of events leading to the ultimate clinical effect. In a simplified form this is sketched out in Figure 5.3 in a sequence due to Barr (1973).

The ultimate clinical significance of a change in formulation behaviour which alters the rate and extent of drug release depends to a large degree on the magnitude of the changes introduced in each of the consequent series of variables leading to the clinical response. It is therefore a function of all other factors which modify each of these variables. Barr pointed out that the variables and the relationships between them may not always be quantifiable but it is still a useful exercise to attempt to define them by mathematical formalism in order to attempt to identify the relationship between the primary variables and secondary factors. For example, if we talk about a dosage form variable (D_f) producing a change in the amount of drug dissolving in the gastro-intestinal tract, and, of course, the rate at which it dissolves, this amount, Q_R, will in turn affect the amount which can be extracted into the systemic circulation, Q_A. Changes in the amount

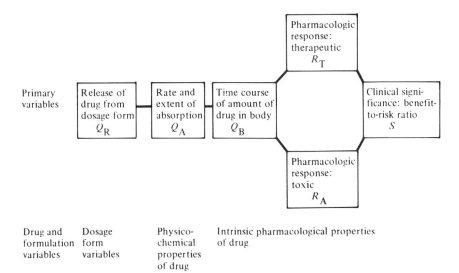

Fig. 5.3.   Sequence of pharmacological events from formulation to clinical effect,
due to Barr (1973).

absorbed may saturate binding sites or influence metabolism mechanisms and this could produce relatively large changes in the amount of drugs in the body. For many drugs, even large fluctuations in the amount of drug in the body will produce relatively few changes in therapeutic effect. Nevertheless, the converse is also true in some situations, and small increases in the body load will increase the therapeutic and/or the toxic effect, depending on the characteristics of the dose-response curve. If this is quantifiable in terms of the pharmacological response associated with the therapeutic (R_T) or adverse effects (R_A), we may be able to measure a clinical significance or benefit-to-risk ratio, S. To illustrate this point, if there was a 50% increase in the amount of a penicillin available to the patient's body it is unlikely that there would be any significant effect on the clinical response since the minimum effective concentration of the drug in the plasma is usually well below the concentrations obtained with normal clinical doses. Penicillin has an exceptionally high benefit-to-risk ratio, and even where toxicity, in the form of an allergenic response, is manifest, this does not appear to be related to the dose. The same is not true for anticoagulant drugs such as warfarin, where a 50% increase in the plasma level may produce profound clinical changes, depending on other factors such as the presence of other drugs which may interfere with protein binding, hereditary factors of the patient and the severity of the condition being treated.

Even though a drug may eventually be completely absorbed, changes in the rate of absorption may have diverse effects on the onset, duration and intensity of the pharmacological and toxicological responses. The magnitude and direction (i.e. increase or decrease) of changes in the pharmacological effects which result from changes in the absorption rate depend in turn on the relationship between the rate processes of absorption and elimination, as well as the relationship involved in the time the drug is present in the body at effective concentrations and the dose-response characteristics. A model may be built up from a stochastic description of the absorption process and the systemic availability as the sum of several sequential and parallel rate processes.

The assessment of drug release behaviour from formulations

Although the most important feature of a formulation is that it should deliver the drug and produce a non-toxic and measurable clinical response in the patient, direct routine clinical testing is not always feasible. Although this is a critical test which must at some stage be carried out, for the purpose of routine batch testing during production and the initial formulation studies, clinical testing is too expensive and the results have superimposed on them all of the other factors mentioned above. For this reason *in vitro* tests have been devised to enable the release patterns of formulations to be studied in isolation. According to Pernarowski (1974), well over 200 such tests have been described, although only a small number have achieved respectability by being incorporated into an official or pharmacopoeial monograph. The experimental factors which influence the results, such as agitation rate and environment have been reviewed elsewhere (Hersey, 1969; Alkan & Groves, 1975). Examples of differences in *in vitro* behaviour are discussed later in this chapter, but care is required when considering the interpretation of results in relation to the *in vivo* situation.

One example is the case of oxytetracycline tablets from various sources,

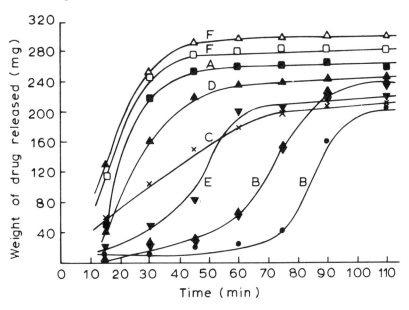

Fig. 5.4. Solution profiles of single tablets of generic brands of 250 mg oxytetracycline tablets. (From Groves, 1973.)

which demonstrated considerable differences in dissolution behaviour *in vitro* (Figures 5.4 and 5.5). However, oxytetracycline is not taken in single doses but rather as repeated doses over a period of time during a course of treatment. As with other antibiotics, it is probable that the clinical dose is far in excess of clinical requirement. Thus, subtle differences in the dissolution profiles *in vitro* may be smoothed out *in vivo* so that the ultimate clinical response may not be significantly affected. If the release is suppressed considerably there may be an increased incidence of clinical 'failure' but, in fact, there are relatively few literature reports suggesting that the formulation of this particular drug represents a problem.

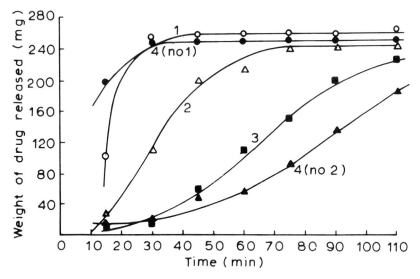

Fig. 5.5.   Solution profiles of single 250 mg oxytetracycline tablets BP from the same
source, manufacturer C, batches 1 to 4.   (From Groves, 1973.)

Examples of drug/formulation interactions

Digoxin

Digoxin is a powerful cardiotonic glycoside which has been in use clinically for nearly 40 years. The daily dose of 0.5-1 mg gives only very small amounts of material circulating in the body, so that the bioavailability studies were not carried out until radio-immune assay techniques became available. In 1971 Lindenbaum *et al.* reported differences between digoxin tablets from different sources. Since there were up to seven-fold differences at the same dose level with material from different sources, it was clear that there was, indeed, a bioavailability problem with this drug. It is a very potent material which represents a hazard to the patient. Lindenbaum *et al.* (1971) produced a good correlation between the dissolution rate of the drug formulation and the bioavailability, but the formulation factors which influence this effect are rather less certain. A re-examination of production material by the major UK manufacturer showed that the bioavailability had halved (Hamer & Grahame-Smith, 1972) due to a change in the method of mixing during the production, which had been introduced in 1969. The old method was brought back in May 1972, after it was obvious that the product had been affected (Johnson *et al.*, 1973). Manninen *et al.* (1972) had earlier pointed to a possible link between tablet disintegration and biological availability, and there may be a relationship with particle size (Shaw *et al.*, 1973) of the crystalline drug. Other factors may be super-imposed on this, since Ampolsuk *et al.* (1974) found that frictional pressure on triturates of digoxin with lactose increased the dissolution rate signifi-cantly. This observation may be related to the work of Florence, Salde & Stenlake (1974), who demonstrated that the infra-red spectrum of crystal-line digoxin changed on grinding due to the formation of an amorphous layer at the surface of the crystal which again had the effect of enhancing at least the initial dissolution rate.

Thus the formulation of digoxin may be quite critical in a biological sense since, as noted by Johnson *et al.* (1973), small alterations in dosage may result in unacceptable loss of effect or, equally unacceptable intoxication. However, superimposed on the actual formulation itself are the factors which can influence the dissolution process, such as the mixing stage of production, which may affect the particle size or result in the production of an amorphous form with a different solution rate. That these two processes are likely to occur, and to varying degrees, during the compression of a tablet formulation may provide a complication when making even very slight changes in the production process. The urgent need for an official dissolution test specification has been recognized and will provide a safe-guard in the future. Other non-tabletted formulations are also being explored clinically, such as soft-gelatin capsules.

Phenytoin

Phenytoin sodium was introduced by Merritt & Putnam in 1938 for the treatment of convulsive disorders, and has remained a drug of first choice in the treatment of major epilepsy since that time. It does however have some disadvantages, in particular a narrow therapeutic ratio (Richens & Dunlop, 1975). Patients on the drug require careful observation since almost all suffer from one or more of the toxic manifestations during their course of treatment. Toxic effects on the central nervous system are the most alarming and include ataxia, tremor, dizziness and even status epilepticus in extreme cases. However, effects on the gastro-intestinal system, especially nausea and vomiting, are common and there are also frequent skin eruptions. These are alarming but not serious and once the patient is stabilized, the drug may be tolerated for very long periods. Phenytoin itself is a weak acid, practically insoluble in water, and the drug is usually given as the sodium salt, although precipitation as the free acid in the stomach might be expected. Differences in bioavailability from various formulations might occur and the possibility of such effects has been subjected to very close scrutiny since a sudden increase in toxicity in Australia in the late 1960s (Tyrer *et al.*, 1970, 1971; Bochner *et al.*, 1972a, b). Since the drug was generally only available through one manufacturer, the sudden increase in toxicity was attributed to a change in formulation of hard gelatin capsules containing the sodium salt. Originally the drug was diluted with calcium sulphate dihydrate, but this was replaced around 1968 in Australia with lactose, apparently producing a rapid increase of the release rate *in vivo*. However, a closer examination has suggested that the effect of the calcium sulphate is to suppress the toxicity of the drug or reduce absorption from the gastro-intestinal tract (Tyrer *et al.*, 1970; Appleton *et al.*, 1972; Bochner *et al.*, 1972b). Tyrer noted that there was increased faecal excretion of phenytoin when the drug was administered in the presence of calcium sulphate, and this may also indicate a direct interaction. Although a calcium phenytoin salt has been described, the formation of an insoluble calcium salt *in vivo* by a simple reaction between the soluble sodium salt or the precipitated free acid and the calcium sulphate in solution does not appear to have been considered, at least until recently (Bastami & Groves, 1978).

Another factor which might influence the absorption, and hence the toxicity of this drug, is the selection of the sodium salt as opposed to the free acid. The absorption of the sodium salt is known to be non-uniform (Albert *et al.*, 1974) and may extend over a period of at least two days (Jusko, Kemp & Alvan, 1976). The drug itself is extensively protein-bound and the half-life has been estimated to be 22 ± 9 hours (Arnold & Gerber, 1970). Since the sodium salt is likely to be precipitated out as the substantially insoluble free acid at the pH of the stomach contents, a number of investigators have examined the use of the free acid itself, especially as it might have some advantage for use as a sustained-release product. Bochner *et al.* (1972a) found that the acid and sodium salt were absorbed at about the same rate but Lund (1974) considered that the sodium salt was absorbed faster. However, Tammisto, Kanko & Kiukari (1976) reported that the preparations used by Lund had poor bioavailability. Their data suggested that the acid was adequately absorbed and gave better control of the epileptic patient than formulations which employed the sodium salt, confirming an earlier report of Dill *et al.* (1956).

A number of other formulation variables have been reported, including the use of tablets or capsules as delivery systems (Manson *et al.*, 1973) and the influence of particle size (Johansen, 1972; Johansen & Wiese, 1970; Neuvonen, Pentikäinen & Alfring 1977). It is not surprising in view of the pH solubility profile of the drug that the pH of the dissolution medium may influence test results *in vitro*. Neuvonen *et al.* (1977) have recently reported a good correlation between absorption when administered to human volunteers and the dissolution rate at pH 9.0, although it is very unlikely that the pH of the gastro-intestinal tract would ever approach such a high value.

If the formation of insoluble salts between phenytoin and adjuvants containing magnesium or calcium ions can be further substantiated *in vivo*, it may offer a clue to solving the problem of clinical variability of a drug which is inherently toxic but is nevertheless useful.

Drug variables which contribute to the variability in response

The factors which influence the solubility of many crystalline solids have been reviewed elsewhere (Brandstatter-Kuhnert, 1959). Effects due to particle size have been observed with griseofulvin (Atkinson *et al.*, 1962), and the problems with digoxin discussed above lead to the concept that crystal polymorphisms may in some cases be influential. This has been documented for cortisone (Callow & Kennard, 1961) and the crystalline forms of novobiocin which are so poorly absorbed that they are inactive. Only the thermodynamically unstable amorphous form of the latter drug is absorbed and addition of so-called inert fillers such as magnesium stearate may accelerate the conversion of the unstable active drug to the stable but unusable type (Mullins & Macek, 1960).

Formulation variables

The effects of formulation additives on drug bioavailability from oral solutions and suspensions have been well reviewed by Hem (1973). Hem has pointed out how the presence of sugars in a formulation may increase the viscosity of the vehicle. However, sugar solutions alone may delay stomach-emptying time considerably when compared to solutions of the same viscosity prepared with celluloses. This may be due to an effect on osmotic pressure. Sugars of different types may also have an effect on fluid uptake by tissues and this in turn correlates with the effect of sugars such as glucose and mannitol on drug transport. Mayersohn and Gibaldi (1971) have investigated the effect of sugars on the passive transfer of riboflavin, salicylates and sulphanilamide. They considered that the effect of sugars such as glucose on absorption would be expected to vary with each drug and demonstrated that riboflavin was more readily affected than either of the other two drugs. If this effect could be confirmed in humans it would mean that materials previously considered to be inert additives or as sweeteners would have to be selected with greater care in future. It also reinforces the need for drugs to be tested *in vivo* in the complete formulation as well as on their own.

Surfactants have been explored widely for their effects on drug absorption, in particular using experimental animals (Gibaldi, 1976; Gibaldi & Feldman, 1970). It is a little difficult to extrapolate their findings on goldfish to man and most studies with this aim in mind have proved to be negative. Prescott, Steel & Ferrier (1970) found that the plasma level of phenacetin was considerably increased in human volunteers in the presence of 0.1% Tween 80. Both the height of the peak plasma level and the integrated area of the peak were elevated compared to levels of drug given alone, with the same particle size. It was claimed that there was a correlation with the incidence of central nervous effects experienced with some subjects such as lightheadedness, drowsiness and headache.

Surfactants may increase the solubility of the drug by incorporation into micelles, but the amounts of material required to increase solubility significantly are such that at least orally the laxative effects are likely to be unacceptable. The competition between the surfactant micelles and the absorption sites is also likely to reduce any useful effect and make difficult any prediction of net overall effect. However, if a surfactant has any effect at all, it is likely to be in the realm of dispersing agents which help suspensions of insoluble materials to be more readily dispersed and available for solution. Natural surfactants, in particular bile salts, may enhance absorption of poorly soluble materials (Gibaldi & Feldman, 1970) and are certainly involved in fat absorption processes.

The use of complexing agents to influence drug solubility, e.g. caffeine, has been studied extensively. For example, Goto, Tsuzuki & Iguchi (1969) found that the caffeine-*p*-aminobenzoic acid complex had a higher lipid-solubility than the free acid alone and was more readily absorbed, at least from the rabbit stomach. Hem (1973) commented that in general this concept has proved promising in theory but disappointing in practice since many of the complexes formed failed to cross test membranes, probably because of their resulting increased molecular size.

The inadvertent formation of complexes or other interactions may have occurred in some formulations and always requires consideration when devising a new product. There have been attempts to improve the bio-availability of poorly absorbed drugs such as griseofulvin using eutectic solutions in materials such as urea or polyethylene glycols (Mayersohn & Gibaldi, 1966). In this formulation the ultimate particle size of the dispersion *in vivo* should be approaching molecular dimensions, but there appears to be no product on the market which uses this concept.

Interactions between drugs and/or vehicles have been very extensively documented when considering solutions for intravenous administration (Neil 1977). Even the relatively simple addition of potassium or sodium chloride solution to a 20 or 25% solution of mannitol may result in the precipitation or salting out of the mannitol. Solutions containing calcium ions cannot be added to bicarbonate or phosphate solution. A common observation is the immediate precipitation of hydrocortisone sodium succinate and tetracycline hydrochloride when mixed together in dilute solution. The reactions of gentomicin sulphate with cloxacillin, cephalothin, aminophylline or heparin are other examples of this type of response where the active ingredient is rendered useless and potentially hazardous to the patient. These reactions are very common and have to be avoided at the point of administration rather than by formulation although, in one sense, they are a side effect caused by formulation.

The stability of formulations

If the drug in a formulation is not stable, the direct toxicity does not usually increase, although tetracycline and neoarsphenamine are exceptions to this general rule. However, the fact that the activity of the drug will go down as the degradation proceeds is a very important point which requires consideration.

The main routes of degradation are those of hydrolysis and oxidation, and both are affected by catalysts to a marked degree. In the first case, if a drug such as aspirin is affected by water, the shelf life of an anhydrous product will obviously be influenced to a considerable degree by the pack the product is marketed in. Moisture left in a product during the manufacturing stage or trace quantities of heavy metals will initiate and accelerate degradation. Similarly, catalysts such as copper or iron will accelerate oxidative reactions, which often are affected by pH. Hence the stability of a product is often influenced quite markedly by the presence of inadvertent traces of metal catalysts or additives which affect the microenvironment around a solid particle to produce pH-controlled degradation.

The point requires to be made again, with emphasis, that the formulation must give optimum drug release at all times during normal shelf storage. This will be achieved only if the likely degradative reactions have been studied carefully, all predisposing factors identified and isolated and the package designed to prevent access of gases, contaminants and light. In other words, the drug formulation has to be considered as a whole since the interactions are so complex.

Physical parameters which influence the behaviour of tabletted drugs

Drugs compressed into pharmaceutical tablets represent a rapid and economical means of dispensing since they can be prepared with an acceptable degree of accuracy, dose-to-dose, by mass production methods on machines which have high efficiencies and output.

However, compressed tablets must satisfy two opposing criteria since, in the physical sense, there must be sufficiently strong binding forces between the particles to achieve overall cohesiveness for the tablet to resist shock from outside forces, from the time of manufacture to the time of use. This will depend on the compressional force applied during manufacture. However, the binding forces must be fundamentally modified in the presence of body fluids so that the tablet breaks up into its constituent particles to allow solution and release of the active component.

The knowledge of the physical nature of the binding forces involved is scanty. Most formulation work on tablets has been to a large extent empirical — some materials work better under certain conditions and others under different conditions. For example, some tablet formulations are perfectly satisfactory when run on single punch tablet machines but are unsatisfactory when transferred to rotary presses since the rate at which the compression is applied and the time for which the material is under compression are different.

Nevertheless, some general conclusions may be drawn. Figure 5.6 gives a simple scheme to illustrate the effect of compression on a powder or granule bed. The bar represents a constraint offered by the tablet punch in the die or the top cap of a hard gelatin capsule, since many of the problems of a compressed powder or granule bed are also experienced when preparing capsules, although usually to a lesser degree. As the bar descends, decreasing the volume of the space between the particles, there is at first little effect and if the situation were reversed the particles would still exist in their

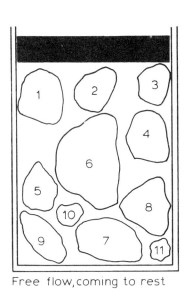
Free flow, coming to rest

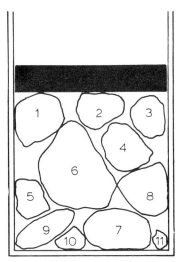
Initial compaction

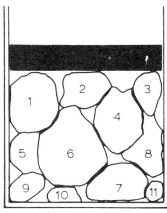
Initial, cohesion

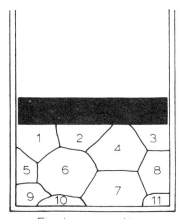
Final compaction

Fig. 5.6. Four stages in compaction of a powder.

original shape. At the second stage some rearrangement is beginning to occur and some surfaces are beginning to adhere. In this situation the shape and volume of the space would be retained if the bar were removed but the compact would probably break up without difficulty since the forces of adhesion would be relatively weak. This would often be the state of the contents of a hard gelatin capsule, but the tablet could probably be represented by the third stage. Here there has been some distortion and flow of the component particles and the binding forces are now stronger. The area of contact is also larger although there will still be some free spaces or pores between the particles. In the final stage of compression all the surfaces are in contact by breakage and distortion of the original shapes, and all the void spaces have been squeezed out. This final stage is only reached if very high compressional forces are used or if the formulation contains a large amount of plastic material such as wax which flows under pressure to fill the spaces at lower pressures. Here the product is a matrix and in general it will only release the drug held in its interior by progressive erosion of the surface, unless channelling agents are added to assist the breakdown.

We have recently examined the physical properties of a model, non-matrix formulation containing lithium carbonate. The critical parameter involved in the subsequent release of drug appears to be the penetration of liquid down the pores remaining in the compressed tablet. This suggests that the scheme proposed originally for the break-up of a tablet by Wagner (1971) requires to be modified by the addition of another block, as shown in Figure 5.7.

Since water has a high dielectric constant it is very effective in disrupting

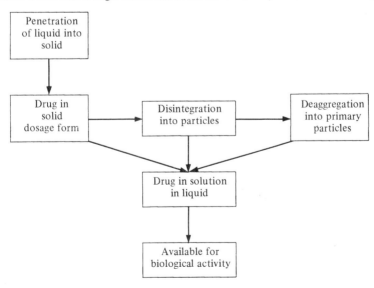

Fig. 5.7.   Sequence of events in release of a drug from a tablet.

the various bond forces between particles. Hence, the faster the water penetrates into a tablet the faster it is likely to disintegrate and release the drug. This process may be critically influenced by changes in the pore size brought about by manufacturing variables, in particular the compressional force and time for which it may be held (i.e. differences between single and rotary punch machines) and by formulation variables which will influence the constitution and, hence, polarity of the pore walls.

Sustained drug release formulations

Lithium salts, used in the treatment of manic depression, are rapidly absorbed and may produce symptoms of overdosage if administered in conventional tablets or capsules. They therefore represent a good example of the type of drug where there is a need for slowing down and controlling release patterns. This has been attempted in a number of commercial products, with apparent clinical success. Another example of a simple salt, readily soluble, which can be troublesome is potassium chloride. The epithelial tissues of the gastro-intestinal tract are subjected to a great deal of insult from a variety of noxious materials, probably more than any other part of the body. These include strong acid, powerful proteolytic enzymes, effective surfactants, micro-organisms, and other irritant materials in food and drink. The tissues are fitted with a protective mechanism which involves flooding the walls with mucus and a rapid replacement of the cells constituting the wall lining. Nevertheless, the system is easily affected by drugs or substances which it comes in contact with for any length of time.

The earlier products of hydrochlorthiazide combined with potassium chloride produced stenotic ulcers, leading to a number of deaths. The ulcers were very formulation-dependent, and resulted from local contact of solid masses which held a reservoir of saturated potassium chloride solution in immediate contact with a small area of the mucosal wall. Over a period of time this could cause lysis of the rapidly forming intestinal cells and ulcer formation. This problem was overcome by careful attention to the formulation, waxy matrices being more useful since they were not prone to adhere to the mucosal walls in the first place.

Levodopa

The treatment of Parkinsonism with levodopa is well established but has some drawbacks. The drug is rapidly absorbed but may be affected by decarboxylases in the gut lumen. It is also rapidly metabolized but will frequently produce symptoms of overdosage, in particular chorea, which may be very distressing for the patient. There are often signs of progressive tolerance to the drug, requiring increased doses at more frequent intervals. This suggests a need for a sustained-release type of preparation in which a lower, non-toxic dose could be administered for a longer period of time between doses. Clinically the drug is given in 500 mg quantitites, either as tablets or capsules, or in 100 mg doses with a suitable decarboxylase inhibitor. A recent examination of some commercially available preparations *in vivo* (Morris *et al.*, 1976) showed that concurrent administration of levo-dopa with a decarboxylase inhibitor produced a plasma concentration-time curve which was comparable with 1/4 to 1/5 of the dose of the drug given alone, suggesting that the gut decarboxylases cause considerable loss of drug before absorption. A slow-release preparation under the same conditions produced much lower plasma concentrations, but which were not sustained. This may have been due to inactivation of the drug before absorption, although administration with a decarboxylase inhibitor did not increase the plasma levels, suggesting that this was unlikely. Absorption of the drug occurs in the proximal small intestine which is a relatively small area. This means that unless all the levodopa has been released before the tablet has reached this vicinity, absorption will be reduced and plasma levels will be diminished. In this case, the idea of using a sustained-release product was reasonable, but the formulation was unsuitable.

A parallel investigation *in vitro* (Alkan & Groves, 1977) showed that the conventional tablets and capsules of the drug released most of their contents within a few minutes, whereas the sustained-release product not only had a considerably increased disintegration time but released the drug in a predictable fashion (Figure 5.8). However, the matrix formulation used

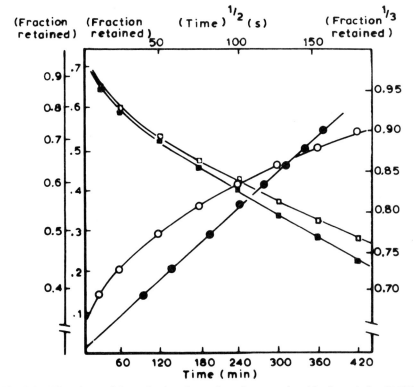

Fig. 5.8. The release of Brompheniramine maleate from matrix tablet formulation V (25% w/w casein) in 0.1 M hydrochloric acid: ○—○ zero order; ■—■ first order; □—□ cube root law; ●—● diffusion-controlled kinetics. (From Groves & Galindez, 1976.)

here appeared to contain a quantity of wax or fat, and the addition of a crude lipase to the dissolution medium resulted in a speeding up of the dissolution process. If this effect occurred *in vivo* it would be undesirable since the quantity of lipases in the gut will be variable, depending on the age of the patient and the diet, leading to an unpredictable rate of drug release.

Brompheniramine

Brompheniramine maleate is more potent than other antihistamines with the same activity and has a shorter duration of action, since it is rapidly absorbed and equally rapidly excreted. Clinically it is usually administered orally as a slow-release preparation. One commercial preparation consists of a slow-release core containing 8 mg of the drug with an additional 4 mg loading dose in a surrounding coat with rapid-release properties. In common with most antihistaminics, a side-effect of the drug is to produce drowsiness, especially at the high dosage levels. One patient became drowsy some 12 hours after taking one of these preparations, as the side effect occurred almost immediately after a fatty meal (Tempel, private communication). A model slow-release formulation was prepared by making an insoluble matrix with waxes to which were added increasing proportions of casein. This is an amphoteric phospho-protein, insoluble in acid but dissolving in alkali or in the presence of proteolytic enzymes such as pepsin or trypsin. An examination of the dissolution data according to the various kinetic models suggested that the diffusion-controlled model postulated by Higuchi was markedly superior (Figure 5.8). This enabled the physical parameters of the matrix model to be evaluated with reasonable precision,

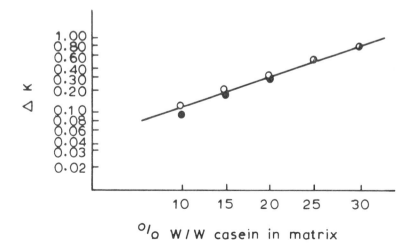

Fig. 5.9.   Increment in the release rate of brompheniramine maleate when the dissolution medium contains proteolytic enzymes: ○—○ buffer pH 8 + trypsin; ●—● 0.1 M hydrochloric acid + pepsin.   (From Groves & Galindez, 1976.)

allowing the tortuosity of pores in the formulation to be calculated as a resistance to diffusion. In turn this enabled the influence of dissolution environment, in particular the effect of enzymes in the dissolution medium, to be measured. As shown in Figure 5.9, there is a marked increase in the drug release rate under acid or alkaline conditions if there is the appropriate proteolytic enzyme present in the dissolution medium.

Although the formulation studied here (Groves & Galindez, 1976) is not necessarily related to any commercial product, it is similar in constitution to patented formulations (Colbert, 1974), and has some clinical advantages since, in principle, the release rate of the drug would be increased as the pH of the gut lumen surrounding the matrix increased and the solubility of the drug decreased. However, whilst it might be argued that the drug is released by physical means, there is some danger that biological factors might intervene if part of the tablet matrix can be affected by proteolytic enzymes, as appears to be the case. This suggests that this type of preparation may not be entirely successful *in vivo* since it involves digestible components which control the drug release rate, and digestive processes in patients are themselves inherently variable (Bell, Davidson & Scarborough, 1968).

Newer formulations designed to influence activity

The most promising type of formulation of the future may be the micro- or macro-capsules in which particles of a product are covered with a coacervate material to protect it from an environment or to influence its solution rate. This approach has been used very successfully for carbon-less copying paper but it is less certain whether it will work with pharmaceutical products. The idea was first explored in the early 1960s, but problems of mechanical strength, integrity of the coating and possible toxicity of components and/or treatments during processing appear to have slowed the development of applications (Nixon, 1976; Nixon & Walker, 1971).

The enhancement of solubility of small ($>1 \mu m$) particles from the Gibbs-Kelvin effect is well recognized (Levi, 1963b) but has received scant attention. The surface forces associated with such solid particles are very considerable so that powders of this size range are usually aggregated and difficult to handle. However, this is not true for oil-in-water emulsions. A way of presenting a rapid release oral formulation may be from a self-emulsifying oil presented in a soft gelatin capsule formulation (Groves & de Galindez, 1976; Groves, 1978).

Liposomes have been of interest recently since they can be made to pass through cell walls and may offer the prospect of delivering drugs to specific tissues (Gregoriadis, 1977; Tyrrell *et al*, 1976). Delivery to the liver appears to be possible although it is not known whether pharmaceutical production of these systems on a sufficiently large scale could be accomplished.

Reverse emulsions (water-in-oil) have been used to deliver anticancer drugs, into the lymphatics (Hashida *et al.*, 1977) and this forms an area where, with established technology, drug therapy may take a further step forward.

A specialized type of emulsion consisting of water emulsified in oil and this in turn emulsified in water — the so called 'double emulsions' or 'liquid membranes' may also offer some scope for future activity. These emulsions may be used to administer labile materials or to form sustained-release products. Recently Chiang *et al.* (1978) have described the potential use of liquid membrane absorbing systems in cases of barbiturate intoxication. The results *in vitro* indicated that a buffer in the internal aqueous phase removed barbiturate in the external aqueous region, thereby preventing it from being absorbed by the organism. Here again there are a number of potentially useful clinical applications of this type of formulation, but there remain a number of practical problems.

Conclusion

Formulation may exercise a considerable influence on the biological activity of a drug. It is rare for a formulation adjuvant to be directly toxic, but such is the complexity of the chemical and physical nature of the materials used that drug release may be enhanced or retarded. Careful study at all stages of the drug properties themselves may only indicate a potential interaction. Testing of the complete product, including the final package, both *in vitro* and *in vivo*, are required to ensure that the patient is not placed in hazard by deliberate or inadvertent changes in the product which may ultimately influence its clinical effectiveness.

References

Albert, K.S., Sakmar, E., Hallmark, M.R., Weidler, D.J. and Wagner, J.G. (1974). *Clin. Pharmac. Ther.*, 16, 727.
Alkan, M.H. and Groves, M.J. (1975). *Manuf. Chem.*, 46 (5), 37.
Alkan, M.H. and Groves, M.J. (1977). *Proc. 1st Int. Cong. Pharm. Technol. Paris, V,* 22.
Ampolsuk, C., Mauro, J.V., Nyhuis, A.A., Shan, N. and Jarowski, C. (1974). *J. Pharm. Sci.*, 63, 117.
Appleton, D.B., Eadie, M.J., Hooper, W.D., Lucas, B., Sutherland, J.M. and Tyrer, J.H. (1972). *Med. J. Aust.*, 1, 410.
Arnold, K. and Gerber, N. (1970). *Clin. Pharmac. Ther.*, 11, 121.
Atkinson, R.M., Bedford, C., Child, K.J. and Tomich, E.G. (1962). *Nature (Lond.).* 193, 188.
Barr, W.H. (1973). *Current Concepts in Pharmaceutical Sciences: Dosage Form, Design and Bioavailability,* ed. Swarbrick, J., p. 31. Philadelphia: Lea & Febiger.
Bastami, S.M. and Groves, M.J. (1978). *Int. J. Pharmaceutics*, 1, 151.
Bell, G.H., Davidson, J.N. and Scarborough, H. (1968). *Textbook of Physiology and Biochemistry* (7th Edit.). Edinburgh: Livingstone.
Bochner, F., Hooper, W.D., Tyrer, J.H. and Eadie, M.J. (1972a). *Neurol. Neurosurg. Psychiatry*, 35. .
Bochner, F., Hooper, W.D., Tyrer, J.H. and Eadie, M.J. (1972b). *Neurol. Sci.*, 16, 481.
Brandstatter-Kuhnert, M. (1959). *Oester. Apoth. Ztg.*, 13, 297.
Callow, R.K. and Kennard, O. (1961). *J. Pharm. Pharmac.*, 13, 723.
Calvary, H.O. and Klumpp, T.G. (1939). *Southern Med., J.*, 32, 1105.
Chiang, C.W., Fuller, G.C., Frankenfeld, J.W. and Rhodes, C.T. (1978). *J. Pharm. Sci.*, 67, 63.
Colbert, J.C. (1974). *Controlled Action Drug Forms, Chem. Technol. Review*, Vol. 24, Noyes, New Jersey.
Dill, W.A., Kazenko, A., Wolf, L.M. and Glazko, A.J. (1956). *J. Pharmac. exp. Ther.*, 118, 270.

Flaum, I. (1978). *J. Pharm. Sci.*, 67, 1.

Florence, A.T., Salde, E.G. and Stenlake, J.B. (1974). *J. Pharm. Pharmac.*, 26, 479.

Garvan, J.M. and Gunner, B.W. (1964). *Med. J. Aust.*, 2, 1.

Gibaldi, M. (1976). *Biopharmaceutics in the Theory and Practice of Industrial Pharmacy* (2nd Edit.), Editors: Lachman, L., Lieberman, H.A. and Kanig, J.L. Philadelphia: Lea & Febiger.

Gibaldi, M. and Feldman, S. (1970). *J. Pharm. Sci.*, 59, 579.

Goto, S., Tsuzuki, O. and Iguchi, S. (1969). *Chem. Pharm. Bull.*, 17, 837.

Gregoriadis, G. (1977). *Nature (Lond.)*. 265, 407.

Groves, M.J. (1966). *Reps. Progr. applied Chem.*, 51, 151.

Groves, M.J. (1973). *Pharm. J.*, 210, 318.

Groves, M.J. (1973). *Parenteral Products*. London: Heinemann Medical.

Groves, M.J. (1977). *Cronache Farm.*, 20, 212.

Groves, M.J. (1978). *Chemy Ind.* (12) June 17, 417.

Groves, M.J. and Alkan, M.H. (1978). *Particle Size Analysis*, Ed. Groves, M.J. London: Heyden.

Groves, M.J. and de Galindez, D.A. (1976). *Acta Pharm. Suecica*, 13, 353.

Groves, M.J. and Galindez, F.E. (1976). *Acta Pharm. Suecica*, 13, 373.

Groves, M.J. and de Malke, S.R. (1976). *Drug Dev. Commun.*, 2, 285.

Haag, H.B. and Ambrose, A. (1937). *Am. J. Pharmac.*, 59, 93.

Hagenbusch, O.E. (1937). *J. Am. med. Ass.*, 109, 1531.

Hamer, J. and Grahame-Smith, L. (1972). *Lancet*, 2, 325.

Hashida, M., Egawa, M., Muranishi, S. and Sezaki, H. (1977). *J. Pharmacokin. Biopharm.*, 5, 225.

Hem, S.L. (1973). *Current Concepts in Pharmaceutical Sciences: Dosage Form, Design and Bioavailability*, Editor: Swarbrick, J. Philadelphia: Lea & Febiger.

Hersey, J.A. (1969). *Manuf. Chem.*, Feb. 32.

Hess, H. (1977). *Drug Dev. Ind. Pharm.*, 3, 491.

Holick, H.G.O. (1937). *J. Am. med. Ass.*, 109, 1517.

Johansen, H.E. (1972). *Arch. for Pharm. og Chemi*, 79, 209.

Johansen, H.E. and Wiese, C.F. (1970). *Arch. for Pharm. og Chemi*, 77, 243.

Johnson, B.F., Fowle, A.S.E., Ladar, S., Fox, J. and Munro-Faure, A.D. (1973). *Br. med. J.*, 4, 323.

Jusko, W.J., Kemp, J.R. and Alvan, G. (1976). *J. Pharmacokin. Biopharm.*, 4, 327.

Levi, G. (1963a). *Prescription Pharmacy*, Editor: Sprowls, J.B. Philadelphia: Lea & Febiger.

Levi, G. (1963b). *Am. J. Pharm.*, 135, 78.

Lindenbaum, J., Mellow, M.H., Blackstone, M.O. and Bulther, V.P. (1971). *New Engl. Med.*, 285, 1344.

Lund, L. (1974). *Eur. J. clin. Pharmac.*, 7, 119.

Manninen, V., Melin, J. and Reissel, P. (1972). *Lancet*, 1, 490.

Manson, J.I., Beal, S.M., Magarey, A., Pollard, A.C., O'Reilly, W.J. and Swanson, L.N. (1975). *Med. J. Aust.*, 2, 590.

Mayersohn, M. and Gibaldi, M. (1966). *J. Pharm. Sci.*, 55, 1324.

Mayersohn, M. and Gibaldi, M. (1971). *J. Pharm. Sci.*, 60, 225.

Merritt, P. and Putnam, J. (1939). *J. Am. med. Ass.*, 711, 1068.

Morris, J.G.L., Parsons, R.L., Trounce, J.R. and Groves, M.J. (1976). *Br. J. Clin. Pharmac.*, 3, 983.

Mullens, J.D. and Macek, T.J. (1960). *J. Am. Pharm. Ass. Sci. Ed.*, 49, 245.

Neil, J.M. (1977). *The Prescribing and Administration of I.V. Additive to Infusion Fluids*. Thetford: Travenol.

Neuvonen, P.J., Pentikainen, P.J. and Elfving, S.M. (1977). *Int. J. clin. Pharmac.*, 15, 84.

Nixon, J.R. (Ed.) (1976). *Microencapsulation*. Drugs of Pharmaceutical Science, Vol. 3. New York: Marcel Dekker.

Nixon, J.R. and Walker, S.E. (1971). *J. Pharm. Pharmac.*, 23 (Suppl.), 147S.

Pernarowski, M. (1974). *Dissolution Technology*, Ed. Leeson, L.J. and Carstensen, J.T. Washington: Academy of Pharmaceutical Science.

Phillips, I., Meers, P.D. and D'Arcy, P.F. (1976). *Microbial Hazards of Infusion Therapy*. Lancaster: M.T.P. Press.

Prescott, L.F., Steel, R.F. and Ferrier, W.R. (1970). *Clin. Pharmac. Ther.*, 11, 496.

Richens, A. and Dunlop, A. (1975). *Lancet*, 2, 247.

Shaw, T.R.D., Carless, J.E., Howard, M. and Raymond, K. (1973). *Lancet*, 2, 209.

Tammisto, P., Kanko, K. and Kiukari, M. (1976). *Lancet*, 1, 254.

Tyrer, J.H., Eadie, M.J. and Hooper, W.D. (1971). *Proc. Aust. Assoc. Neurol.*, 8, 37.

Tyrer, J.H., Eadie, M.J., Sutherland, J.M. and Hooper, W.D. (1970). *Br. med. J.*, 2, 271.

Tyrrell, D.A., Heath, T.D., Collos, C.M. and Ryman, B.E. (1976). *Biochem. Biophys. Acta*, 457, 260.

Wagner, J.G. (1971). *Biopharmaceutics and Relevant Pharmacokinetics*. Hamilton, Illinois: Drug Intelligence Publications.

Winding, O. (1977). *Am. J. Hosp. Pharm.*, 34, 705.

Winding, O. (1978). *Angiography* (in the press).

6.   Free radical aspects of hepatotoxicity

T. F. Slater

The drug-metabolizing enzyme system (DMES) (for reviews see Parke, 1968; Briggs & Briggs, 1974) is located mainly in the liver, in terms of activity per whole organ (Knecht, 1966; see Slater, 1972); within the liver the DMES is firmly associated with the lipoprotein membranes of the endoplasmic reticulum (for reviews on endoplasmic reticulum structure and fluidity see Claude, 1969; Stier, 1978). The DMES consists of an NADPH-specific flavoprotein (often measured and described as NADPH-cytochrome c reductase, as cytochrome c may be used as an 'artificial' acceptor for the enzyme), a phospolipid component (e.g. phosphatidyl choline) and a terminal cytochrome (P-450 or P-448); there may also be a small amount of a non-haem iron protein closely associated with the DMES (Salerno & Ingledew, 1975). Several groups of investigators have succeeded in separating and purifying the major DMES components and in reconstituting overall drug-metabolizing activity (see Coon *et al.*, 1977; Levin *et al.*, 1977; Ingelman-Sundberg & Glaumann, 1977). Although, in whole organ terms, the major activity occurs in liver endoplasmic reticulum, many other tissues possess low levels of drug-metabolizing enzyme activity that may be of considerable biological significance in relation to tissue injury and cancer produced by exposure to toxic agents (Orrenius & Ernster, 1974; Benedetto, Slater & Dianzani, 1976).

Although the general result of the metabolism of a foreign substance by the DMES is a decrease in toxicity, occasionally a substance is converted through interaction with the DMES to a product that has very much greater toxicity; this is one aspect of what Sir Rudolph Peters (1963) has called 'lethal synthesis'.

Some examples of agents that are metabolized by interaction with the DMES to yield highly toxic products are illustrated in Figure 6.1: among the products of such metabolism are free radicals, epoxides, and carbonium-ions or ion-radicals.

The formation of free radical products can arise either by direct electron transfer from the DMES to the parent compound, or by prior metabolism to the hydroxylated derivative followed by further oxidation (Figure 6.2).

In this article, emphasis will be placed upon the formation and chemical

(i) $CCl_4 \longrightarrow CCl_3^{\bullet}$

(ii) $CH_2\!=\!CHCl \longrightarrow H_2\overset{\displaystyle O}{\underset{}{C-CHCl}}$

(iii) $\overset{CH_3}{\underset{CH_3}{\gtrless}} N\!-\!N\!=\!O \longrightarrow CH_3\!-\!\underset{H}{N}\!-\!N\!=\!O \longrightarrow CH_3^{+}$

(iv)   Flagyl $\longrightarrow$ Flagyl$^{-\bullet}$

(v)

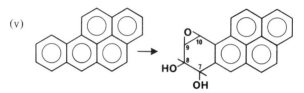

Fig. 6.1. Examples of foreign substances that are metabolized by the liver endoplasmic reticulum-cytochrome P-450 complex to highly toxic products. For references to the examples quoted see: (i) Slater (1972); (ii) and (iii) Connors (1978); (iv) Willson (1977); (v) King *et al.* (1976) and Yang *et al.* (1976).

reactivities of free radicals formed as a result of DMES-associated activity, in relation to toxic events that result within the cell (see Slater, 1972; Pryor, 1976).

Generally speaking, free radicals are chemically highly reactive, and the formation of such metabolic products within the membranes of the endoplasmic reticulum due to DMES activity can lead to a variety of damaging events. (i) There may be hydrogen-atom abstraction from a thiol group that is thereby converted to a thiyl radical; two such thiyl radicals may then dimerize to yield the disulphide bond:

$$R^{\bullet} + X\text{-}SH \longrightarrow RH + X\text{-}S^{\bullet}$$

(i) $CCl_4 \longrightarrow [CCl_4]^{-\bullet} \longrightarrow CCl_3^{\bullet} + Cl^{-}$

(ii) $BP \longrightarrow BP^{+\bullet} \xrightarrow{\text{Pyr}} BP\,Pyr^{+\bullet}$

(iii) $R\text{-}NH_2 \longrightarrow R\text{-}\underset{OH}{N}H \longrightarrow R\text{-}\underset{O^{\bullet}}{N}H$

Fig. 6.2. Formation of free radical products from foreign substances by (i) electron transfer; (ii) and (iii) oxidation of either the parent substance as in (ii), or of a metabolite as in (iii). For references see (i) Willson & Slater (1975); (ii) Cavalieri & Roth (1976); (iii) Stier *et al.* (1972).

Since many enzymes require thiol groups for full metabolic activity, such free-radical oxidation of essential thiol groups may lead to considerable changes in enzyme activity. (ii) The reactive free radical may attack double bonds in lipids, proteins and nucleotides, or hydroxyl or thiol groups to result in covalent binding of the free radical group to the biological component. Covalent binding may (and may not) significantly modify the biological properties of the materials involved (see Uehleke, 1973). (iii) The free radical may abstract a hydrogen atom from a neighbouring polyunsaturated fatty acid (PUFAH) to initiate the process known as lipid peroxidation (Figure 6.3). The latter process can result in major structural damage to biomembranes (e.g. the endoplasmic reticulum) and to changes

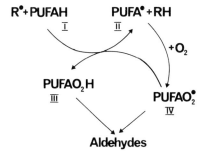

Fig. 6.3.   The initial events in the process of lipid peroxidation. A reactive free radical (R·) abstracts a hydrogen-atom from a polyunsaturated fatty acid (PUFAH I) producing a fatty acid radical (II). This reacts rapidly with oxygen to yield the peroxy-radical (III), which can abstract a hydrogen atom from another molecule of I to form the hydroperoxide (IV). In so doing, a further molecule of II is generated, thereby continuing the chain process. The species III and IV can undergo complex breakdown paths to yield low molecular weight peroxides and aldehydes as indicated. For background references see Slater (1972) and Ugazio and Dianzani (1978).

in metabolic function and in membrane fluidity. Many types of tissue injury are now known to involve the formation of reactive free radicals as a primary stage, followed by a stimulation of lipid peroxidation as a secondary event (Slater, 1972; Plaa & Witschi, 1976). Generally, an increase in the rate and extent of lipid peroxidation in a tissue is indicative of the local formation of reactive free radicals and of the likelihood of significant biological damage.

Lipid peroxidation is a complex process and its extent may be experimentally assessed in various ways (Slater, 1975; Figure 6.4). However, the only procedures that are convenient and practicable for measuring lipid peroxidation in tissue samples or intracellular fractions are diene conjugation, malonaldehyde production, fluorescence changes and, perhaps, ethane production.

It is evident from what has been outlined above that some substances are metabolized by the DMES to free radical products and that these may initiate a variety of damaging reactions within the cell. Much work has been devoted over the last 10 years or so to understanding the detailed sequence of events that occur in such types of chemically induced tissue injury; to

(i) $\underline{PUFA(H)}$ + R$^{\bullet}$ $\longrightarrow$ PUFA$^{\bullet}$ + RH

(ii) PUFA$^{\bullet}$ + $\underline{O_2}$ $\longrightarrow$ PUFAO$_2$$^{\bullet}$

(iii) PUFAO$_2$$^{\bullet}$ + PUFA(H) $\longrightarrow$ $\underline{PUFAO_2H}$ + PUFA$^{\bullet}$

(iv) PUFAO$_2$$^{\bullet}$ $\longrightarrow$ $\underline{diene\ conjugation}$

(v)   PUFAO$_2$$^{\bullet}$ $\longrightarrow$ $\underline{aldehydes,\ hydroxy\text{-}alkenals,\ ethane}$

(vi) Lipid peroxidation $\longrightarrow$ $\underline{Fluorescence\ changes}$

Fig. 6.4.   The various methods that may be used to study the rate of lipid peroxidation are indicated by an underlining of the relevant components measured. The process, which involves a peroxidative degradation of polyunsaturated fatty acid (PUFAH), can be measured by following the disappearance of PUFAH (see Horning *et al.*, 1962) by the uptake of oxygen (see Slater, 1968), or by the formation of lipid peroxide (Johnson & Siddiqi, 1970; Heath & Tappel, 1976). During the overall process there is a re-arrangement of double bonds (diene-conjugation) that can be used to follow the course of the reaction. Among the breakdown products are malonaldehyde (for references see Slater, 1972) and ethane (Riely *et al.*, 1974) which may also be measured as indices of peroxidation. Under biological conditions, peroxidation is accompanied by cross-linking of proteins and characteristic changes in the lipid fractions that produce detectable alterations in fluorescence (Fletcher *et al.*, 1973). An additional fluorescence technique has recently been described by Waller & Recknagel (1977).

illustrate the variety of experimental approaches that have been used I will concentrate on one main example, the hepatotoxic action of carbon tetra-chloride (see Recknagel, 1967; Slater, 1972, 1978).

A single dose (1-2 ml/kg body wt.) of carbon tetrachloride when administered to a rat (or to many other animal species) produces an acute liver injury: centrilobular necrosis and fatty degeneration. A number of other tissues are also affected by the toxic agent (e.g. kidney) but the most serious and extensive damage is located in the liver. Although many other tissues accumulate higher concentrations of carbon tetrachloride than appear in the liver (Slater, 1966) the fact that the major damage is produced in liver suggests that carbon tetrachloride has to undergo some metabolic modification before exerting its full toxic effects. A large amount of evidence now supports the view that carbon tetrachloride is metabolized in liver (and to a small extent in some other tissues) endoplasmic reticulum to a highly reactive product (Slater, 1966; Recknagel, 1967; Recknagel & Glende, 1973) or products of which the major one is probably the trichloro-methyl radical ($CCl_3 \cdot$).

The trichloromethyl radical is chemically very reactive (Willson & Slater, 1975) and may be expected to bind covalently to neighbouring proteins and lipids, and initiate lipid peroxidation. In fact, covalent binding of these radicals occurs very early in liver endoplasmic reticulum after oral dosing with carbon tetrachloride (Recknagel & Glende, 1973) and this is followed a short time later by a large stimulation of lipid peroxidation (Figure 6.5). It can be seen in Figure 6.5 that two different methods for estimating lipid peroxidation (diene conjugation and malonaldehyde measurement) give very similar results; measurement of ethane in expired air has also recently been used to detect lipid peroxidation produced by carbon tetrachloride in rats (Riely, Cohen & Lieberman, 1974; Hafemann & Hoekstra, 1975; Lindstrom & Anders, 1978).

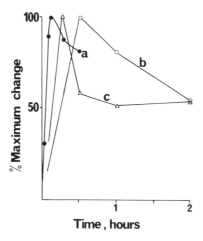

Fig. 6.5. Some early effects on liver microsomal components produced by oral dosing with carbon tetrachloride in the rat. The changes in covalent binding (*a*) are from Recknagel & Glende (1973); for diene conjugation (*b*) from Klaassen & Plaa (1969); and for malonaldehyde content (*c*) from Jose, P.J. & Slater, F.T. (1972 and also unpublished).

When sections of liver are examined under the electron microscope at various times after dosing rats with carbon tetrachloride, the earliest morphological disturbances are apparent in the endoplasmic reticulum of cells in the centrilobular zone of the liver lobules (Oberling & Rouiller, 1956; Smuckler, Iseri & Benditt, 1962). This localization of damage in the early stages to the membranes of the endoplasmic reticulum is consistent with metabolism to the toxic radical taking place in the DMES located in the endoplasmic reticulum. The localization of the necrosis to the centrilobular zone of the liver lobules can best be explained by a concentration of the DMES in that zone relative to other zones such as the mid-zone and the periportal zone. In fact, recent studies have demonstrated a relative concentration of cytochrome P-450 in the central zone by the use of microdensitometric analysis of single cells (Gooding *et al.*, 1978; Figure 6.6).

The detailed investigation of the reactions of the trichloromethyl radical is made difficult by the high chemical reactivity of this electrophilic species, and hence its short life-time in biological environments. One approach to the study of the kinetic behaviour of such short-lived intermediates is the use of pulse radiolysis (Willson, 1978) to generate transient quantities of specific free radical species and then to follow their subsequent decay. Using this procedure, Willson and Slater (1975) found that the trichloromethyl radical reacted rapidly with a number of biologically important substances; its biological half-life has been calculated to be about $100\,\mu s$ (Slater, 1976). The short life-time of this radical under conditions *in vivo* shows that it cannot be expected to diffuse very far from its site of formation in the endoplasmic reticulum: in essence, the very high chemical reactivity of the trichloromethyl radical ensures that it is trapped in its micro-environment (Figure 6.7). However, secondary products resulting from the interaction of the radical with neighbouring polyunsaturated fatty

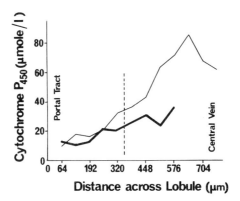

Fig. 6.6. The distribution of cytochrome P-450 in individual liver cells (as measured by micro-densitometry) across a rat liver lobule. The variation from the portal tract to the central vein can be seen in the control situation (thick line) and after induction of cytochrome P-450 with phenobarbital (see Gooding *et al.*, 1978).

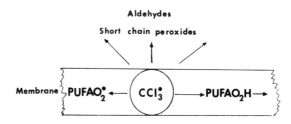

Fig. 6.7. The relative magnitudes of diffusion after 'activation' of carbon tetrachloride to the trichloromethyl radical in rat liver endoplasmic reticulum. The reactive primary radical is essentially trapped in its micro-environment due to its lipophilicity and very short half-life. Secondary species, such as the lipophilic long-chain lipid peroxides, can diffuse in the plane of the membrane. Tertiary species, low molecular weight peroxides and derived aldehydes, can escape from the membrane and can produce damaging effects far distant from the initial locus of carbon tetrachloride activation (see Slater, 1976).

acids (e.g. lipid hydroperoxides) can diffuse within the membrane as a result of their longer life-times (i.e. lower reactivity) and hydrophobic character. Tertiary products resulting from the breakdown of lipid hydroperoxides (e.g. short chain lipid peroxides, aldehydes and unsaturated aldehydes) may escape from the membrane environment and produce damaging effects at a considerable distance from the site of formation of the trichloromethyl radical itself. Aldehydes such as 4-hydroxypent-2-en-1-al, which are products of lipid peroxidation (Schauenstein, 1967) have life-times *in vivo* of several minutes (Conroy *et al.*, 1975) and so can escape from the liver and cause systemic effects. As shown by Ugazio *et al.* (1976) and Roders, Glende & Recknagel (1978), lipid peroxides and unsaturated aldehydes that result from lipid peroxidation can cause a variety of deleterious effects on capillary permeability, erythrocyte integrity, and platelet aggregation.

With such highly reactive products as the trichloromethyl radical it is difficult to be absolutely sure that this species is actually produced *in vivo*, since the rather limited extent of metabolism of carbon tetrachloride that occurs, combined with the high chemical reactivity and short biological half-life ensure that the steady-state concentration of the radical in the liver will be almost vanishingly small. The most direct way of demonstrating the occurrence of trichloromethyl radicals in liver samples after exposure to carbon tetrachloride is to rapidly freeze-clamp a piece of liver with tongs cooled in liquid nitrogen (–196°C) and then to analyse the frozen sample with electron spin resonance (ESR) spectroscopy (Ingram, 1969; Swartz, Guterrez & Reichling, 1978). Several attempts using ESR have been made to detect trichloromethyl radicals in liver samples (Slater, 1972; Calligaro, Congiu & Vannini, 1970) but no clear-cut evidence has been obtained; in the author's view this is due largely to the very low concentrations of the radical that occur in the liver after oral dosing with carbon tetrachloride.

Failing *direct* demonstration of trichloromethyl radicals using ESR, the available course is to use a variety of indirect approaches that cumulatively would constitute a powerful argument in favour of the formation of this radical *in vivo*. For example, using $^{14}CCl_4$, a number of studies have shown covalent binding that is consistent with the formation of trichloromethyl radicals (Reynolds & Lee, 1967, 1968; Gordis, 1969). Moreover, analysis of expired air and of tissue samples by gas-liquid chromatography have shown that small amounts of hexachloroethane and chloroform are produced from carbon tetrachloride (Butler, 1961; Fowler, 1969); these data are consistent with dimerization of the radical and with hydrogen atom abstraction. A more recent but still indirect attempt to demonstrate the formation of trichloromethyl radicals in liver has involved so-called free radical traps (Perkins, Ward & Horsfield, 1970). In this technique (Figure 6.8), a transient reactive radical is trapped by a substituted nitrone which in the

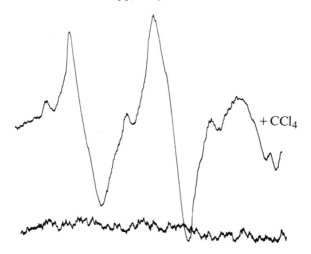

Fig. 6.8.   The results of incubating liver microsomes, NADPH and nitrosobutane (spin trap) with and without carbon tetrachloride on the electron spin resonance spectrum. Incubation was for 5 min at 37°C. For experimental details see Ingall *et al.* (1978).

ensuing process is converted to a relatively stable nitroxyl radical having a characteristic triplet ESR spectrum. In consequence, a very low but continuous production of trichloromethyl radicals would be demonstrable as a steadily increasing accumulation of nitroxyl radicals having a characteristic ESR hyperfine structure. When this technique was tried with liver microsomes (Ingall *et al.*, 1978) treated with carbon tetrachloride, a triplet signal rapidly appeared; however, it is probable that this particular signal results from secondary radical species (e.g. peroxy radicals) rather than the primary trichloromethyl species. It is known that the latter reacts very quickly with O_2 to yield a radical adduct CCl_3O_2˙ (Packer, J., Slater, T.F. and Willson, R.L., unpublished results).

Another area of study that is closely related to topics already discussed, and which is equally complex in its nature, is the study of mechanisms of protection against cellular injury produced by such toxic species (see Slater, 1978). Only a very brief survey of protective mechanisms will be given here and obvious protective measures such as decreasing exposure to, or absorption of a toxic material, and attenuating its subsequent metabolism to a toxic intermediate will be not mentioned. Emphasis will be placed here only on procedures that result in scavenging or trapping the reactive free radical intermediates. We shall again use the trichloromethyl radical as an example.

Three criteria for a radical scavenger *in vivo* can be deduced. Firstly, the reactivity of the trichloromethyl radical is so high that its biological life-time is extremely short; this means that any effective scavenger must be present preferably at the time of formation of the radical in order to scavenge the toxic species before it causes damage to its local environment. It would be no good administering a scavenger several hours after exposure to carbon tetrachloride for example; the damage would already have occurred. Secondly, the high reactivity of the trichloromethyl radical means that its radius of diffusion from the site of formation will be very small; in consequence, any effective scavenger must get very close to the actual locus of radical formation in order to react with it. Thirdly, since the trichloromethyl radical is chemically very reactive, it interacts readily with a variety of neighbouring biomolecules (lipids, proteins, nucleotides, etc.) that are present locally in a high concentration; thus any effective scavenger must be present in a high enough concentration to compete successfully with these neighbouring molecules. In other words, a suitable scavenger must get to the right place, at the right time, and in a high enough concentration in order to be effective. These are demanding criteria and of fifty or so free radical scavengers tested in my laboratory, only a few have satisfied the requirements mentioned above. One scavenger that is effective in scavenging trichloromethyl (and other electrophilic) radicals at low concentrations *in vivo* and *in vitro* is the phenothiazine derivative Promethazine. When given either just before or together with carbon tetrachloride, Promethazine protects the rat against the necrogenic action of the hepatotoxic agent (Rees, Sinha & Spector, 1961). Promethazine (0.1-10 μM) inhibits the stimulation of lipid peroxidation *in vitro* that normally results from exposure to carbon tetrachloride with liver microsomal suspensions (Slater & Sawyer, 1971) or with isolated hepatocytes (Poli *et al.*, 1978). Using pulse radiolysis techniques, Willson and Slater (1975) showed that Promethazine reacts very rapidly with trichloromethyl radicals; recent work, however, has shown that this interaction is dependent on oxygen and probably involves a scavenging of the radical adduct $CCl_3O_2\cdot$ by Promethazine (Packer, J., Slater, T.F. and Willson, R.L., unpublished data).

Many toxic reactions can arise by the metabolism of a foreign compound to a highly reactive intermediate. The study of such damaging reaction sequences and of related protective mechanisms, is of obvious relevance to improving our knowledge of the mechanisms of tissue injury in general, and also to the disturbances associated with chemical carcinogenesis in particular.

References

Benedetto, C., Slater, T.F. and Dianzani, M.U. (1976). *Biochem. Trans.*, 4, 1094.

Briggs, M. and Briggs, M. (1974). In *The Chemistry and Metabolism of Drugs and Toxins.* London: Heinemann Medical Books.

Butler, T.C. (1961). *J. Pharmac. exp. Ther.*, 134, 311.

Calligaro, A., Congiu, L. and Vannini, V. (1970). *Rass. med. Sarda.*, 73, 365.

Cavalieri, E. and Roth, R. (1976). *J. org. Chem.*, 41, 2679.

Claude, A. (1969). In *Microsomes and Drug Oxidations.* Editors: Gillette, J.R., Conney, A.H., Cosmides, G.J., Estabrook, R.W., Fouts, J.R. and Mannering, G.J., pp. 3-39. New York: Academic Press.

Connors, T.A. (1978). In *Biochemical Mechanisms of Liver Injury.* Editor: Slater, T.F. New York: Academic Press.

Conroy, P.J., Nodes, J.T., Slater, T.F. and White, G.W. (1975). *Eur. J. Cancer*, 11, 231.

Coon, M.J., Ballou, D.P., Hangen, D.A., Krezoski, S.O., Nordblom, G.D. and White, R.E. (1977). In *Microsomes and Drug Oxidations*, pp. 82-94. Eds. Ullrich, V., Roots, I., Hildebrandt, A., Estabrook, R.W. and Conney, A.H., pp. 82-94. Oxford: Pergamon Press.

Fletcher, B.L., Dillard, C.J. and Tappel, A.L. (1973). *Analyt. Biochem.*, 52, 1.

Fowler, J.S.L. (1969). *Br. J. Pharmac. Chemother.*, 37, 733.

Gooding, P.E., Chayen, J., Sawyer, B.C. and Slater, T.F. (1978). *Chem. Biol. Interact.*, 20, 299.

Gordis, E. (1969). *J. clin. Invest.*, 48, 203.

Hafemann, D.G. and Hoekstra, W.G. (1975). *Fedn Proc.*, 34, 939.

Heath, R.L. and Tappel, A.L. (1976). *Analyt. Biochem.*, 76, 184.

Horning, M.G., Earle, M.J. and Maling, H.M. (1962). *Biochim. biophys. Acta,* 56, 175.

Ingall, A., Finch, S., Lott, K., Slater, T.F. and Stier, A. (1978). *Biochem. Trans.* (in the press).

Ingelman-Sundberg, M. and Glaumann, H. (1977). *FEBS Letters*, 78, 72.

Ingram, D.J.E. (1969). *Biological and Biochemical Applications of Electron Spin Resonance.* London: Hilger.

Johnson, R.M. and Siddiqi, I.W. (1970). *The Determination of Organic Peroxides.* Oxford: Pergamon.

Jose, P.J. and Slater, T.F. (1972). *Biochem. J.,* 128, 141P.

King, H.S.W., Osborne, M.R., Beland, F.A., Harvey, R.G. and Brookes, P. (1976). *Proc. Natl. Acad. Sci. (U.S.A.),* 73, 2679.

Klaassen, C.D. and Plaa, G.L. (1969). *Biochem. Pharmac.*, 18, 2019.

Knecht, N. (1966). *Naturforsch.*, 21, 799.

Levin, W., Ryan, D., Huang, M.T., Kawalek, J., Thomas, P.E., West, S.B. and Lu, A.Y.H. (1977). In *Microsomes and Drug Oxidations,* Editors: Ullrich, V., Roots, I., Hildebrandt, A., Estabrook, R.W. and Conney, A.H., pp. 185-191. Oxford, Pergamon.

Lindstrom, T.D. and Anders, M.W. (1978). *Biochem. Pharmac.*, 27, 563.

Oberling, C. and Rouiller, C. (1956). *Annals Anat. Path.*, 1, 401.

Orrenius, S. and Ernster, L. (1974). In *Molecular Mechanisms of Oxygen Activation*, pp. 215-244. Editor: Hayaishi, O. New York: Academic Press.

Drug toxicity

Parke, D.V. (1968). *The Biochemistry of Foreign Compounds.* Oxford: Pergamon.

Perkins, M.J., Ward, P. and Horsfield, A. (1970). *J. chem. Soc.* (B), 395.

Peters, R.A. (1963). In *Biochemical Lesions and Lethal Synthesis.* Oxford: Pergamon.

Plaa, G.L. and Witschi, H. (1976). *Ann. Rev. Pharmac. Tox.*, 16, 125.

Poli, G., Chiono, M.P., Slater, T.F., Dianzani, M.U. and Gravela, E. (1978). *Biochem. Trans.* (in the press).

Pryor, W.A. (1976). In *Free Radicals in Biology,* Vols. I and II. New York: Academic Press.

Recknagel, R.O. (1967). *Pharmac. Rev.*, 19, 145.

Recknagel, R.O. and Glende, E.A. (1973). *C.R.C. Critical Reviews in Toxicology,* 2, 263.

Rees, K.R., Sinha, K.P. and Spector, W.G. (1961). *J. Path. Bact.*, 81, 107.

Reynolds, E.S. and Lee, A.G. (1967). *Lab. Invest.*, 16, 591.

Reynolds, E.S. and Lee, A.G. (1968). *Lab. Invest.*, 19, 272.

Riely, C.A., Cohen, G. and Lieberman, M. (1974). *Science,* 183, 208.

Roders, M.K., Glende, E.A. and Recknagel, R.O. (1978). *Biochem. Pharmac.*, 27, 437.

Salerno, J.C. and Ingledew, W.J. (1975). *Biochem. biophys. Res. Commun.*, 65, 618.

Schauenstein, E. (1967). *J. Lipid Res.*, 8, 417.

Slater, T.F. (1966). *Nature,* 209, 36.

Slater, T.F. (1968). *Biochem. J.*, 106, 155.

Slater, T.F. (1972). In *Free Radical Mechanisms in Tissue Injury.* London: Pion.

Slater, T.F. (1975). In *Pathogenesis and Mechanisms of Liver Cell Necrosis.* Editor: Keppler, D. Lancaster: M.T.P.

Slater, T.F. (1976). *Panminerva Medica,* 18, 381.

Slater, T.F. (1978). *Biochemical Mechanisms of Liver Injury.* London: Academic Press.

Slater, T.F. and Sawyer, B.C. (1971). *Biochem. J.*, 123, 823.

Smuckler, E.A., Iseri, O.A. and Benditt, E.P. (1962). *J. exp. Med.*, 116, 55.

Stier, A. (1978). In *Biochemical Mechanisms of Liver Injury*, Editor: Slater, T.F. London: Academic Press.

Stier, A., Reitz, I. and Sackmann, E. (1972). *Naunyn-Schmiedeberg's Arch. Pharmac.*, 274, 189.

Swartz, H., Guterrez, P. and Reichling, B. (1978). In *Biochemical Mechanisms of Liver Injury*, Editor: Slater, T.F. London: Academic Press.

Uehleke, H. (1973). In *Experimental Model Systems in Toxicology and their Significance in Man,* p. 119. (Proc. Eur. Soc. Study Drug Toxicity, Vol. 15.).

Ugazio, G., Torrielli, M.V., Burdino, E., Sawyer, B.C. and Slater, T.F. (1976). *Biochem. Trans.*, 4, 353.

Ugazio, G. and Dianzani, M.U. (1978). In *Biochemical Mechanisms of Liver Injury*, Editor: Slater, T.F. London: Academic Press.

Waller, R.L. and Recknagel, R.O. (1977). *Lipids,* 12, 914.

Willson, R.L. (1977). *Chem. Ind.*, pp. 183-193.

Willson, R.L. (1978). In *Biochemical Mechanisms of Liver Injury*, Editor: Slater, T.F. London:Academic Press.

Willson, R.L. and Slater, T.F. (1975). In *Fast Processes in Radiation Chemistry*, Editors: Adams, G.E., Fielden, E.M. and Michael, B.D., pp. 147-161. Chichester: John Wiley.

Yang, S.K., McCourt, D.W., Roller, P.P. and Gelboin, H.V. (1976). *Proc. Natl. Acad. Sci. (U.S.A.)*, 73, 2594.

7. Toxicological consequences of enzyme induction and inhibition

Dennis V. Parke

Introduction

Drugs and other environmental chemicals are deactivated and detoxicated by the drug-metabolizing enzymes of the liver, including especially the mixed-function oxidases of the endoplasmic reticulum. It is perhaps less well known that the same mixed-function oxidases can catalyse the converse reaction and so metabolically activate drugs and environmental chemicals to make them more toxic. Indeed, this is the way many carcinogens are metabolized within the cell to yield the proximate and ultimate carcinogens, and the way in which many toxic chemicals are biologically activated.

Repeated dosing with many drugs, or with certain environmental chemicals, leads to enhanced activity of these microsomal enzymes as a result of increased enzyme synthesis. Enzyme induction may result from either excess substrate or from the effect of hormones; glucagon and cyclic $3',5'$-AMP may act as second messengers. In the case of induction of the liver microsomal drug-metabolizing enzymes, it is believed that high substrate concentration, and not hormonal regulation, is responsible for the increased enzyme synthesis. However, high substrate concentration will lead initially to inhibition of these enzymes, and consequently we find that inhibition and induction are related phenomena (Figure 7.1). If a drug is slowly metabolized, or is present at high concentration, the enzyme active site will be occupied by substrate for long periods of time, and this will lead to competitive inhibition of the enzyme, which may last for several hours. This lack of available enzyme leads to genomal derepression, accelerated synthesis of enzyme protein and enhanced enzymic activity. Hence, with slowly metabolized substrates, such as phenobarbitone, enzyme inhibition occurs for the first 12 hours or so, and this is later followed by a period of enzyme induction.

The mixed-function oxidases of the endoplasmic reticulum of the liver, including the terminal oxygenase cytochrome P-450, obviously have a more fundamental biological role than the detoxication of drugs. This other role is probably concerned with the synthesis of proteins and glycoproteins for export from the cell, and it would seem that this synthesis may occur only when the ribosomes are attached to the endoplasmic reticulum. The ribosomes are probably attached to the endoplasmic reticulum through

Drug toxicity

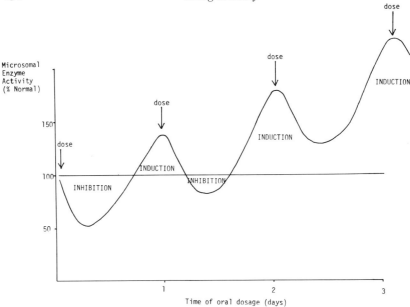

Fig. 7.1.   Relationship of enzyme inhibition and enzyme induction on repeated dosage of enzyme-inducing drugs.

cytochrome P-450. This cytochrome is also concerned with the synthesis of other molecules such as cholesterol and the steroid hormones, functions which make this enzyme essential to life. Hence, it is perhaps not surprising that cytochrome P-450 and the mixed-function oxidases are subject to a feed-back regulatory system (enzyme induction) far superior to those for most other enzymes and markedly more effective than that regulating haemoglobin synthesis. It is also not surprising that induction and inhibition of this enzyme system have far more profound consequences than mere alteration of the rates of detoxication of drugs, and appear to be involved in many toxic processes and disease states, including carcinogenicity.

Inhibition of the drug-metabolizing enzymes may be the result of high levels of substrate, leading to competitive inhibition which is followed by enzyme induction, or to non-competitive inhibition in which the enzyme is more permanently inhibited by binding of the inhibitor at or near the enzyme active site. The activity of the hepatic microsomal mixed-function oxidases may be inhibited by a wide range of compounds including the classic inhibitor SKF 525-A (2-diethylaminoethyl 2,2-diphenylvalerate HCl, which subsequently induces the enzymes), imidazole derivatives (Wilkinson, Hetnarski & Yellin, 1972), benzimidazole, benzoxazole and benzothiazole derivatives (Holder *et al.*, 1976; Gil & Wilkinson, 1977), methylenedioxy-aryl compounds (Fujii *et al.*, 1970) and thiono sulphur-containing compounds (Hunter & Neal, 1975). Many hydroxylated products of drugs may lead to inhibition of the hydroxylation of their precursors, or of other substrates, as for example, the hydroxylated metabolites oxyphenbutazone (phenylbutazone), 4-hydroxyantipyrine (antipyrine) and 2-hydroxydesmethylimipramine (imipramine) which competitively inhibit the oxidative metabolism of their precursors and the oxidative metabolism of other drugs (Soda & Levy, 1975). Other types of inhibition of the mixed-function oxidases include the inhibition of haem and cytochrome P-450 synthesis by cobalt (De Matteis & Gibbs, 1977), inhibition by cyclic 3′,5′-AMP or dibutyryl cyclic 3′,5′-AMP (Weiner, Buterbaugh & Blake, 1972), or by various agents, such as the antiviral compound tilorone, which induces the production of interferon (Renton & Mannering, 1976). The phenomenon of ligand complex formation between certain chemicals and cytochrome P-450, leading to inhibition of cytochrome P-450 and the mixed-function oxygenases, destruction of P-450, and toxic phenomena such as hepatic necrosis and hepatocellular carcinogenesis, has recently been recognized.

Induction of cytochrome P-450 and the mixed-function oxygenases is believed to be the consequence of the slow rate of metabolism of a drug, so consequently, drugs most slowly metabolized are the more potent enzyme-inducing agents; the extents of microsomal enzyme induction produced by a series of barbiturates were directly related to the plasma half-lives of the drugs and to their rates of metabolism (Pelkonen & Kärki, 1973; Valerino *et al.*, 1974; Ioannides & Parke, 1975).

Three classes of inducer of the drug-metabolizing enzymes are now recognized:
1. Drugs — which lead to an increase of cytochrome P-450 and of the coupled reductase(s).
2. Carcinogenic polycyclic hydrocarbons — yield an increase of cytochrome P-448, but not to any significant increase of reductase(s), and
3. Catatoxic steroids — which give no increase of cytochrome(s), but lead to a substantial increase in NADPH-cytochrome c reductase.

The effect of the carcinogenic polycyclic hydrocarbons, and indeed of many other carcinogenic species, appears to be to convert cytochrome P-450 to cytochrome P-448. This conformational change of cytochrome P-450 into cytochrome P-448 occurs in a short period of time, probably less than one hour, does not involve protein synthesis, but is followed by increased *de novo* synthesis, or true enzyme induction, of cytochrome P-448 some 24-48 hours afterwards. This change is accompanied by degranulation of the endoplasmic reticulum with consequent interference in the synthesis of glycoproteins, which may be related to the initiation of carcinogenesis.

Differences between drugs and carcinogens as enzyme inducers

The carcinogenic polycyclic aromatic hydrocarbons, such as benzo(*a*)-pyrene and 3-methylcholanthrene, are rather slow inducers of the microsomal enzymes compared with drugs such as phenobarbitone. The carcinogens yield cytochrome P-448 instead of cytochrome P-450, with no increase in the reductase. The increase in *de novo* protein synthesis is slow and with methylcholanthrene does not reach a maximum for several days or weeks, whereas with phenobarbitone the maximum increase in enzyme synthesis occurs within 2 or 3 days.

In contrast to drugs, polycyclic hydrocarbons lead to no marked hepatic

Table 7.1. Differences between phenobarbital and carcinogenic polycyclic hydrocarbon inducers.

Biological parameter	Phenobarbital	Polycyclic hydrocarbons
Liver enlargement	Marked hepatic hypertrophy	No marked hypertrophy
Enzyme components	Cytochrome P-450 increased; NADPH-cytochrome c reductase increased	Cytochrome P-450 replaced by cytochrome P-448; no marked increase of reductase
Protein synthesis	Increased; inhibition of microsomal ribonuclease	Increased; inhibition of microsomal ribonuclease; immediate appearance of cytochrome P-448 is independent of protein synthesis
Phospholipid synthesis	Marked increase in microsomal phospholipid; UDP-glucuronyl transferase increase is latent	No marked increase in phospholipid; UDP-glucuronyl transferase is expressed
Substrate binding	Increased type I and type II bindings	Increased type II binding only
Substrate metabolism	Increased ethylmorphine N-demethylation, hydroxylation of hexobarbital, and 4-hydroxylation of biphenyl	Increased de-ethylation of ethoxyresorufin, hydroxylation of benzo(a)pyrene, and 2-hydroxylation of biphenyl

(See Parke, 1975)

hypertrophy, no marked inhibition of microsomal ribonuclease, and to no marked increase in microsomal phospholipid, all suggesting lesser increases in *de novo* synthesis (see Table 7.1). In addition there are substantial differences between drugs and carcinogens in the changed preference for substrate, and of the products of oxygenation. Whereas phenobarbital increases the binding of Type I and Type II substrates, carcinogens increase

Table 7.2. Differences in substrate specificity.

Liver parameter or substrate	Pretreatment with		
	Phenobarbital	3-Methylcholanthrene (% normal)	Pregnenolone 16α-carbonitrile
Cytochrome P-450	230	[180]†	180
NADPH-cytochrome c reductase	190	110	230
Ethylmorphine N-demethylase	460	230	1040
Benzphetamine N-demethylase	730	90	350
Benzo(a)pyrene hydroxylase	400	1400	640
Aniline hydroxylase	120	170	—
Testosterone 7α-hydroxylase	100	200	—
Testosterone 16α-hydroxylase	550	50	—

† Cytochrome P-448.
(From Lu *et al.*, 1972 and 1973)

only the binding of Type II substrates, for example, the hydroxylation of hexabarbital and phenobarbital are increased by drugs but show no marked increase following treatment with carcinogen inducers. An even more fundamental difference is seen with the metabolism of biphenyl, for whereas drugs enhance the 4-hydroxylation of biphenyl, the 2-hydroxylation is increased only by carcinogens. This distinct difference between these two types of enzyme-inducing agent has been made the basis of a short-term test for chemical carcinogenicity (McPherson, Bridges & Parke, 1974).

Differences in substrate specificity are listed in Table 7.2 and it should be noted that after pretreatment with methylcholanthrene the demethylation of benzphetamine and the 16α-hydroxylation of testosterone are actually decreased. Benzo(a)pyrene hydroxylation is significantly increased as are also the 7α-hydroxylation of testosterone and the hydroxylation of aniline — a Type II substrate. The most marked increase produced by treatment with the catatoxic steroid, pregnenolone-16α-carbonitrile, is the demethylation of ethylmorphine which seems to be more dependent on the level of reductase than on cytochrome P-450.

Drug interactions due to enzyme inhibition

A list of some drug-interactions resulting from the inhibition of the drug-metabolizing enzymes are shown in Table 7.3. From this it is seen that alcohol inhibits the metabolic deactivation of chloral hydrate leading to tachycardia, hypotension and marked vasodilation due to the heightened activity of the chloral hydrate. The competitive inhibition of the deactivation of pethidine by phenelzine and other monoamine oxidase inhibitors leads to severe respiratory depression associated with the excessive activity of the pethidine. Similarly, sulphonamides, like sulphamethizole, inhibit drug metabolism, increasing the half-lives of phenytoin (11.8 to 19.6 hours), tolbutamide (5.7 to 9.2 hours), and warfarin (65 to 93 hours), so

Table 7.3.   Drug interactions due to microsomal enzyme inhibition.

Inhibiting agent	Observed drug	Effect	Reference
Alcohol	Chloral hydrate	Tachycardia, hypotension, marked vasodilation	Sellers *et al.* (1972 a, b)
Phenelzine and other monoamine oxidase inhibitors	Pethidine	Severe respiratory depression and death	Clark & Thompson (1972); Jounela (1968)
Disulfiram (Antabuse)	Phenytoin	Ataxia, nystagmus, cerebellar damage	Stripp *et al.* (1969); Vesell *et al.* (1971)
Sulphamethizole and other sulphonamides	Phenytoin, tolbutamide, warfarin	Increased plasma half-lives and therapeutic response	Lumholtz *et al.* (1975)
Prednisolone	Cyclophosphamide	Increased plasma half-life, decreased cytotoxic activity	Faber *et al.* (1975)

potentiating their pharmacological activity (Lumholtz *et al.*, 1975). The anti-alcoholic drug, disulfiram, and the volatile anaesthetic halothane, both lead to non-competitive inhibition of cytochrome P-450 and the drug-metabolizing enzymes, and thus prolong and intensify the effects of phenytoin administered simultaneously, leading to ataxia, nystagmus and cerebella damage. Drug-metabolizing ability seems to be impaired in women taking oral contraceptive steroids and the plasma half-lives of drugs are increased (antipyrine, 10.8 to 14.1 hours; phenybutazone, 71 to 80 hours) (O'Malley, Stevenson & Crooks, 1972), which is in accord with observations that drug metabolism is inhibited in animals in late pregnancy or by progesterone and progestogens (Soyka & Long, 1972).

Conversely, if the drug is activated by metabolism, inhibition will impair that activation. Prednisolone administered simultaneously with cyclophosphamide inhibits the activation of this cytotoxic, anti-cancer drug. Similarly, chloramphenicol after 12 days' continuous treatment increases the plasma half-life of cyclophosphamide from 7.6 to 11.4 hours with consequent loss of cytotoxic activity (Faber, Mouridsen & Skovsted, 1975).

Drug interactions due to enzyme induction

Drug interactions due to induction of the drug-metabolizing enzymes are shown in Table 7.4. The barbiturate phenobarbitone, which is metabolized only very slowly in man, leads to marked enzyme induction which lowers

Table 7.4.   Drug interactions due to microsomal enzyme induction.

Inducing agent	Observed drug	Effect	Reference
Phenobarbitone	Prednisolone	Impaired respiration in asthmatics	Brooks *et al.* (1972)
Phenobarbitone	Chloramphenicol	Decreased plasma half-life and antibacterial activity	Palmer *et al.* (1972)
Rifampicin	Tolbutamide	Decreased plasma half-life and diminshed hypo-glycaemic effect	Zilly *et al.* (1975)
Phenytoin	Oral contraceptive steroids	Break-through bleeding, and pregnancy	Hempel & Klinger (1976)
Spironolactone and other catatoxic steroids	Bishydroxycoumarin	Prothrombin levels return to normal	Solymoss *et al.* (1970)
Prednisolone	Cyclophosphamide	Enhanced cytotoxic action	Faber *et al.* (1974)

the toxicity of strychnine, decreases the plasma half-life of chloramphenicol and enhances the metabolic deactivation of prednisone with deterioration of respiratory control in asthmatics. Rifampicin, the antitubercular antibiotic, is another potent enzyme-inducing drug, and lowers the plasma half-lives of hexobarbital (325 to 122 min) and tolbutamide (418 to 183 min) in healthy volunteers (Zilly, Breimer & Richter, 1975). In combination with isoniazid, rifampicin greatly increased the potential hepatotoxicity of this other antitubercular agent and precipitated acute hepatitis with hepatic encephalopathy in a number of patients (Pessayre *et al.*, 1977).

Corticosteroids also bring about enzyme induction in man, and prolonged treatment with prednisone leads to an increased rate of metabolism of cyclophosphamide, with the consequent enhancement of the cytotoxic action of this anti-cancer drug (Faber, Mouridsen & Skovsted, 1974). The administration of spironolactone and other catatoxic steroids similarly enhances the rate of deactivation of anticoagulant drugs such as bishydroxycoumarin, restoring prothrombin levels to normal.

Many enzyme-inducing drugs result in break-through bleeding in women on hormone contraception and in extreme cases many result in ineffective contraceptive cover and pregnancy. Drugs particularly associated with interactions with oral contraceptives are the antitubercular agent rifampicin, and the anti-epileptic drugs phenobarbitone, phenytoin and carbamazepine (Hempel & Klinger, 1976).

Cigarette smoking also leads to induction of the hepatic drug-metabolizing enzymes; the half-life of antipyrine was significantly shorter in smokers (10.6 hours) than in non-smokers (12.4 hours), but increased significantly on stopping smoking (Hart *et al.*, 1976). Smoking is therefore yet another factor affecting the metabolism of drugs and contributing to the variation in human pharmacokinetics.

Many naturally occurring substances are both inhibitors and inducers of the microsomal drug-metabolizing enzymes, and none has been studied more than alcohol. There are many claims that ethanol induces the drug-metabolizing enzymes of the liver and specifically increases one particular form of cytochrome P-450 (Khanna *et al.*, 1976; Kalant *et al.*, 1976). However, this is a matter of considerable controversey and many laboratories, including our own (Ioannides, Lake & Parke, 1975) have been unable to demonstrate enzyme induction except after very high dosage (>12 g/kg body wt./day) (Parke, 1975). From our own studies we concluded that moderate ingestion of alcohol was unlikely, through enzyme induction, to affect the toxicity or therapeutic effects of drugs or toxic chemicals. However, the ingestion of alcohol does have a pronounced *inhibitory* effect upon the drug-metabolizing enzymes of the liver, especially when the rate of consumption is high and the microsomal enzymes become involved in its metabolism. Thus the simultaneous ingestion of alcohol markedly increases the plasma half-life of pentobarbitone in rats, whereas this is unaltered in animals previously given alcohol for several weeks.

Effects of enzyme induction and inhibition on toxicity

Some examples of the effects of enzyme induction and inhibition on the toxicity of chemicals are listed in Table 7.5. Pretreatment of animals with the enzyme inducing agents, phenobarbitone, phenaglycodol or thiopental increase the 2-hydroxylation and conjugation of strychnine and thus decrease its toxicity. Similarly, pregnenolone-16α-carbonitrile decreases the acute hepatotoxicity of dimethylnitrosamine.

Where drugs or toxic chemicals are activated (see Chapter 1) instead of being detoxicated by metabolism, enzyme induction will lead to increased toxicity. For example, pretreatment with phenobarbitone leads to increased toxicity of phenacetin and paracetamol, and markedly increases the hepatotoxicity of carbon tetrachloride. The centrilobular hepatic necrosis produced by bromobenzene is also markedly increased in the rat following stimulation of metabolism by phenobarbitone but is decreased following pretreatment with 3-methylcholanthrene. Unlike phenobarbitone, the 3-methylcholanthrene does not markedly accelerate the metabolism of bromobenzene, but shifts the pattern of metabolism away from the more

Table 7.5. Effects of microsomal enzyme inhibition and induction on toxicity.

Toxic chemical	Inhibitor or inducing agent	Effect	Reference
Induction-decreased toxicity			
Strychnine	Thiopental, phenaglycodol	Increased hydroxylation and conjugation, decreased acute toxicity	Kato (1961)
Dimethylnitrosamine	Pregnenolone-16α-carbonitrile	Loss of acute hepato-toxicity	Somogyi *et al.* (1972)
Induction-increased toxicity			
Bromobenzene	Phenobarbitone	Increased hepatic necrosis	Zampaglione *et al.* (1973)
Monocrotaline	Phenobarbitone	Increased hepatic necrosis and lung lesions	Allen *et al.* (1972)
Inhibition-decreased toxicity			
Benzo(*a*)pyrene	7,8-Benzoflavone	Decreased covalent binding binding to DNA	Selkirk *et al.* (1974)
2-Acetamidofluorene	*p*-Hydroxyacetanilide	Increased glucuronylation, decreased *N*-hydroxy-lation and carcinogenicity	Mohan *et al.* (1976)
Inhibition-increased toxicity			
2-Acetamidofluorene	Piperonyl butoxide	Increased *N*-hydroxy-lation and carcinogenicity	Friedman & Woods (1977)
Pentobarbitone	Ethanol	Increased plasma half-life, narcosis and acute toxicity	Ioannides *et al.* (1975)

toxic pathways, increasing the amounts of bromophenyldihydrodiol and 2-bromophenol formed and decreasing the amount of 4-bromophenol and bromophenylmercapturic acid (Zampaglione *et al.*, 1973).

Similarly, whereas the hepatotoxicity produced by carbon tetrachloride is increased by phenobarbital (see Table 7.6), pretreatment with methylcholanthrene decreases the toxicity (Suarez *et al.*, 1972; Suarez, Carlson & Fuller, 1975). This has been attributed to the absence of any increase in NADPH-cytochrome c reductase accompanying the increase of cytochrome P-450/P-448. The activation of carbon tetrachloride to the toxic trichloromethyl radical (see Chapter 6) probably requires reductive dechlorination by cytochrome P-450, but, following the damage of the endoplasmic reticulum membranes by this radical, leakage of electrons from the micro-somal transport chain at the point of the cytochrome c reductase appears to occur. There is now increasing evidence that cytochrome P-448 is not able to catalyse mono-oxygenation, but subsequent to an uncoupling of the microsomal mixed-function oxygenase system the NADPH-cytochrome c reductase functions as an oxygenase, leading to increased lipid peroxida-tion. Hence, it would seem that carbon tetrachloride hepatotoxicity requires the mediation of both cytochrome P-450 (reductive dechlorination) and NADPH-cytochrome c reductase (lipid peroxidation), and conversion by methylcholanthrene of cytochrome P-450 to P-448 with no increase in the reductase consequently leads to a diminution of toxicity.

Table 7.6. The effects of phenobarbital and 3-methylcholanthrene on carbon tetrachloride hepatotoxicity in rats.

Pre-treatment	Malonaldehyde formed (nmol/mg microsomal protein 15min)		NADPH-cytochrome c reductase (nmol reduced/mg microsomal protein/min)		Cytochrome P-450 ($E_{450-500}$/mg microsomal protein $\times 10^4$)		Acute hepato-toxicity
	CCl_4	Control	CCl_4	Control	CCl_4	Control	CCl_4
Control (saline)	3.5	2.2	85	95	105	130	++
Pheno-barbital	6.9	2.2	165	175	105	270	+++
Control (corn oil)	5.5	2.7	–	–	–	–	++
3-Methyl-cholanthrene	4.3	2.7	95	120	195	[325]*	–

* Cytochrome P-448

(Suarez *et al.*, 1972, 1975)

The acute lethality and hepatotoxic effects of the pyrrolizidine alkaloids, monocrotaline, lasiocarpine and heliotrine, are also markedly affected by microsomal enzyme inducers such as phenobarbitone, phenytoin, spirono-lactone and pregnenolone-16α-carbonitrile (Tuchweber *et al.*, 1974), and whereas the lethality and toxicity of monocrotaline and heliotrine are greatly increased, the lethality and hepatic lesions produced by high doses of lasiocarpine are greatly diminished by the enzyme-inducing agents. Since the inducing agents increase the rates of formation of pyrrolic metabolites from all three alkaloids, it is suggested that pyrrole derivatives cannot be solely responsible for the toxicity of the pyrrolizidine alkaloids, as has been suggested.

Microsomal enzyme induction may also affect testosterone biosynthesis, and, in contrast to the effect on the liver cytochrome, pretreatment of rats with 3-methylcholanthrene leads to a *decrease* of cytochrome P-450 in the testis (50%), decreased progesterone 17α-hydroxylase activity (40%), decreased testosterone biosynthesis (40%), and decreased weight of the seminal vesicles (Stripp, Menard & Gillette, 1974). In contrast, pretreatment with phenobarbitone had no effect on testicular cytochrome P-450 or any other of these parameters affecting male fertility.

Many studies have been made of the effects of microsomal enzyme inhibitors on the activation of carcinogens, obviously with a view to decreasing their potential carcinogenicity. 7,8-Benzoflavone, an inhibitor of aryl hydrocarbon hydroxylase, non-selectively inhibits the rat liver hydroxylation of benzo(*a*)pyrene and also inhibits the covalent binding of these to DNA (Selkirk *et al.*, 1974). 1,2-Epoxy-3,3,3-trichloropropane, which also inhibits benzo(*a*)pyrene hydroxylase activity, inhibits epoxide hydrase in addition, and consequently increases the binding to DNA with complete elimination of dihydrodiol formation. Retinol and various vitamin A derivatives, which are related to 7,8-benzoflavone, together with the anti-antioxidant butylated hydroxytoluene, also inhibit epoxidation of benzo-(*a*)pyrene and other carcinogenic hydrocarbons, leading to decreased binding of the active carcinogen metabolites to DNA (Hill & Shih, 1974).

Inhibition may also increase the activity of carcinogens; for example, piperonyl butoxide administered to hamsters inhibits the 7-hydroxylation of 2-acetamidofluorene by 61% but simultaneously stimulates the *N*-hydroxylation 10-fold, leading to a marked increase in binding of this carcinogen to RNA and DNA (Friedman & Woods, 1977).

Inhibition of metabolic pathways other than hydroxylation may also lead to marked changes in the activity of carcinogens. Pretreatment of rats with *p*-hydroxyacetanilide leads to no significant change in microsomal aryl hydroxylase but increases the glucuronyl transferase 3-fold, resulting in a marked protection against tumour induction by 2-acetamidofluorene or its *N*-hydroxy metabolite (Mohan *et al.*, 1976).

Enzyme induction in extrahepatic tissues

Enzyme induction and inhibition are not confined to the microsomal enzymes of the liver, but also occur in the lungs, the gastro-intestinal tract and several other tissues, and may lead to increased or decreased toxicity as with the liver enzymes.

One of the major anomalies concerning extrahepatic enzyme induction is the induction of certain specific mixed-function oxidases of the mammalian placenta. Although the placenta contains a very small amount of cytochrome P-450, it does exhibit certain mixed-function oxygenase activity, especially that concerning the synthesis of oestrogens by the aromatization of androgens. Attempts to induce this cytochrome P-450 system by the administration of various drugs have been largely unsuccessful, but benzopyrene hydroxylase, 3-methyl-4-monomethylaminoazobenzene-*N*-demethylase, and phenacetin de-ethylase activities, and cholesterol metabolism, are markedly affected by the mother smoking cigarettes. From Table 7.7, a dose-response to smoking is apparent, and there is a marked increase in benzpyrene hydroxylation and a decrease in cholesterol metabolism in the placenta as the number of cigarettes smoked per day increases. What effect this has on the unborn infant is still unknown, except that low weight-for-date babies are associated with cigarette smoking. As smoking decreases the

Table 7.7.   Effect of cigarette smoking on microsomal mixed-function oxidation
in human term placenta.

Cigarettes per day	Benzpyrene hydroxylation (nmol phenol/g protein/15 min)	Cholesterol metabolism (nmol pregnenolone/g protein/h)
0	4.5 ± 3.7	43 ± 12
5-15	29 ± 6	35 ± 7
15-25	240 ± 20	33 ± 8
> 25	2200 ± 210	22 ± 6

(Juchau *et al.*, 1974)

metabolism of cholesterol to pregnenolone, it is possible that this would decrease the placental synthesis of progestational hormones and oestrogens, which are essential for the maintenance of the pregnancy.

Long-term drug therapy and folate deficiency

One of the major toxic effects of enzyme induction occurs with long-term drug therapy. Studies in our laboratory, on institutionalized patients receiving a number of different drugs, indicate that the extent of enzyme induction, and the consequent adverse side effects, are determined more by the duration of the treatment than by the chemical or pharmacological nature of the drug (Labadarios *et al.*, 1977). From Table 7.8, it can be seen that during the period of 2-5 years of drug therapy, there is a marked

Table 7.8.   Effects of duration of treatment with enzyme-inducing drugs
(anticonvulsants, phenothiazines, or tricyclics) on enzyme induction and folate status.

Duration of drug treatment (years)	Enzyme induction as measured by urinary excretion of *D*-glucarate (mol/24 h)	Folate status as measured by urinary excretion of formiminoglutamate in the FIGLU test (mg/9 hours)
none	9 ± 2	7.1 ± 1.6
2-5	108 ± 32	12.4 ± 1.4
5-10	46 ± 20	18.7 ± 2.2
>10	38 ± 10	20.2 ± 1.4

(Labadarios *et al.*, 1977)

enzyme induction as measured by the urinary *D*-glucarate excretion, and this is matched by only a modest increase in the urinary formiminogluta-mate (FIGLU) excretion, which is taken as an index of the folate status of these patients. However, after five years there is a progressive increase in the FIGLU excretion with simultaneous depression of the plasma and erythrocyte folate concentrations, and this is accompanied by a progressive fall of *D*-glucarate excretion and enzyme induction. Our explanation of this phenomenon is that the continuous administration of enzyme-inducing drugs results in a continued high rate of microsomal enzyme synthesis which makes a high demand on folate. The dietary intake of folate of these people is limited and consequently their folate status progressively declines until, after about 5 years, the dietary folate is no longer adequate to support enzyme induction. Consequently, induction decreases and toxic side effects appear, due to the continued high dosage of the anticonvulsant, phenothiazine or tricyclic drugs.

In an animal study to substantiate these clinical observations, rats maintained on low-folate, normal folate and folate-supplemented diets, were given phenytoin plus phenobarbitone in comparable dosage to the human therapeutic dose over their life span. The offspring born to rats on the low-folate diet, had low birth weights, but those on this diet which also received the phenobarbitone plus phenytoin showed marked deformities of the bones and soft tissues. Similarly, those animals on the normal folate diet receiving the drugs also produced litters with bone and soft tissue deformities and low birth weights. Only those animals maintained on the folate-supplemented diet showed no adverse effects from the continued administration of phenobarbitone plus phenytoin (Labadarios, 1975). These experiments confirmed the previous findings that long-term treatment with enzyme-inducing drugs can, through folate deficiency, result in teratogenicity in the progeny of the patients.

A similar experiment in which rats maintained on these three folate diets were given phenobarbitone, phenytoin or imipramine, in high dosage, also confirmed the folate demands of enzyme-inducing drugs (Labadarios, 1975). From Table 7.9, it may be seen that animals on the low-folate diet given phenobarbitone did not show the normal response of induction of

Table 7.9.   The effects of drugs and folate supplementation on enzyme induction and folate status of rats.

Treatment	RBC folate (ng/ml)	Cytochrome P-450 (nmol/g liver)	FIGLU (mg/h)
Low-folate diet			
Controls	56 ± 1	19 ± 1.4	0.5 ± 0.02
Phenobarbitone	43 ± 3	20 ± 1.7	8.6 ± 0.1
Phenytoin	49 ± 3	20 ± 0.9	1.2 ± 0.1
Imipramine	44 ± 1	15 ± 0.9	1.3 ± 0.1
Folate-supplemented diet			
Controls	98 ± 3	18.2 ± 0.6	0.1 ± 0.01
Phenobarbitone	96 ± 3	49 ± 3.0	0.1 ± 0.01
Phenytoin	99 ± 1	22 ± 0.9	0.1 ± 0.01
Imipramine	99 ± 4	29 ± 2.0	0.1 ± 0.01

Drugs were administered daily for 12 weeks at 0.5 g/kg/day for phenobarbitone or phenytoin, or 0.25 g/kg/day for imipramine.

(Labadarios, 1975)

cytochrome P-450, but that the effort to produce this enzyme induction had led to a much more marked deterioration of the folate status, as indicated by the high FIGLU excretion. On the folate-supplemented diet, the animals were able to exhibit enzyme induction following administration of phenobarbitone, phenytoin or imipramine, and no animals showed any folate depletion on this diet.

The prolonged administration of anticonvulsant drugs (phenobarbitone, phenytoin, primidone, pheneturide), and other enzyme-inducing drugs, may also result in vitamin D deficiency and osteomalacia. Cholecalciferol (vitamin D_3) requires hydroxylation in the liver to 25-hydroxycholecalciferol and further hydroxylation in the kidney to form 1,25-dihydroxycholecalciferol, the biologically active co-enzyme. Anticonvulsant drugs appear to disturb this mechanism, presumably by the enhancement of deactivating mechanisms of 1,25-dihydroxycholecalciferol, since inducers such as phenobarbitone accelerates the 25-hydroxylation and do not alter the rate of the subsequent conversion to 1,25-dihydroxycholecalciferol (Burt, Freston & Tolman, 1976).

Safrole, enzyme induction and hepatic toxicity

In an extensive study of natural chemicals as potential inducing agents of the microsomal drug-metabolizing enzymes, we found two potent inducers, namely, safrole and iso-safrole. Safrole is a weak liver carcinogen which is probably activated by hydroxylation of the allyl side-chain and 1′-acetoxy-safrole, 1′-hydroxysafrole-2′,3′-oxide, and other hydroxylated products have been shown to be mutagenic and tumorigenic (Wislocki *et al.*, 1977).

Prolonged repeated administration of safrole leads to an increase in the 2-hydroxylation of biphenyl with a simultaneous and progressive decrease in the 4-hydroxylation of biphenyl, and also in the hydroxylation of most other substrates (Parke & Gray, 1978). This results from a type of non-competitive enzyme inhibition resulting from ligand complex formation of an active metabolite of safrole with cytochrome P-450 (see Figure 7.2).

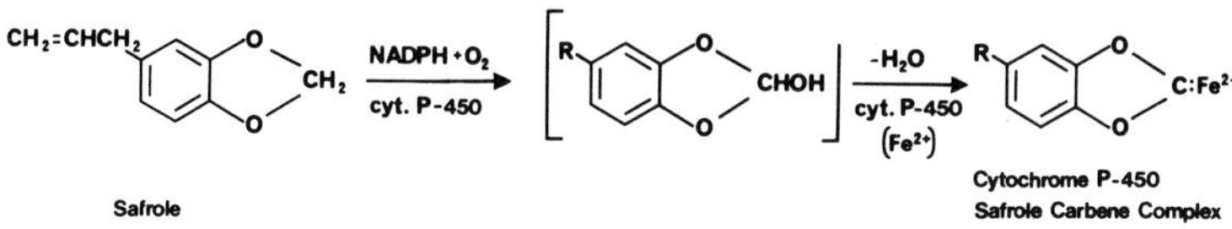

Fig. 7.2. Formation of carbene complex of safrole metabolite with cytochrome P-450.

Safrole and many other methylenedioxyaryl compounds, such as piperonyl butoxide, are metabolized by oxidation of the methylenedioxy group. The highly reactive intermediate so formed interacts with cytochrome P-450 to form a ligand complex which results in the appearance of a redox difference spectrum at 455 mm. The consequence of this ligand binding is that cytochrome P-450 loses its enzymic activity and is converted to cytochrome P-448. This loss of cytochrome P-450 activity leads to a marked induction of the microsomal oxidases, which metabolize safrole further to reactive metabolites, followed by ligand complexing of the metabolites to the newly formed cytochrome P-450. In this way, continuous administration of safrole results in marked enzyme induction of the hepatic microsomal enzymes but with concomitant loss of cytochrome P-450 enzyme activity. Hence, we have the apparent paradox of enzyme induction accompanied by simultaneous enzyme inhibition.

Treatment of animals with safrole or isosafrole, either orally or intra-peritoneally, results in immediate (10 min) enhancement of the activity of biphenyl 2-hydroxylation, which lasts for a period of several hours and is then followed by true enzyme induction (*de novo* protein synthesis). As biphenyl 2-hydroxylation is a specific measure of cytochrome P-448, and is not shown by cytochrome P-450, it appears that treatment of animals with safrole or isosafrole leads to conversion of cytochrome P-450 to cyto-chrome P-448 before *de novo* protein synthesis has time to occur. This again confirms that the conversion of cytochrome P-450 to cytochrome P-448 by carcinogens is initially a conformational change, which is followed by increased synthesis of cytochrome P-448. This is supported by kinetic studies, which show that although pretreatment with phenobarbitone increases the V_{max} of both biphenyl 2- and 4-hydroxylation, the V_{max} values are not substantially increased after pretreatment with the carcino-gen, 3-methylcholanthrene. The carcinogen appears to increase the 2-hydroxylation of biphenyl by decreasing the K_m value, whereas pheno-barbitone pretreatment leads to its increase (see Table 7.10).

Table 7.10. Apparent kinetic constants of biphenyl hydroxylation by liver microsomes from normal rats and rats pretreated with phenobarbitone or 3-methylcholanthrene.

	2-Hydroxylation		4-Hydroxylation	
	$K_m \times 10^{-4}$M	V_{max}	$K_m \times 10^{-4}$M	V_{max}
Untreated, control	4.7 ± 0.4	2.2 ± 0.1	1.4 ± 0.1	3.5 ± 0.1
Phenobarbitone-pretreated	37.6 ± 9.9	7.3 ± 1.6	0.4 ± 0.05	18.8 ± 1.7
Methylcholanthrene-pretreated	2.2 ± 0.3	2.3 ± 0.1	1.0 ± 0.2	5.9 ± 0.3

(Burke & Bridges, 1975)

Ligand complexes of cytochrome P-450, enzyme inhibition and toxicity

This formation of ligand complexes of cytochrome P-450 is now known to be a general phenomenon involving lipophilic amines, phosphines, carbanions, carbenes, organic sulphides and organic thiols. These sub-strates of cytochrome P-450 are metabolized to highly reactive inter-mediates which then form a ligand complex with the cytochrome, generally resulting in its conversion to cytochrome P-448 with a simultaneous loss of normal mixed-function oxygenase activity.

Numerous thiocarbonyl compounds (disulfiram) and thiophosphonyl compounds (parathion) are converted into their oxygen analogues by the microsomal mixed-function oxidases, and in consequence of this, sulphur is transferred onto the cytochrome P-450, resulting in inhibition of hydroxy-lase activity, lipid peroxidation, and destruction of cytochrome P-450. This is probably similar to ligand complex formation by reactive metabolites.

Many halogenated compounds, such as carbon tetrachloride, chloro-form, halothane, Freons, etc., form ligand complexes with cytochrome

P-450. They undergo dehalogenation by cytochrome P-450 operating in the anaerobic mode. The resultant, highly reactive, dehalogenated radicals then bind with cytochrome P-450 to form a carbene complex, as occurs in the formation of other ligand complexes of cytochrome P-450 (see Figure 7.3).

The non-competitive inhibition of the mixed-function oxidases by SKF 525-A is also due to ligand complex formation, resulting initially in

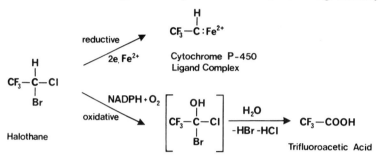

Fig. 7.3.   Reductive and oxidative microsomal metabolism of halothane.

inhibition of cytochrome P-450 activity, followed later by induction of the microsomal enzymes (Buening & Franklin, 1976). Amphetamine and its *N*-substituted analogues also give rise to ligand complex formation, but this is very slow or non-existent in normal rats, whereas with phenobarbital-treated animals, ligand complex formation with amphetamine increases 10-fold; with 3-methylcholanthrene-treated animals, the rate of complex formation falls even below that for normal animals (Franklin, 1974). Ligand complex formation, with its consequent inhibition of the mixed-function oxygenases, manifestation of cytochrome P-448 (biphenyl 2-hydroxylase) activity, lipid peroxidation, destruction of cytochrome P-450, and the associated cytotoxicity, therefore appears to be dependent on a particular species of cytochrome P-450, which is preferentially induced by treatment with phenobarbitone, and does not occur with cytochrome P-448. As this complex formation may lead to several processes of cellular toxicity, including tissue necrosis and tumour formation, enzyme induction by drugs may in itself constitute a toxic hazard by favouring ligand complex formation with ubiquitous environmental chemicals, such as the halogenated hydrocarbons and the thiophosphonyl and thiocarbonyl pesticides (see Figure 7.4).

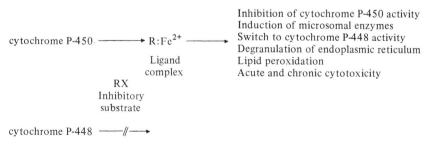

Fig. 7.4.   Ligand complex formation with cytochrome P-450 microsomal enzyme induction, enzyme inhibition and cytotoxicity.

The conversion of cytochrome P-450 to cytochrome P-448, when irreversible, is associated with damage to the endoplasmic reticulum, and impairment of the synthesis of proteins and glycoproteins. It may result in damage to the tissues concerned, i.e. hepatic necrosis, and might also give rise to tumour formation (see Figure 7.5). Indeed, ligand complex formation has been postulated as a possible mechanism of the carcinogenic action of chloroform, and many other chemicals, in certain animal species (Parke, 1978). The amount of damage to the endoplasmic reticulum and the conversion of cytochrome P-450 to cytochrome P-448 depends on the extent

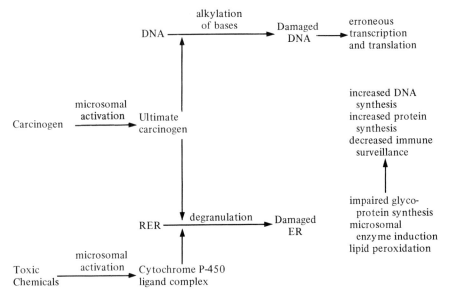

Fig. 7.5.   Postulated mechanisms of carcinogenicity and cytotoxicity involving microsomal activation and cytochrome P-450 ligand complex formation.

of ligand complex formation and on the rate of metabolic activation of the chemicals involved. Hence, it is not surprising that chloroform, and several other halogenated chemicals, recently classified as carcinogens, are carcinogenic only in the mouse, a species which exhibits a very high rate of metabolic activation (Parke, 1978). It is therefore likely that the toxic hazard to man from ingestion of the numerous chemicals which can lead to ligand complex formation with cytochrome P-450 and to degranulation of the endoplasmic reticulum, is not great if dosage is low. However, as so many different chemicals are known to participate in this phenomenon, the accumulated dosage of all of these has to be considered, and their total effects on the endoplasmic reticulum evaluated. This evaluation is now a major health and socio-economic problem of concern to all toxicologists.

References

Allen, J.R., Chesney, C.F. and Frazee, W.J. (1972). *Toxic appl. Pharmac.*, 23, 470.

Brooks, S.M., Werk, E.E., Ackerman, S.J., Sullivan, I. and Thrasher, K. (1972). *New Engl. J. Med.*, 286, 1125.

Buening, M.K. and Franklin, M.R. (1976). *Drug Metab. Disp.*, 4, 244.

Burke, M.D. and Bridges, J.W. (1975). *Xenobiotica*, 5, 357.

Burt, R., Freston, J.W. and Tolman, K.G. (1976). *J. clin. Pharmac.*, 16, 393.

Clark, B. and Thompson, J.W. (1972). *Br. J. Pharmac.*, 44, 89.

De Matteis, F. and Gibbs, A.H. (1977). *Biochem. J.*, 162, 213.

Faber, O.K., Mouridsen, H.T. and Skovsted, L. (1974). *Acta pharmac. tox.*, 35, 195.

Faber, O.K., Mouridsen, H.T. and Skovsted, L. (1975). *Br. J. clin. Pharmac.*, 2, 281.

Franklin, M.R. (1974). *Drug Metab. Disp.*, 2, 321.

Friedman, M.A. and Woods, S. (1977). *Res. Commun. Chem. Path. Pharmac.*, 17, 623.

Fujii, K., Jaffe, H., Bishop, Y., Arnold, E., Mackintosh, D. and Epstein, S.S. (1970). *Toxic. appl. Pharmac.*, 16, 482.

Gil, D.L. and Wilkinson, C.F. (1977). *Pest. Biochem. Physiol.*, 7, 183.

Hart, P., Farrell, G.C., Cooksley, W.G.E. and Powell, L.W. (1976). *Br. med. J.*, 2, 147.

Hempel, E. and Klinger, W. (1976). *Drugs*, 12, 442.

Hill, D.L. and Shih, T.-W. (1974). *Cancer Res.*, 34, 564.

Holder, G.M., Little, P.J., Ryan, A.J. and Watson, T.R. (1976). *Biochem. Pharmac.*, 25, 2747.

Hunter, A.L. and Neal, R.A. (1975). *Biochem. Pharmac.*, 24, 2199.

Ioannides, C., Lake, B.G. and Parke, D.V. (1975). *Xenobiotica*, 5, 665.

Ioannides, C. and Parke, D.V. (1975). *J. Pharm. Pharmac.*, 27, 739.

Jounela, A.J. (1968). *Annls. Med. exp. Biol. Fenn.*, 46, 531.

Juchau, M.R., Zachariah, P.K., Colson, J., Symms, K.G., Krasner, J. and Yaffe, S. (1974). *Drug Metab. Disp.*, 2, 79.

Kalant, H., Khanna, J.M., Lin, G.Y. and Chung, S. (1976). *Biochem. Pharmac.*, 25, 337.

Kato, R. (1961). *Arzneimittel-Forsch.*, 11, 797.

Khanna, J.M., Kalant, H., Yee, Y., Chung, S. and Siemens, A.J. (1976). *Biochem. Pharmac.*, 25, 329.

Labadarios, D. (1975). Studies on the effects of drugs on nutritional status. Ph.D. thesis, University of Surrey, England.

Labadarios, D., Dickerson, J.W.T., Lucas, E.G., Obuwa, G.H. and Parke, D.V. (1977). *Br. J. clin. Pharmac.*, 5, 167.

Lumholtz, B., Siersback-Nielsen, K., Skovsted, L., Kampmann, J. and Hansen, J.M. (1975). *Clin. Pharmac. Ther.*, 17, 731.

Lu, A.Y.H., Somogyi, A., West, S., Kuntzman, R. and Conney, A.H. (1972). *Arch. Biochem. Biophys.*, 152, 457.

Lu, A.Y.H., Levin, W., West, S., Jacobson, M., Ryan, D., Kuntzman, R. and Conney, A.H. (1973). *Ann. N.Y. Acad. Sci.*, 212, 156.

McPherson, F., Bridges, J.W. and Parke, D.V. (1974). *Nature (Lond.)*, 252, 488.

Mohan, L.C., Grantham, P.H., Weisburger, E.K., Weisburger, J.H. and Idoine, J.B. (1976). *J. Nat. Cancer Inst.*, 56, 763.

O'Malley, K., Stevenson, I.H. and Crooks, J. (1972). *Clin. Pharmac. Ther.*, 13, 552.

Palmer, D.L., Despopoulos, A. and Rael, E.D. (1972). *Antimicrob. Agents Chemother.*, 1, 112.

Parke, D.V. (1975). In *Enzyme Induction.* Editor: Parke, D.V., pp. 207-271. London and New York: Plenum.

Parke, D.V. (1978). *Ecotoxicology and Envir. Safety* (in the press).

Parke, D.V. and Gray, T. (1978). In *Primary Liver Tumours,* Editors: Remmer, H. and Bolt, H. Lancaster: MTP Press.

Pelkonen, O. and Kärki, N.T. (1973). *Chem.-Biol. Interact.*, 7, 93.

Pessayre, D., Bentata, M., Degott, C., Nouel, O., Miguet, J.-P., Rueff, B. and Benhamou, J.-P. (1977). *Gastroenterology*, 72, 284.

Renton, K.W. and Mannering, G.J. (1976). *Biochem. Biophys. Res. Commun.*, 73, 343.

Selkirk, J.K., Croy, R.G., Roller, P.P. and Gelboin, H.V. (1974). *Cancer Res.*, 34, 3474.

Sellers, E.M., Lang, M., Koch-Weser, J., Le Blanc, E. and Kalant, H. (1972a). *Clin. Pharmac. Ther.*, 13, 37.

Sellers, E.M., Carr, G., Bernstein, J.G., Sellers, S. and Koch-Weser, J. (1972b). *Clin. Pharmac. Ther.*, 13, 50.

Soda, D.M. and Levy, G. (1975). *J. Pharm. Sci.*, 64, 1928.

Solymoss, B., Varga, S., Krajny, M. and Werringloer, J. (1970). *Thromb. Diath. haemorrh.*, 23, 562.

Somogyi, A., Conney, A.H., Kuntzman, R. and Solymoss, B. (1972). *Nature, New Biology*, 237, 61.

Soyka, L.F. and Long, R. (1972). *J. Pharmac. exp. Ther.*, 182, 320.

Stripp, B., Greene, F.E. and Gillette, J.R. (1969). *J. Pharmac. exp. Ther.*, 170, 347.

Stripp, B., Menard, R.H. and Gillette, J.R. (1974). *Life Sci.*, 14, 2121.

Suarez, K.A., Carlson, G.P., Fuller, G.C. and Fausto, N. (1972). *Toxic appl. Pharmac.*, 23, 171.

Suarez, K.A., Carlson, G.P. and Fuller, G.C. (1975). *Toxic appl. Pharmac.*, 34, 314.

Tuchweber, B., Kovacs, K., Jago, M.V. and Beaulieu, T. (1974). *Res. Commun. Chem. Path. Pharmac.*, 7, 459.

Valerino, D.M., Vesell, E.S., Aurori, K.C. and Johnson, A.O. (1974). *Drug Metab. Disp.*, 2, 448.

Vesell, E.S., Passananti, G.T. and Lee, C.H. (1971). *Clin. Pharmac. Ther.*, 12, 785.

Weiner, M., Buterbaugh, G.G. and Blake, D.A. (1972). *Res. Commun. Chem. Path. Pharmac.*, 4, 37.

Wilkinson, C.F., Hetnarski, K. and Yellin, T.O. (1972). *Biochem. Pharmac.*, 21, 3187.

Wislocki, P.G., Miller, E.C., Miller, J.A., McCoy, E.C. and Rosencrantz, H.S. (1977). *Cancer Res.*, 37, 1883.

Zampaglione, N.G., Jollow, D.J., Mitchell, J.R., Stripp, B., Hamrick, M. and Gillette, J.R. (1973). *J. Pharmac. exp. Ther.*, 187, 218.

Zilly, W., Breimer, D.D. and Richter, E. (1975). *Eur. J. clin. Pharmac.*, 9, 219.

8.   Neurological toxicity of drugs

Peter Jenner and C. David Marsden

Introduction

The nervous system differs from most other tissues in that each of its individual elements is specialized for a specific but different task. It is feasible to destroy a large proportion of the liver without compromising overall liver function, for remaining liver cells will cope adequately. However, destruction of small sections of the nervous system inevitably causes deficit, the nature of which depends on the specialized function of that part. Thus damage to a restricted area of the dominant left cerebral hemisphere of man will prevent speech, while a lesion confined to one side of the cerebellum will cause incoordination of the ipsilateral limbs.

The central nervous system, that is the brain and spinal cord, also differs from most other tissues in that its neurones cannot regenerate, so damage once done cannot be repaired. Such recovery as may occur depends on factors other than regrowth of nerve cells. Peripheral nerves, on the other hand, can regenerate, although very slowly.

Further, the central nervous system is uniquely protected from many metabolic or drug insults by a highly effective blood-brain barrier. The blood-brain barrier is both physical and metabolic. Large molecules find difficulty penetrating it, and only lipid-soluble agents enter easily. Specific metabolic systems pump out certain electrolytes such as calcium and potassium, to maintain the concentration of these substances that are critical to keep nerve transmission constant. Specific enzymic systems destroy toxins and circulating pharmacologically active agents so as to prevent entry into the central nervous system. Thus active amines such as noradrenalin and dopamine are destroyed by monoamine oxidase residing in the capillary walls that comprise part of the blood-brain barrier. Inevitably, diseases causing a breakdown of the blood-brain barrier may provoke excessive drug entry with resulting toxicity. For example, meningitis allows much easier entry of penicillin into brain, with the risk of provoking epileptic fits if given systemically in massive dosage. Of course, drugs injected directly into the cerebrospinal fluid at lumbar puncture by-pass the blood-brain barrier with the corresponding risk of overdosage. Penicillin again is an example; two or three patients annually die from status epilepticus due to failure to realize that the dose of intrathecal penicillin required to treat meningitis is only a fraction of that given systemically.

These general introductory comments serve to illustrate that the nervous system is, in a number of ways, a unique organ. Its response to toxic agents inevitably differs in certain respects from that of other organs. Against this background, we propose first to review the ways in which the nervous system can react to toxic agents, and then to discuss the manner in which drugs can affect the nervous system.

Clinical syndromes of neurotoxicity

Despite its complexity the nervous system can respond to toxic agents in only a limited number of ways. These are best considered anatomically, starting at the head and working down to the muscles.

Toxic actions affecting the brain

Diffuse encephalopathy. The brain usually is affected diffusely by toxic drugs or poisons. The presenting features of a drug-induced encephalopathy are due to progressive loss of higher intellectual functions culminating in a global dementia, with, if acute or sub-acute, a clouding of consciousness, visual hallucinations and motor restlessness. Such an acute toxic confusional state or delirium is typical of drug-induced encephalopathies. Untreated, it will be accompanied by epileptic fits and will progress to drowsiness, coma and death.

Drugs may provoke such an encephalopathy either by an indirect systemic effect on some other factor essential to brain metabolism, or by a direct action on the brain itself.

Examples of the former mechanism include hypoglycaemia provoked by anti-diabetic agents such as insulin, hyponatraemia provoked by diuretics in those with liver failure, or hypercalcaemia caused by vitamin D intoxications. A more subtle example is the encephalopathy provoked by isoniazid therapy in tuberculosis, which is attributed to drug-induced vitamin B_6 deficiency. Examples of the latter mechanism include the acute toxic confusional states provoked by anticholinergic drugs or anticonvulsants.

Certain drugs may provoke diffuse cerebral oedema causing the syndrome of benign intracranial hypertension characterized by headache, papilloedema and raised intracranial pressure. Such drugs include steroids (and steroid withdrawal) and oral contraceptives, as well as lead to which children who indulge in the habit of sucking paints (pica) are particularly at risk.

Focal brain lesions. Damage to a restricted area of brain may occur non-specifically due to stroke provoked by drugs. Such strokes may be due to intracerebral haemorrhage as a result of anticoagulant therapy, or to cerebral infarction secondary to vascular occlusion following thrombosis (as in those rare women taking the contraceptive pill who have a stroke) or hypotension (caused by over-enthusiastic therapy with drugs that lower blood pressure).

A rare problem of drug-induced focal brain pathology is the appearance of brain tumours in those on long-term immuno-suppression, such as those with kidney transplants.

Another form of focal brain damage provoked by drugs or toxic agents is due to the specific susceptibility of a selected portion of the brain to drug action. Examples include the loss of memory due to vitamin B_1 deficiency in alcoholics associated with selective damage to limbic areas, the cerebellar syndrome of incoordination of limbs and unsteadiness of gait provoked by chronic phenytoin or alcohol, or the variety of movement disorders due to basal ganglia action of neuroleptic antipsychotic drugs.

The cerebellum is particularly susceptible to a range of drugs, and unsteadiness is one of the sensitive symptoms of overdosage with drugs such as anticonvulsants, benzodiazepines, tricyclic antidepressants and the like.

The neuroleptic antipsychotic drugs, which include phenothiazines, butyrophenones and thioxanthenes, may by their action on the basal ganglia provoke a variety of extrapyramidal side effects including acute dystonic reactions, Parkinsonism, akathisia and tardive dyskinesia (which are discussed at greater length below).

Epilepsy. Many drugs may provoke epileptic fits without other evidence of brain injury. Otherwise normal individuals have a fit if given specific convulsant drugs such as metrazole or ergot, or may have fits during withdrawal of drugs such as alcohol, amphetamines, anticonvulsants, etc. Those with a tendency to epilepsy anyway may be susceptible to less obvious drug triggers such as phenothiazines or tricyclic anti-depressants.

Psychiatric syndromes. Certain drugs may provoke psychiatric illness with no evidence of physical brain dysfunction. Thus depression is a well-recognized unwanted effect of treatment of hypertension with α-methyl-dopa or reserpine. Indeed, such observations were the stimulus to the development of various amine hypothesis of affective disorders.

Other drugs such as lysergic acid and mescaline may provoke acute psychotic states, and chronic amphetamine abuse has caused a psychiatric illness remarkably similar to schizophrenia. This latter observation led to the dopamine hypothesis of schizophrenia.

Neuro-endocrine syndromes. Drugs interfering with the release or action of hypothalamic releasing or inhibiting factors, or with pituitary function, may provoke a range of endocrine disturbances. For example, galactorrhoea and secondary amenorrhoea caused by hyperprolactinaemia produced by phenothiazines.

Toxic actions affecting the spinal cord and peripheral nervous system

Myelopathy. Damage to the spinal cord to cause weakness and stiffness of the legs — a spastic paraplegia — is an uncommon unwanted effect of drugs. Perhaps the best known example was the appearance of such a syndrome accompanied by optic nerve damage amongst large numbers of Japanese in the 1960s — so-called subacute myelo-opto-neuropathy, or SMON for short. Epidemiological evidence has suggested that this epidemic may have been due to the predilection of the Japanese to ingest large quantities of the anti-diarrhoea agent clioquinol (Enterovioform). The anti-tuberculosis agent ethambutol may cause a similar syndrome.

Also, the spinal cord is particularly vulnerable to toxic agents introduced into the cerebrospinal fluid at lumbar puncture, for it is inevitably bathed by the highest concentration of drugs so applied. Intra-thecal methotrexate, employed to combat leukaemia, may cause spinal cord damage in this manner.

Peripheral neuropathy. Many drugs may damage peripheral nerves. Most do so indiscriminately, affecting motor nerves to muscle, sensory nerves, and autonomic nerves. The resulting clinical picture is that of weakness and wasting of the distal muscles of arms and legs, especially of the hands and feet, paresthesia and sensory loss distally over fingers and toes spreading up the arms and legs if progressive, and symptoms of autonomic neuropathy such as postural fainting, impotence and lack of sweating.

The number of drugs known to cause such a peripheral neuropathy is legion and includes chloral, chloroquine, clioquinol, vincristine, disulphiram, emetine, glutethamide, isoniazid, nitrofurantoin, phenytoin, stilbamidine, streptomycin, sulphonamides, thalidomide, and most recently, perhexiline. In addition to drugs, many other toxic agents damage peripheral nerves, including insecticides such as DDT, acrylamide, heavy metals such as lead, arsenic, mercury and thallium, solvents such as trichloroethylene, and, of course, alcohol.

In general, such neurotoxic agents damaging peripheral nerves do so in one of two ways. Either they kill the neurone itself, in which case the nerve fibre or axon dies back from its tip furthest from the cell body in spinal cord or posterior root ganglion; or they damage the myelin sheath investing the nerve fibres, so-called demyelinating neuropathies. Most toxins cause axonal degeneration, with secondary loss of myelin.

Drugs may also provoke peripheral nerve damage indirectly. For example, barbiturates may provoke a florid subacute neuropathy in patients suffering from hereditary porphyria, while the neuropathy produced by isoniazid in slow acetylators with tuberculosis is due to secondary vitamin B_6 deficiency.

Myopathy

In considering neurotoxicity anatomically, drug-induced muscle disease, or myopathy, must be discussed.

A few drugs provoke myasthenic weakness, that is weakness produced by exercise and relieved by rest, in those with myasthenia gravis. Such drugs, which include the aminoglycosides, further compromise transmission from nerve to muscle at the muscle end-plate.

Other drugs may actually damage the muscle's contractile machinery, for example, steroids, ACTH, chloroquine and emetine. Such patients present with painless weakness of proximal muscles of arms and legs, making it difficult to raise the arms above the head, or to climb stairs and get out of a low chair.

The ubiquitous alcohol rarely may provoke an acute painful muscle necrosis during a heavy bout.

Other drugs may cause profound weakness by effects on electrolytes, particularly potassium. Diuretics, and carbenoxolone employed in peptic ulceration, may produce such a large urinary potassium excretion as to cause hypokalaemic paralysis.

Finally, a small proportion of the population inherit an abnormality of muscle rendering them unduly susceptible to all anaesthetic agents. The latter cause hyperpyrexia, rigidity, respiratory and cardiac distress and often death in such individuals — the malignant hyperpyrexia syndrome.

Drug-induced neurotoxicity

In considering specific types of neurotoxins which affect the central nervous system we have included not only drugs, but also compounds which the population at large may meet inadvertently.

We will first consider compounds which produce neurotoxicity that has occurred in epidemic proportions in either isolated pockets of the population or throughout the general population. Second, consideration of the neurotoxicological problems which can arise through the widespread clinical use of drugs will be discussed by reference to two specific drug groups, the anticonvulsants and the neuroleptic antipsychotics.

Neurotoxic epidemics

There have been a large number of extensive epidemics of neurotoxicity due to specific poisons which have occurred for a variety of reasons. Organophosphate insecticides have been responsible for many outbreaks of neurotoxicity and cause a vicious peripheral neuropathy. For example, the largest disaster occurred in 1930 in the United States when the organophosphate insecticide TOCP was accidentally added to a soft drink 'Ginger Jake' and involved some 20 000 individuals. Similarly, an outbreak in 1959 in Morocco in which a lubricant containing TOCP was used to dilute olive oil resulted in some 10 000 cases of peripheral nerve paralysis. Insecticides are now, in this country at least, tightly controlled, with careful monitoring of those who work with such compounds. However, in only one third of all patients presenting with a peripheral neuropathy can the cause be identified. In the other two-thirds of the patients, no firm conclusion can be drawn although there is a strong suspicion amongst neurologists that since, in those where the cause can be identified, drugs (or other foreign compounds) are the commonest offender, many of those in whom a cause cannot be identified may have developed a peripheral neuropathy secondary to exposure to agents which remain unknown.

Mercury toxicity can cause a severe and often lethal peripheral neuropathy as well as affecting the brain by producing an encephalopathy. The main outbreak of organic mercury poisoning occurred by the eating of fish that had taken up mercury compounds discharged into a bay district around Minimata in Japan. A similar epidemic of mercury poisoning is believed to be occurring at the present time among Canadian Indians due to the discharge of organic mercury into the Great Lakes. The fish-eating Indians who live around these lakes are now exhibiting signs of peripheral nerve disease.

The most disastrous epidemic of mercury poisoning to occur in modern times occurred in Iraq as a result of attempts to relieve famine. Mercury-dressed seed intended for agricultural use was mistakenly used by the starving population as food.

This type of example serves to illustrate the sort of rare large epidemics occurring in relatively isolated areas. However, other neurotoxicity appears as a smaller problem since the incidence is spread throughout the population.

For example, acrylamide which is used as a flocculator for soil produces a peripheral neuropathy. Similarly, the excessive use of skin cleansers containing hexachlorophane on areas of damaged skin can lead to central nervous system damage due to large-scale absorption through the skin.

A similar problem can be seen in the clinical use of drugs. For example, vincristine is one of the most widely used anticancer agents and is highly effective in the control of Hodgkin's disease and leukaemia. However, many patients so-treated develop some degree of peripheral neuropathy.

Anticonvulsant drugs

Epilepsy is a common illness. One in two hundred of the population suffers from recurrent fits while one in five may have a fit at some time during their life. In 40% of those suffering recurrent fits the disease is lifelong and therefore requires drug treatment for life to suppress symptoms.

A wide range of drugs such as diphenylhydantoin, phenobarbitone and ethosuximide are used to treat epilepsy, but none of them is entirely effective. The occurrence of toxicity problems is not surprising if drugs are administered for a lifetime. However, the incidence of toxicity produced by antiepileptic drugs has become apparent only in the last decade. The major drugs used to treat epilepsy, diphenylhydantoin and phenobarbitone, have been used since the 1950s but recognition of their long-term side effects has only become widespread in the last decade.

On acute administration, the commonly used antiepileptic drugs produce acute intoxication exemplified by fluttering eyes, double vision, unsteadiness, slurring of speech, drowsiness, confusion, coma and death. Chronic intoxication may involve many systems of the body. The effects produced include overgrowth of connective tissue, hairiness, acne and a variety of metabolic problems such as folic acid deficiency and altered calcium metabolism. Damage also occurs to peripheral nerves and to the cerebellum. Anticonvulsants cause profound enzyme induction which may be responsible for many of the side effects of long-term treatment.

The acute toxic side effects of drugs like diphenylhydantoin are clearly dose-dependent and the use of serum level measurements of anticonvulsants has been of considerable help to clinicians in order to assess the significance of patients' complaints in relation to drug toxicity.

Neuroleptic antipsychotic drugs

Neuroleptic antipsychotic drugs appear to act by blocking dopamine receptors in the brain. Such drugs are exemplified by phenothiazines, such as chlorpromazine, which were the original group to be introduced into long-term therapy and have latterly been joined by butyrophenones such as haloperidol and pimozide. The major side effects produced by such drugs are involuntary movement disorders caused by their action on the extra-pyramidal motor system of the brain. Acute administration of neuroleptic antipsychotic drugs causes the onset of acute dystonic reactions in some 2% of susceptible individuals within 48 h of starting treatment. Patients exhibiting this syndrome frequently present with the neck thrown back by muscle spasm, the mouth forced open, the tongue pushed out and the eyes turned up to the ceiling. The syndrome produces extreme discomfort and can be lethal if the muscle spasms affect the throat to restrict air entry.

Such drugs may all cause Parkinsonism, characterized by poverty of movement, stiffness of muscles, a flexed posture and tremor at rest, in anyone if given in large enough dose. Such drug-induced Parkinsonism is often accompanied by motor restlessness or akathisia. On chronic adminis-tration, some 20-40% of those treated with these drugs for two or more years may develop the syndrome of tardive dyskinesia. This syndrome is characterised by abnormal movements of the mouth, trunk and limbs, may persist in as many as 50% of cases even though the offending drug is stopped. Indeed, tardive dyskinesias often appear only when therapy is reduced or even withdrawn.

Neuroleptic antipsychotic drugs also serve to illustrate how carefully one has to examine differences between types of side effect when considering mechanisms and appropriate methods of treatment. Thus, the production of acute dystonic reactions, drug-induced Parkinsonism, akathisia and tardive dyskinesias are all due to an abnormality of one part of the brain, the extrapyramidal nervous system. However, in all probability each syndrome involves a different mechanism. For example, while anticholiner-gic drugs are commonly prescribed to counteract the Parkinsonian side effects of neuroleptic antipsychotic therapy, the administration of anti-cholinergics to patients with tardive dyskinesias worsens the abnormal movement disorder. Here we have a difficult dilemma of one group of agents, the neuroleptic antipsychotic drugs, producing side effects one of which may be improved by a concurrent drug administered, the other of which may be made worse.

The mechanisms involved in the production of side effects by neuroleptic antipsychotic agents revolve around dopamine receptors in the brain and dopamine in general, and provide an illustration of how one group of drugs can produce a wide range of problems by an action on one part of the nervous system.

Predisposing factors to drug-induced neurological disease

It is important to realize when considering neurotoxicity that a number of factors can cause a predisposition to drug-induced neurological disease. For example, it is readily apparent that drug over-dosage is more likely to result in neurotoxicity than the administration of therapeutic amounts of drug. Also, the way in which the drug is metabolized within the body may influence the incidence of toxicity. Thus, the higher concentrations of isoniazid observed in patients with tuberculosis who are slow acetylators may provoke a peripheral neuropathy. Indeed, the disease state itself may induce susceptibility to neurological disease, as seen by the occurrence of fits during porphyria where patients are rendered unduly sensitive to barbiturates. In some cases diet may be of importance. The example is well known of the administration of monoamine oxidase inhibitors for depression combining with a large dietary tyramine intake, such as from cheese, to produce vicious hypertension which may lead to intracerebral haemorrhage. Interactions between drugs can also lead to problems. Thus, the co-administration of sulthiame with diphenylhydantoin serves to potentiate the anticonvulsant-induced side effects by inhibition of the metabolism of diphenylhydantoin. Lastly, as we have already mentioned, the route of administration as in the case of intrathecal penicillin and the presence of damage to the blood-brain barrier can provide the factor necessary to elicit drug-induced neurological disease where normally none might be observed.

The part played by predisposing factors serves to highlight the care which must be used in attempting to identify the causative agent or factor in this type of disorder.

Conclusion

This is a relatively simple framework for thinking of the spectrum of problems that drugs can produce in the nervous system. But there are really a very restricted number of mechanisms or number of ways in which the nervous system can respond to drug damage. Obviously, some drugs will produce admixtures of damage to various portions of the nervous system, whereas others produce relatively pure pictures of damage to one portion of the nervous system. Some drugs are just simply good neurotoxic agents. For example, alcohol will produce an encephalopathy — if you take too much of it you become drowsy, you may develop fits, you may become unconscious and indeed you may die of alcohol poisoning. Alcohol will produce a cerebellar syndrome — it makes you drunk, you stagger along and although this usually stops when the blood alcohol level drops, you may develop permanent cerebellar damage from prolonged drinking. Alcohol damages the spinal cord — it may produce a myelopathy, it may make you go blind, it may produce a peripheral nerve neuropathy and it may also produce an acute primary muscle problem.

Other drugs are, however, more specific in their action. Some can specifically affect the optic nerve to produce blindness or apparently only affect the auditory nerve to produce deafness. Indeed, one of the most intriguing remaining problems is why certain drugs specifically affect certain parts of the nervous system and not others.

With regard to the mechanism by which neurotoxicity is brought about, we understand very little. For example, at present at least fourteen chemical neurone transmitter systems are known to be operating in the brain. There are far more chemical substances in the brain that may be acting as neuronal transmitters, although this remains to be proved. If one takes the example of a single neurone in the brain which forms part of the nigro-striatal dopamine-containing pathway and build up what is known of the inter-relationship between this neurone and connecting neuronal systems, the degree of complexity is grossly apparent. Thus it has been demonstrated that events in the nigro-striatal pathway can be influenced at least by the involvement of other neurones containing acetylcholine, GABA, 5HT, noradrenalin, substance P, encephalins and glutamate. Thus even in the limited collection of neurones forming the nigro-striatal pathway the controlling influences on the operation of one unit in the brain are enormous.

Such a situation presents a fair range of possible ways in which drugs can influence one neurone, let alone the intact working nervous system.

Bibliography

Bradford, H.F. and Marsden, C.D. (1976). *Biochemistry and Neurology*. London: Academic Press.

Marsden, C.D., Tarsy, D. and Baldessarini, R.J. (1975). In *Psychiatric Aspects of Neurologic Disease*, Editors: Benson, D.F. and Blumer, D., p. 219. New York: Grune & Stratton.

Reynolds, E.H. (1975). *Epilepsia*, 16, 319.

Roizon, L., Shiraki, H. and Grcevic, N. (1977). *Neurotoxicology*, Vol. 1. New York: Raven Press.

Walton, J.N. (1977). *Brain's Diseases of the Nervous System*. 8th Ed. Oxford: Oxford University Press.

9. The induction of cancer by drug therapy

T. A. Connors

Introduction

Iatrogenic cancer is of increasing concern because of the demonstration over the past ten years that chemicals previously thought to be innocuous, because of their low acute toxicity, may on chronic administration have serious long term effects, including cancer induction. The potential carcinogenicity of pharmaceuticals has thus been recognized well after the period of expansion of the drug industry between 1935 and 1965. Man, for the past forty years, may have been exposed to medicaments which have not been adequately tested for carcinogenicity. This must be regarded as a serious problem, since the level of exposure during medication may be high and continuous compared with say, the exposure from potential carcinogens occurring as contaminants of foodstuffs.

There are a number of problems involved in assessing the carcinogenic hazards arising from the use of medicaments at recommended therapeutic levels:

1. The risks involved cannot be readily quantified by comparison with a control population because of the lack of good epidemiological studies or even adequate documentation of the case histories of patients who have developed cancer after exposure to a particular drug. In many publications it is difficult to interpret the results because the total numbers of patients treated cannot be identified nor their duration of treatment. The absolute incidence of cancer cannot therefore be calculated or compared with identical populations not undergoing treatment. There is a need for registries (similar to those that have been set up for kidney transplant patients and for children surviving intensive therapy for malignant disease) which record the incidence of tumours in humans treated chronically with widely used medicaments. Case reports should be organized to include all relevant details, especially dosage, the latent period of tumour induction and the type of tumour. Details should also be available of the number of people so treated.
2. The pathological condition for which the drug is being used may actually predispose towards cancer. The increased cancer risk of patients suffering from xeroderma pigmentosa and Fanconi's anaemia is well known. There also appears to be an association between malaria

and Burkitt's lymphoma, and between schistosomiasis and bladder cancer. Hence in the absence of proper controls, drugs used to treat these conditions might be suspected of increasing the incidence of cancer, where this is due in fact to some property of the disease. A further complication is that a drug non-carcinogenic in normal animals may be carcinogenic in animals suffering from a particular pathological condition. Hycanthone (I) for example does not cause

I

HYCANTHONE

cancer in normal mice. However, when used to treat mice infected with *S. Mansoni cercariae*, it caused a significant increase in hepatocellular carcinomas when compared to mice infected with the schistosome only (Haese, Smith & Bueding, 1973). A further major factor preventing assessment of risk has been the finding that compounds normally non-carcinogenic or carcinogenic only at high doses in mammals may be greatly potentiated by a whole variety of extrinsic and intrinsic factors.

3. An undetected cancer may be responsible for the pathological condition for which the drug is being used. Brain tumours may cause epileptic seizures and hence co-exist with the disease at a higher than expected rate (Clemmesen, Fuglsang-Frederiksen & Plum, 1974). Any assessment of the carcinogenicity of anti-epileptics by studies in humans is therefore made difficult because of this association. It is also possible that a particular pathological state may increase the chances of a very early diagnosis of cancer.

4. The therapeutic treatment by prolonging the survival of patients with a hitherto incurable and lethal disease may allow previously unknown features of the natural disease to be manifest. With the improved survival of patients with acute lymphoblastic leukaemia and Hodgkin's disease treated with powerful combinations of drugs, it has been recognized that there is, in the long term, an increase in secondary malignancies (*Lancet*, 1977; Arseneau *et al.*, 1977). Thus, Brody, Schottenfeld & Reid (1977) have shown that for Hodgkin's disease patients treated between 1950 and 1954, there is a lower cumulative probability of a second cancer compared with patients treated between 1960 and 1964, whose probability of getting a second cancer was in turn less than those patients treated between 1968 and 1972. Over these periods there has been an increase in the intensity of therapy, for example the use of radiotherapy combined with chemotherapy and the development of multiple drug combinations used at high dose

levels. At the same time the median survival time of patients with Hodgkin's disease has increased considerably. Whether the increased incidence of second cancers is due to a natural progression of the disease, to better follow-up of patients or to the treatment is still debatable. However, more and more cases of second malignancies arising in patients treated with chemotherapy are now being reported (Einhorn, 1978) and it seems likely that there is some increase in risk of developing a second cancer (particularly leukaemias and lymphomas) after intensive drug treatment. It will prove difficult to estimate the risk for individual drugs because of the complexity of modern treatment schedules which involve combinations of anti-cancer agents, sometimes with irradiation, plus a whole range of supportive measures, such as administration of analgesics and antiemetics.

Cytotoxic agents

This rather misleading term is the general name given to several classes of chemicals originally used as anti-cancer agents but then later used as immunosuppressants and antipsoriatics and in the treatment of 'auto-immune' disease and diseases of collagen. They have also been investigated for their potential as insect male chemosterilants and as epilatory agents. Cytotoxic agents have in common the property of killing cells in cycle by interfering specifically at certain stages of the synthesis of DNA, RNA or protein. Their use as anti-cancer agents is a reflection of their ability to inhibit the proliferation of tumours, but in most cases their use is associated with damage to the proliferating cells of the bone marrow and gut mucosa. They have been used as immunosuppressants to prevent the rejection of kidney homografts, because of their effects on dividing lymphocytes, and as chemosterilants, because of their toxicity to developing spermatogonia and spermatocytes. It has also been known for many years that some of these chemicals are carcinogenic in animals and man. Sulphur mustard gas (II) for example, which was first used as a chemical warfare agent, was also used to treat cancer as early as 1934. There is a strong association between

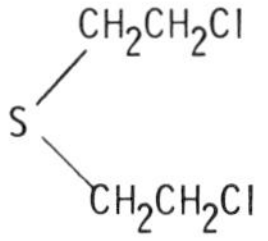

$$S \begin{cases} CH_2CH_2Cl \\ CH_2CH_2Cl \end{cases}$$

II
SULPHUR MUSTARD

$$CH_3 \, N \begin{cases} CH_2CH_2Cl \\ CH_2CH_2Cl \end{cases}$$

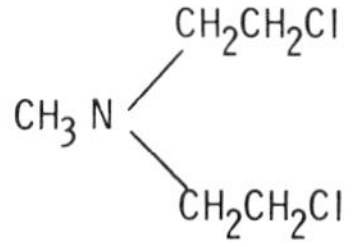

III
NITROGEN MUSTARD

workers exposed to sulphur mustard gas during its manufacture and cancers of the respiratory tract (Yamada, 1963). Nitrogen mustard (the hydrochloride of methyl-N,N-di-2-chloroethylamine (III)) was introduced as an anti-cancer agent in 1943 and is in widespread use today, although it was shown to be carcinogenic in animals as early as 1949 (Boyland & Horning, 1949).

Three main classes of cytotoxic agent contain members of proven carcinogenicity, the alkylating agents, antitumour antibiotics and the antimetabolites.

Alkylating agents

Expressed in simple terms, an alkylation is any reaction in which the hydrogen group of a molecule is substituted by an alkyl radical. The alkyl radical may be quite a complex structure, the sole requirement being that the alkyl group is linked to the molecule by a fully saturated carbon atom. For example

$$RSCH_2CH_2Cl + HOOCR' \rightarrow RSCH_2CH_2OOCR' + HCl$$

Many different chemicals can alkylate given the appropriate conditions, but the major classes used medicinally are the nitrogen mustards, sulphonoxyalkanes (methane sulphonates), ethyleneimines (aziridines) and the epoxides (oxiranes). Some antitumour agents such as the bromohexitols are converted into alkylating agents *in vitro*. The majority of the alkylating agents act by an S_N2 mechanism involving the formation of an intermediate transition complex between the alkylating agent and the molecule with which it reacts. However, their mechanism of reaction and the molecules with which they react can be best understood if they are considered to act by an S_N1 mechanism which involves the formation of a positively charged and highly reactive carbonium (or carbenium) ion. Figure 9.1 shows the hypothetical reactive species of the four common types of alkylating agent. Positively charged carbonium ions (which are one form of an electrophilic reactant) will react with negatively charged molecules or with molecules containing uncharged nitrogen atoms (because of their high electron density). When an alkylating agent is administered, many different molecules will be alkylated, since negatively charged centres (nucleophilic sites) are a common feature of many biological molecules. The thiols of proteins and amino acids are particularly reactive, as are ionized carboxylic and phosphoric acids. In nucleic acids there are many sites susceptible to alkylation including ring and exocyclic nitrogen atoms, ionized phosphate groups and the exocyclic oxygen atoms of guanine and thymine. Following covalent binding of alkylating agents to macromolecules, especially DNA, cells in cycle do not divide normally, developing into giant cells with abnormal amounts of proteins and nucleic acids. These giant cells die before entering mitosis. At lower dose levels much of this damage may be repaired and the cells may survive. However in some cases, possibly because of faulty DNA repair, a somatic cell undergoes a mutation which is

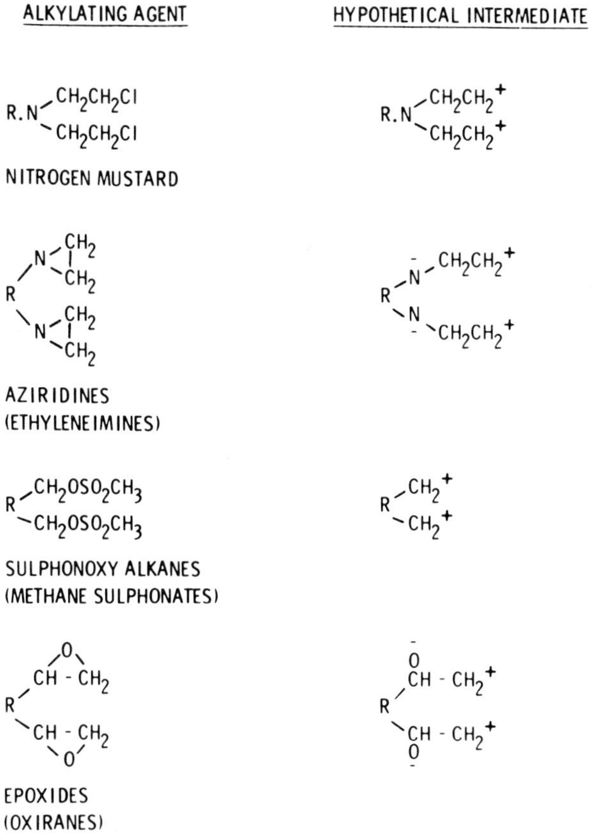

ALKYLATING AGENT   HYPOTHETICAL INTERMEDIATE

$$R.N \overset{\displaystyle CH_2CH_2Cl}{\underset{\displaystyle CH_2CH_2Cl}{}} \qquad\qquad R.N \overset{\displaystyle CH_2CH_2^+}{\underset{\displaystyle CH_2CH_2^+}{}}$$

NITROGEN MUSTARD

AZIRIDINES
(ETHYLENEIMINES)

$$R \overset{\displaystyle CH_2OSO_2CH_3}{\underset{\displaystyle CH_2OSO_2CH_3}{}} \qquad\qquad R \overset{\displaystyle CH_2^+}{\underset{\displaystyle CH_2^+}{}}$$

SULPHONOXY ALKANES
(METHANE SULPHONATES)

EPOXIDES
(OXIRANES)

Fig. 9.1.   Examples of few types of alkylating agent used in the treatment of
cancer and their reactive species.

responsible for the subsequent malignant transformation.

The following are the most widely used alkylating agents in medicine for
which there is some evidence of carcinogenicity.

Melphalan (*L*-Sarcolysine, *L*-PAM, phenylalanine mustard, Alkeran)
Melphalan (IV) is an aromatic nitrogen mustard used in the treatment of
various cancers, especially ovarian carcinoma and multiple myeloma. More
recently it has been used in the adjuvant chemotherapy of stage ii and iii
breast cancers treated by surgery. As with most other therapeutic agents,
there have been no epidemiological studies in man on the long-term effects
of melphalan treatment. However, it has been given over a long period of

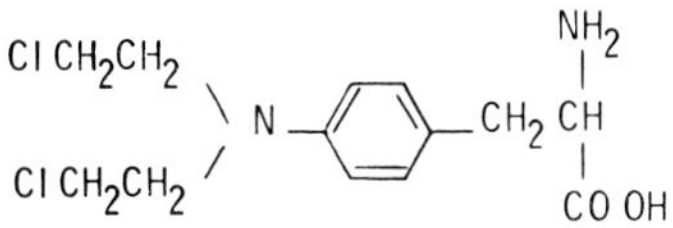

IV
MELPHALAN

time to patients suffering from myeloma or ovarian carcinoma and in both cases there is evidence that an increased risk from acute leukaemia exists (Karchmer *et al.*, 1974; Kyle, Pierre & Bayrd, 1975; Einhorn, 1978). Although in some of the cases described, melphalan was only one agent of many including other alkylating agents and radiotherapy, in other cases mephalan was the only treatment; it is reasonable to assume that prolonged treatment increases the incidence of leukaemia, but the degree of risk is unknown at present.

Melphalan and other alkylating agents mentioned below (e.g. cyclophosphamide, nitrogen mustard, thioTEPA and chlornaphazine) are mutagenic in assays using *Salmonella* strains (Benedict *et al.* 1977). There is also ample evidence that melphalan is carcinogenic in rodents. In one experiment using groups of 60 mice of both sexes, melphalan caused a significant increase in lung tumours 39 weeks after thrice-weekly intraperitoneal injections for four weeks of dose levels above 1.07 mg/kg (Shimkin *et al.*, 1966). Melphalan may be administered to humans daily over a period of months sometimes approaching a total dose of 8.0 mg/kg. More recently even higher doses of melphalan have been used in clinical cancer chemotherapy.

Nitrogen Mustard (Mustine, HN2, Mechlorethamine). Nitrogen mustard hydrochloride (III) is still in wide use today in the treatment of a variety of cancers, especially Hodgkin's disease where it is part of a widely used four-drug combination usually administered after radiotherapy. It has also been investigated as a potential therapeutic agent for the treatment of rheumatoid arthritis and other non-malignant diseases.

There is no direct evidence for the carcinogenicity of HN2 in humans, but the possibility of an increased cancer incidence, especially acute non-lymphocytic leukaemia as a result of intensive chemotherapy using drug combinations containing nitrogen mustard has been discussed (Arsenau *et al.*, 1977). In rats, nitrogen mustard caused a variety of malignant tumours (Schmähl & Oswald, 1970). In mice, administration of weekly intravenous doses of HN2 for long periods led to an increased incidence of thymic lymphomas and pulmonary adenomas (Conklin, Upton & Christenberry, 1965).

Chlorambucil (Leukeran). Chlorambucil (V) was previously used in the treatment of many cancers but especially chronic lymphocytic leukaemia

$$Cl\,CH_2CH_2 \diagdown N - \langle \rangle - CH_2CH_2CH_2CO\,OH$$
$$Cl\,CH_2CH_2 \diagup$$

V
CHLORAMBUCIL

$$Cl\,CH_2CH_2 \diagdown N - P \diagup O \diagdown O - CH_2 \diagdown CH_2$$
$$Cl\,CH_2CH_2 \diagup \qquad NH - CH_2 \diagup$$

VI
CYCLOPHOSPHAMIDE

and malignant lymphomas. Leukaemia and other tumours have been reported as second malignancies in patients treated with chlorambucil (Catovsky & Galton, 1971) but there is insufficient evidence to decide whether it is a carcinogen in man. In rats and mice there is definite evidence of its carcinogenicity causing lung tumours and lymphomas in mice and lymphomas in male rats (Weisburger *et al.*, 1975).

Cyclophosphamide (Cytoxan, Endoxan). Cyclophosphamide (VI) has been used extensively in the past not only in the treatment of a variety of malignancies, but also as a therapeutic agent for many collagen-vascular disorders and 'autoimmune' diseases (IACR Monograph, 1975). Like many other alkylating agents, it has also been tested as an insect chemosterilant (and as a result of its known side effect of alopecia in man, it has been investigated as an epilatory agent for the chemical shearing of sheep (Bakke *et al.*, 1972). Four cases of squamous cell carcinoma have been recorded by Marshall (1974) in patients who were given cyclophosphamide for glomerulonephritis or lupus erythematosus, and other cases have been reported of cancer arising in patients treated with cyclophosphamide for non-malignant disease (Sieber & Adamson, 1975). The strongest evidence that cyclophosphamide is a carcinogen for man comes from studies in patients given high doses of the drug and who subsequently developed bladder cancer. To date there have been a number of publications associating a high incidence of bladder cancer with treatment by cyclophosphamide (Wall & Clausen, 1975; Schmähl *et al.*, 1977). Cyclophosphamide is metabolized to reactive species and with high dose levels it is likely that a much greater concentration of these species (which are probably responsible for the cystitis observed) occurs in the bladder.

In a series of experiments, cyclophosphamide has caused a variety of tumours in mice and rats. In some cases the dose level of the drug was comparable to that used clinically (Schmähl & Osswald, 1970; Schmähl, 1974).

Other nitrogen mustards. The other nitrogen mustards of interest are *N,N*-di-2-chloroethyl-β-naphthylamine (Chlornaphazine) (VII) and phenoxybenzamine (VIII). The former was first used in 1948 in the treatment of Hodgkin's disease and polycythaemia vera. As with

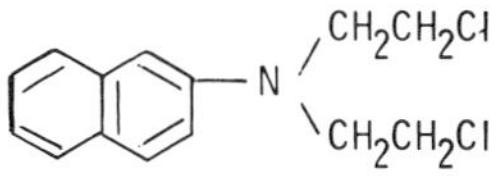

VII
CHLORNAPHAZINE

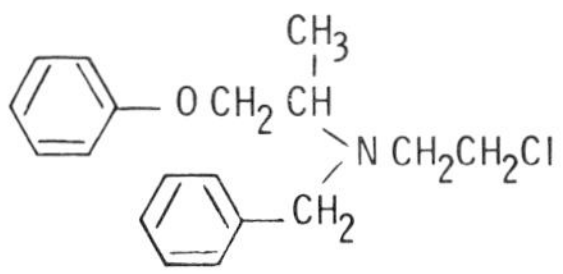

VIII
PHENOXYBENZAMINE

cyclophosphamide, this drug was shown to cause cystitis and was later implicated as a bladder carcinogen in man (Chievitz & Thiede, 1962; Thiede & Christensen, 1969). The assumption has been made that chlornaphazine is carcinogenic after metabolism to the known potent carcinogen, β-naphthylamine. This involves the removal of two chloroethyl groups from the molecule, and while monodechloroethylation is a known biotransformation process for some difunctional nitrogen mustards, the removal of both functional arms has never been demonstrated. However, the possibility that chlornaphazine is not a carcinogen in its own right but requires activation *in vivo* is supported by mutagenic studies on *Salmonella* strains. In these experiments (Benedict *et al.*, 1977), while most alkylating agents were directly acting, chlornaphazine and cyclophosphamide were mutagenic only when incubated with a liver S9 drug-metabolizing fraction. Phenoxybenzamine is of interest because it is an α-adrenergic blocking agent and may be used in acute situations such as in the treatment of acute cardiogenic shoc. or may be given by mouth over long periods in the treatment of periphera. vascular disorders. In some instances, doses up to 240 mg daily have been administered. The long duration of action of phenoxybenzamine is thought to be due to its covalent binding to receptors through its chloroethyl radical. There is no evidence from case reports or epidemiological studies that phenoxybenzamine is carcinogenic in man but it does produce an increased incidence of lung tumours in mice (Stoner *et al.*, 1973).

Other alkylating agents. Many bifunctional aziridines (ethyleneimines) have also been used in the treatment of cancer. The most widely used have been TEM (IX), ThioTEPA (X) and Trenimon (XI). In all cases they have been shown to be carcinogenic in rodents, but their possible carcinogenicity

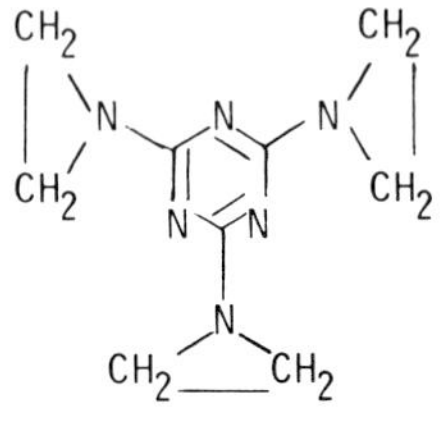

IX
T.E.M

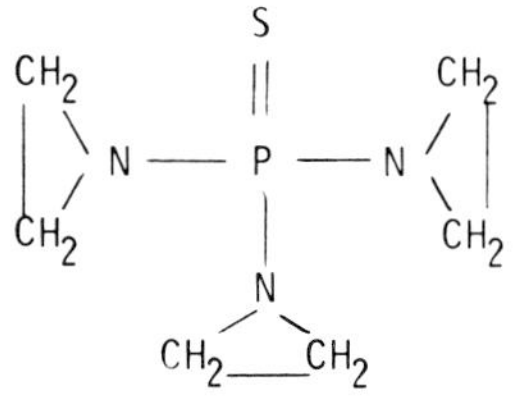

X
Thio - TEPA

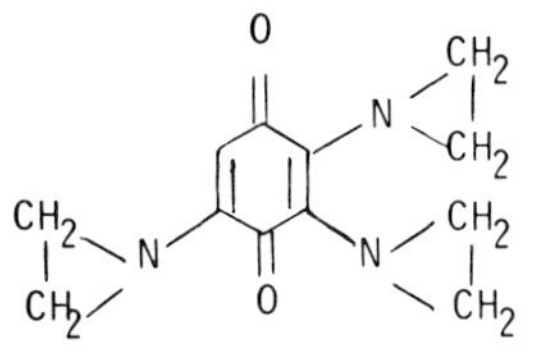

XI
TRENIMON

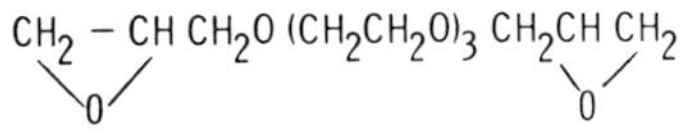

$$CH_2 - CH\ CH_2O\ (CH_2CH_2O)_3\ CH_2CH\ CH_2$$

XII
ETHOGLUCID

$$CH_2 - C - C - C - C - CH_2$$

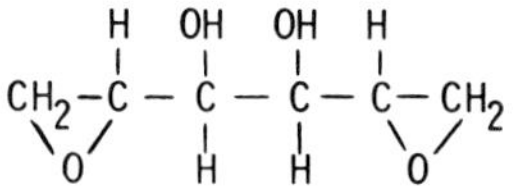

XIII
DIANHYDROGALACTITOL

in man has not been established, although nine cases of acute leukaemia have been reported in patients treated with ThioTEPA for other malignancies (IACR Monograph 1975).

A large number of epoxides were investigated some years ago but very few have had more than limited use as anticancer agents. Ethoglucid (XII) has been used in the treatment of cancer and has caused lung cancer after intraperitoneal injection to mice (Shimkin *et al.*, 1966). Dianhydrogalactitol (XIII) is at present being investigated in the treatment of brain tumours in man, and anguidine, a mycotoxic agent produced by *Fusaria* and containing an epoxide group, is being evaluated as a potential agent in the treatment of colon cancer (Eagan *et al.*, 1977; Corbett *et al.*, 1977). Tricothecenes related to anguidine are irritants and cytotoxic at high doses but have not yet been studied in detail for their carcinogenic action. The role of epoxides in carcinogenesis has of late become an important line of research because of the discovery that many pharmaceuticals have structural features prone to epoxidation *in vivo*. Oesch (1976) lists a number of commonly produced drugs which are transformed *in vivo*, sometimes only by a minor pathway, to epoxides (allobarbital, secobarbital, alphenal, protriptyline, carbamazepine, cyproheptadine, and phylloquinone). A number of products of drug metabolism have also been identified which suggest that an epoxide has been formed as an intermediate (e.g. diethylstilboestrol, diphenylhydantoin, phensuximide, phenobarbital, mephobarbital, methaqualone, lorazepam, imipramine and acetanilide). Among the sulphonoxyalkanes, Myleran (used widely in the treatment of chronic myeloid leukaemia) is a leukaemogen in experimental animals (Harris, 1976; Upton, Wolff & Sniffen, 1961). Koss (1969) has also shown post

$$CH_3SO_2O(CH_2)_4OSO_2CH_3$$

XIV
MYLERAN

mortem many preneoplastic changes in the tissues of patients receiving Myleran over a long period.

More recently some newer classes of alkylating agents have been investigated for their antitumour activity and several are now in clinical use. These agents, like the difunctional alkylating agents, probably kill cells by reacting covalently with DNA, but they are monofunctional and are quite distinct in some of their biological properties. Virtually all of them are suspect carcinogens as measured by short-term tests for carcinogenicity, by carcinogenicity studies in rodents or by an association with the subsequent development of cancer in man. Among these classes of anticancer agent are the nitrosoureas, such as BCNU (XV) (Weisburger, 1977), dialkyltriazenes, such as DIC (XVI) (Skibba, Erturk & Bryan, 1970) and Natulan (XVII) (Kelly *et al.*, 1964). The co-ordination complex of platinum Cis PDD (XVIII), now being increasingly used in the treatment of a number of

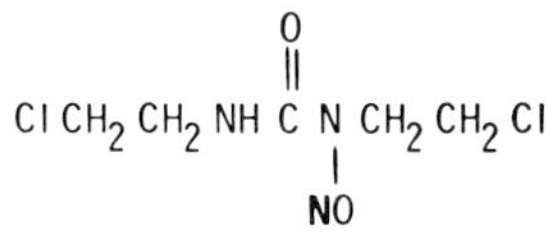
O
Cl CH2 CH2 NH C N CH2 CH2 Cl
NO

XV
BCNU

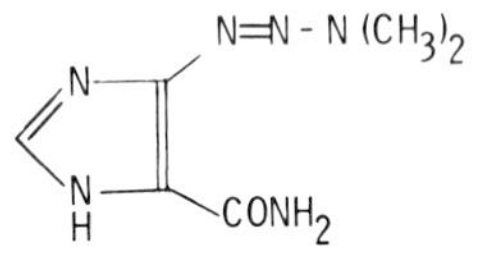
N=N - N (CH3)2
N
N
H
CONH2

XVI
DIC

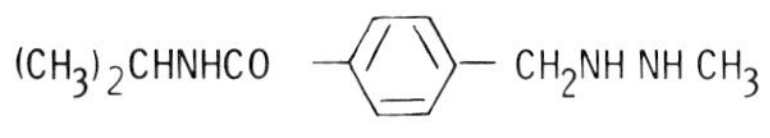
(CH3)2CHNHCO
CH2NH NH CH3

XVII
NATULAN

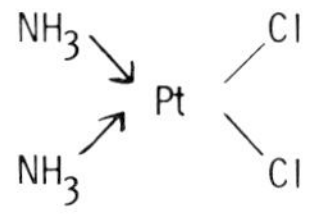
NH3
Cl
Pt
NH3
Cl

XVIII
Cis PDD

cancers, particularly ovarian carcinoma and teratoma, has not been investigated in detail for its carcinogenic activity but has been shown to be mutagenic in *Salmonella* (Benedict *et al.*, 1977).

Other anticancer agents

Three other major classes of chemical have been used in cancer chemotherapy. The antitumour antibiotics, a diverse group of products isolated from soil micro-organisms, usually inhibit cell proliferation by some form of interaction with DNA. This is often the result, not of covalent binding, but of a very strong non-covalent binding to specific areas of DNA. With some of these agents cytotoxicity may be the result of DNA breaks. The most commonly used antibiotics in the treatment of cancer are adriamycin, actinomycin, bleomycin, streptozotocin, mitomycin C and daunomycin. Although actinomycin D and bleomycin are negative in bacterial mutagenicity tests (which are claimed to correlate well with animal carcinogenesis) there is ample evidence of their carcinogenicity in animals (Benedict *et al.*, 1977). Adriamycin and its less frequently used analogue daunomycin cause breast tumours in rats (Bertazolli, Chieli & Solcia, 1971) and chromosomal damage in humans (Sieber & Adamson, 1975). Mitomycin C and streptozotocin have also been shown to be carcinogenic in rodents (Schmähl & Osswald, 1970; Mauer *et al.*, 1974).

The antimetabolites include analogues of purines, pyrimidines and folic acid and are cytotoxic as a result of their interference with the *de novo* synthesis of purines or pyrimidines or with the polymerization of nucleic acids. Because of the strong possibility that alkylating agents are carcinogenic in man, it has been advocated that antimetabolites should be used where possible instead of alkylating agents in the treatment of cancer (*Lancet*, 1977). There is certainly less evidence that the antifolate methotrexate is a carcinogen. It is inactive in the salmonella mutagenicity test (Benedict *et al.*, 1977) and has given negative results in animals. Life-long feeding, for instance, caused some histological changes in mice and hamsters but did not increase the incidence of tumours (Rustia & Shubik, 1973). However methotrexate has been quite extensively used in the treatment of psoriasis and Sieber & Adamson (1975) record thirteen cases of cancer arising in patients treated with methotrexate for psoriasis. In one case, a psoriatic patient treated for three years with methotrexate developed a hyperplastic lymphoid condition resembling lymphosarcoma. On discontinuation of treatment, the hyperplasia disappeared, implicating methotrexate as the causative agent. Azathioprine breaks down rapidly *in vivo* to form 6-mercaptopurine, which is an inhibitor of purine biosynthesis *de novo*. Both compounds cause human chromosome damage and are carcinogens in rodents (Sieber & Adamson, 1975; Weisburger, 1977). In conjunction with steroids, azathioprine has been widely used as immunosuppressant therapy in patients with kidney transplants and the increased risk of cancer in such patients has previously been mentioned. Immunosuppressive antimetabolites such as azathioprine have also been used to treat 'autoimmune' diseases and there are a number of reports in the literature of unusual types of cancer arising after treatment with these chemicals (Sieber & Adamson.

1975). However whether the increased cancer incidence is the result of a direct effect of the antimetabolite at the cellular level, or whether it is a feature of the chronically immune-depressed patient is not clear. The association between an increased cancer incidence and disorders of the immune system has already been referred to.

The use of cytotoxic agents in the treatment of cancer and non-malignant diseases would thus seem to be associated with an increased incidence of cancer. Some chemicals do seem to be more dangerous in this respect than others, but this may be because they have been more widely used in man or their effects more fully recorded. They may have also been used in instances where the patient may receive prolonged treatment, for example myeloma or chronic leukaemia or non-lethal diseases such as psoriasis. On the other hand, it may be because they have been more fully investigated in laboratory systems. The decision to use these agents must be a positive judgement bearing in mind the poorly quantified risk that each agent represents. In the case of acute lymphoblastic leukaemia, where the prognosis is less than one year without treatment, the use of chemotherapy is clearly justified. In this case, the possibility (not certainty because only the risk is increased) of inducing a second cancer some years later is to be preferred to immediate death. Clearly the least dangerous drugs should be used if there is a choice between equally active treatments but this is rarely the case, since, for each type of cancer which responds to chemotherapy, there is usually a best combination of drugs which has been worked out on a trial and error basis over many years. Where combinations of such drugs have been studied experimentally for their carcinogenesis, there is no evidence of any additive or synergistic effects. In some drug combinations in fact there even appeared to be mutual inhibition of carcinogenicity (Weisburger, 1977). Thus the use of drug combinations in cancer chemotherapy is to be encouraged, while there is still considerable research required to find effective but less dangerous therapeutic agents. In cases where drug therapy is only of limited effectiveness, that is where there is only tumour regression with little increase in survival time, then one must balance the benefits of the treatment against the short-term toxic effects of the treatment rather than against any of its long-term effects. The decision to use chemotherapy is more difficult in situations such as the use of chemotherapy adjuvant to surgery in the therapy of breast cancer. Depending on the staging of the tumour and the status of the patient, some women undergoing surgery for breast cancer will not relapse and will survive many years tumour-free. The percentage of such patients tumour-free for at least three years after the operation can (in premenopausal women at least) be significantly increased if chemotherapy is given immediately after surgery. The dilemma facing the clinician is that some of the patients will have a long-term survival after surgery alone, but since this small group cannot be identified they will be overtreated if adjuvant chemotherapy is given. This is clearly a case where the increased risk of the drug combination should be quantified so that a judgement can be made of the benefits versus the risk.

The use of cytotoxic agents in the treatment of non-malignant disease creates similar difficulties. Obviously they should not be used where there are effective alternatives which have been shown to have no long-term toxicity. However, there may be examples where the quality of life is so poor that it is reasonable to use drugs which will successfully treat the condition but increase the risk from cancer some years later.

Other pharmaceutical agents

The development of short term tests for carcinogenicity and the demonstration that many chemical structures have the potential to be transformed into reactive and possibly carcinogenic metabolites, will mean that many pharmaceutical agents will be reassessed for their carcinogenicity. As with the anticancer agents, there have been few epidemiological studies, while most experimental data are inadequate. The following examples are a few of the more widely used agents.

Arsenic

The carcinogenic effects of arsenic in workers exposed to high levels of the metal were recognized more than 150 years ago. There is also an association between skin cancer and exposure to arsenic (as its oxides or sodium, potassium and calcium salts) in drinking water and insecticides (IACR monograph, 1973). Despite this close connection between arsenic and cancer, especially skin cancer, arsenicals have been used until comparatively recently in the treatment of a number of skin conditions, particularly psoriasis vulgaris (Regelson *et al.*, 1968; Robson & Jelliffe, 1963; Schmähl, Thomas & Auer, 1977). However, most experiments designed to assess carcinogenicity of arsenic in rodents have given negative results. This has prevented detailed studies on its mechanism of action, but arsenic has been found to inhibit DNA polymerase. Since this may lead to faulty repair it may increase the incidence of skin cancer by rendering cells more susceptible to the DNA damaging effects of, for example, u.v. irradiation.

Diethylstilboestrol

A medicament may increase the incidence of a particular type of cancer but not be immediately obvious if the cancer involved is a common one and if the medicament is used generally in a large population. Chemical carcinogens have most chance of being detected if they cause an increased cancer incidence in a specific population, such as the bladder cancer associated with distillers of β-naphthylamine, if they increase the incidence of a rare type of cancer, such as the haemangiosarcomas associated with vinyl chloride, or if the cancer occurs at an atypical age. The carcinogenicity of diethylstilboestrol was first recognised because of the occurrence of an unusual type of vaginal adenocarcinoma in young women aged 15-22 years instead of the expected age of 50 years or more (Herbst & Scully, 1970; Greenwald *et al.*, 1971). Sixty-four cases of diethylstilboestrol-related carcinomas of the vagina and cervix had been recorded by 1972 and by 1976 this number had increased to more than 400 cases. Since stilboestrols were in widespread use between 1950 and 1970 to prevent unwanted abortion, it is likely that there will still be many cases of vaginal cancer in the offspring of women treated with this chemical. It has, for example, been estimated that in the United States some 16 000 women may have been given stilboestrol between 1960 and 1970. This compound is clearly very potent, since some mothers whose offspring developed vaginal carcinoma had received as little as 25 mg per day for one month only. It is likely that the synthetic oestrogen interferes with the proper development of the utero-vaginal tract in the embryo. The increased oestrogen stimulation during puberty may then cause hyperplasia which itself may lead to a malignant transformation, or which may make the tissue sensitive to exogenous carcinogens. It has been shown experimentally that diethylstilboestrol causes hyperplasia in rodents at the age of puberty, but that these changes can be prevented if mice are castrated before they reach the age of puberty.

Diazepam

Diazepam (XIX) (and its metabolite oxazepam) are widely used in the treatment of anxiety. Daily doses of up to 100 mg may be administered over long periods. Many people must have been exposed to diazepam since the annual production figures in Europe run to several thousand kilograms. There is no

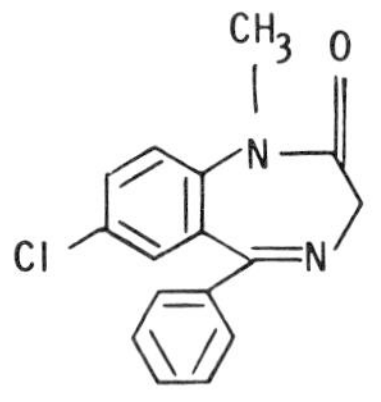

XIX
DIAZEPAM

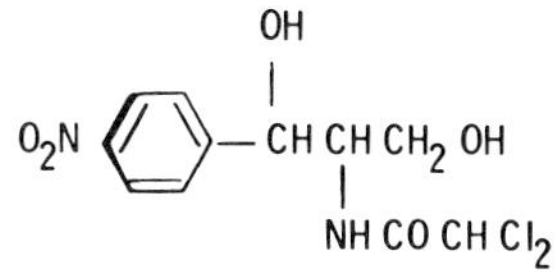

XX
CHLORAMPHENICOL

evidence that diazepam is carcinogenic in humans, but in one experiment in mice liver cell adenomas were associated with the feeding of 0.15% oxazepam in the diet for 12 months. Since diazepam is demethylated to a large extent there is a possibility that intermediate methylols are formed which are possibly the reactive intermediates of some carcinogens (see Chapter 1).

Chloramphenicol

Chloramphenicol (XX) has been used to treat many bacterial infections, and for typhoid fever high doses of up to a 100 g over four weeks may be given. While there are no good animal data on the carcinogenicity of chloramphenicol, there is definite evidence that it induces bone marrow damage (Wallerstein *et al.*, 1969). It has been postulated that following episodes of bone marrow depression caused by chloramphenicol, there may be an increased risk of leukaemia (Fraumeni, 1967). Since chloramphenicol is extensively metabolized in man, it is possible that it is a reactive metabolite that is causing the bone marrow damage.

Metronidazole and related nitro compounds

Metronidazole (XXI) and a number of chemically related nitroheterocyclic derivatives are used in the treatment of a variety of bacterial and protozoal infections. In mice, metronidazole significantly increased the incidence of

$$CH_2CH_2OH$$

$$O_2N \qquad N \qquad CH_3$$

$$N$$

XXI
METRONIDAZOLE

lung tumours and lymphomas and increased the incidence of mammary fibroadenomas in rats (IACR Monograph, 1977). It is mutagenic in bacteria, probably after reduction of the nitro groups which may occur enzymatically or in areas of low oxygen tension (Rosenkranz & Speck, 1975). The urine of human patients receiving 750 mg daily of metronidazole has also been shown to contain substances mutagenic to *Salmonella* (Legator, Connor & Stoeckel, 1975). Chemicals such as misonidazole which are 2-nitro analogues of metronidazole are effective radiation sensitizers and are now being tested clinically in cancer radiotherapy (Urtasun, Band & Chapman, 1976). Misonidazole also has some antitumour action on its own, probably as a result of reduction in the anerobic areas of tumours to reactive species (Stratford & Adams, 1977). Another nitroimidazole, niridazole is also carcinogenic in mice and hamsters. Several thousand derivatives of 5-nitrofurans have also been tested for their antibacterial action and many have been produced commercially.

Phenacetin and paracetamol

Phenacetin (XII) and its *O*-dealkylated metabolite paracetamol are widely used analgesic and antipyretic agents. The abuse of phenacetin has been correlated with papillary necrosis of the kidneys and an association has been claimed between heavy use of phenacetin and carcinoma of the renal pelvis. Schmähl *et al.* (1977) have listed 38 cases of tumours of the renal pelvis thought to have been induced by phenacetin overconsumption. *N*-Hydroxy-phenacetin, a putative metabolite of phenacetin, causes hepatocellular carcinoma in rats after oral administration (Nery, 1971). Both phenacetin and paracetamol are hepatotoxic in high doses and for this reason must be suspect carcinogens, since many compounds acutely toxic to the liver have been shown to cause hepatic cancer on long-term administration. The mechanism of hepatotoxicity of the two chemicals has been studied (Nelson, McMurty & Mitchell, 1978). Phenacetin is converted mainly to paracetamol and the latter may be excreted as a variety of metabolites. Probably at moderate doses the majority are non-toxic products such as *O*-glucuronides and sulphates. However, a small amount of *N*-hydroxy-paracetamol may be formed by microsomal metabolism and this can rearrange to the corresponding iminoquinone which is an electrophilic reactant. If only a small amount of this reactive species is formed, it is detoxified by conjugation with glutathione. However, in very high doses reserves of glutathione may be depleted and the quinone reacts with other essential sites leading to hepatotoxicity.

Phenylbutazone

Phenylbutazone (XXIII) is, like phenacetin, an analgesic and antipyretic but also has inflammatory action. Schmähl *et al.* (1977) have compiled 28 case histories of patients treated with phenylbutazone (mainly for treatment of inflammatory joint pain) who subsequently developed leukaemia.

Isoniazid (*isonicotinic acid hydrazide*)

Isoniazid (XXIV) and its analogues are used in large amounts as anti-tubercular and antileprotic agents. There is no evidence in man from its widespread use in the treatment of tuberculosis that it is carcinogenic. It

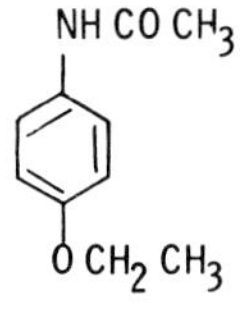

XXII
PHENACETIN

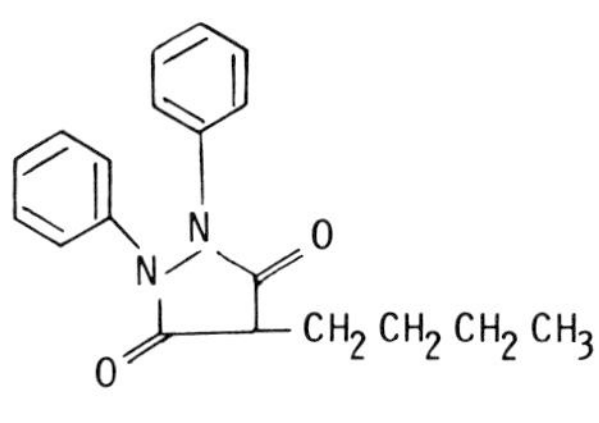

XXIII
PHENYLBUTAZONE

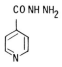

XXIV
ISONICOTINIC ACID HYDRAZIDE

has, however, been shown by a number of authors to be carcinogenic in mice (IACR Monograph 1974). More recently isoniazid has been shown to be converted to a series of reactive and potentially carcinogenic metabolites in both human and rat microsomes (see Chapter 1) (Nelson *et al.*, 1976).

The rudimentary evidence for the carcinogenicity of a whole variety of other pharmaceutical substances is discussed in various monographs of the International Agency for Cancer Research. In addition to the large amount of work involved in assessing the possible carcinogenicity in man of each chemical the problem is made far more difficult because it is now obvious that a variety of factors can influence the carcinogenicity of a particular substance. Thus many substances containing nitrogen may react under physiological conditions with nitrite (which is in foodstuffs or which may arise from bacterial reduction of nitrate) to yield carcinogenic nitrosamines, for example the reaction products of nitrite with pyramidon, chlorpromazine and oxytetracycline (Lijinsky, 1974).

References

Arseneau, J.C., Canellos, G.P., Johnson, R. and De Vita, V. (1977). *Cancer*, 40, 1912.
Bakke, J.E., Feil, V.J., Fjelstul, C.E. and Thacker, E.J. (1972). *J. agric. Fd Chem.*, 20, 384.
Benedict, W.F., Baker, M.S., Haroun, L., Choi, E. and Ames, B.N. (1977). *Cancer Res.*, 37, 2209.
Bertazolli, C., Chieli, T. and Solcia, E. (1971). *Experientia*, 27, 1209.
Boyland, E. and Horning, E.S. (1949). *Br. J. Cancer*, 3, 118.
Brody, R.S., Schottenfeld, D. and Reid, A. (1977). *Cancer*, 40, 1917.
Catovsky, D. and Galton, D.A.G. (1971). *Lancet*, 1, 478.
Chievitz, E. and Thiede, T. (1962). *Acta med. scand.*, 172, 513.
Clemmesen, J., Fuglsang-Frederiksen, V. and Plum, C.M. (1974). *Lancet*, i, 705.
Conklin, J.W., Upton, A.C. and Christenberry, K.W. (1965). *Cancer Res.*, 25, 20.
Corbett, R.H., Griswold, D.P., Roberts, B.J., Peckham, J.C. and Schabel, F.M. (1977). *Cancer*, 40, 2660.
Doll, R. and Kinlen, L. (1970). *Br. med. J.*, 4, 420.
Eagan, R.T., Ingle, J.N., Frytak, S., Rubin, J., Kvols, L.K., Carr, D.T., Coles, D.T. and O'Fallon, J.R. (1977). *Cancer Treatment Repts.*, 61, 1339.
Einhorn, N. (1978). *Cancer*, 41, 444.
Fraumeni, J.F. (1967). *J. Am. med. Assoc.*, 201, 150.
Greenwald, P., Barlow, J.J., Nasca, P.C. and Burnett, W.S. (1971). *New Engl. J. Med.*, 285, 390.
Haese, W.H., Smith, D.L. and Bueding, E. (1973). *J. Pharmac. exp. Ther.*, 186, 430.
Harris, C.C. (1976). *Cancer*, 37, 1014.
Herbst, A.L., and Scully, R.E. (1970). *Cancer*, 25, 745.
IACR Monographs on the evaluation of carcinogenic risk of chemicals to man (1973). International Agency for Research on Cancer, Vol. 2, Lyon 1973.

IACR Monographs on the evaluation of carcinogenic risk of chemicals to man (1974). International Agency for Research on Cancer, Vol. 4, Lyon 1974.

IACR Monographs on the evaluation of carcinogenic risk of chemicals to man (1975). International Agency for Research on Cancer, Vol. 9, Lyon 1975.

IACR Monographs on the evaluation of carcinogenic risk (1977). International Agency for Research on Cancer, Vol. 13, Lyon 1977.

Karchmer, R.K., Amare, M., Larsen, W.E., Mallouk, A.G. and Caldwell, G.G. (1974). *Cancer*, 33, 1103.

Kelly, M.G., O'Gara, R.W., Gadekar, K., Yancey, S. and Oliverio, V. (1964). *Cancer Chemother. Rept.*, 39, 77.

Koss, G.L. (1969). *Ann. N.Y. Acad. Sci.*, 163, 931.

Kyle, R.A., Pierre, R.V. and Bayrd, E.D. (1975). *Arch. Intern. Med.*, 135, 185.

Lancet. Leading article (1977). 1, 519.

Legator, M.S., Connor, T.H. and Stoekel, M. (1975). *Science*, 118, 1118.

Lijinsky, W. (1974). *Cancer Res.*, 34, 225.

Marshall, V. (1974). *Transplantation*, 17, 272.

Mauer, S., Lee, C., Natarian, J. and Brown, D. (1974). *Cancer Res.*, 34, 158.

Nelson, S.D., Mitchell, J.R., Timbrell, J.A., Snodgrass, W.R. and Corcoran, G.B. (1976). *Science*, 193, 901.

Nelson, S.D., McMurty, R.J. and Mitchell, J.R. (1978). In *Biological Oxidation of Nitrogen*. Editor: Gorrod, J.W., p. 319. Amsterdam, New York and Oxford: Elsevier/North Holland Biomedical Press.

Nery, R. (1971). *Xenobiotica*, 1, 339.

Oesch, F. (1976). *Biochem. Pharmac.*, 25, 1935.

Regelson, W., Kim, U., Ospina, J. and Holland, J.F. (1968). *Cancer*, 21, 514.

Robson, A.O. and Jelliffe, A.M. (1963). *Br. med. J.*, 2, 207.

Rosenkranz, H.S. and Speck, W.T. (1975). *Biochem. Biophys. Res. Commun.*, 66, 520.

Rustia, M. and Shubik, P. (1973). *Toxic. appl. Pharmac.*, 26, 329.

Schmähl, D. and Osswald, H. (1970). *Arzneimittel-Forsch.*, 20, 1461.

Schmähl, D. (1974). *Z. Krebsforsch.*, 81, 211.

Schmähl, D., Thomas, C. and Auer, R. (1977). *Iatrogenic Carcinogenesis*. Berlin, Heidelberg, New York: Springer-Verlag.

Shimkin, M.B., Weisburger, J.H., Weisburger, E.K., Gubareff, N.K. and Suntzeff, V. (1966). *J. Nat. Cancer Inst.*, 36, 915.

Sieber, S.M. and Adamson, R.H. (1975). *Adv. Cancer Res.*, 22, 57.

Skibba, J., Erturk, E. and Bryan, G. (1970). *Cancer*, 26, 1000.

Stoner, G.D., Shimkin, M.B., Kniazeff, A.J., Weisburger, J.H., Weisburger, E.G. and Gori, G.B. (1973). *Cancer Res:*, 33, 3069.

Stratford, I.J. and Adams, G.E. (1977). *Br. J. Cancer*, 35, 307.

Thiede, T. and Christensen, B. (1969). *Acta med. scand.*, 185, 133.

Upton, A.C., Wolff, F.F. and Sniffen, E.P. (1961). *Proc. Soc. exp. Biol. Med.*, 108, 464.

Urtasun, R.C., Band, P. and Chapman, J.D. (1976). *New Engl. J. Med.*, 294, 1364.

Wall, R.L. and Clausen, K.P. (1975). *New Engl. J. Med.*, 293, 271.

Wallerstein, R.O., Condit, P.K., Kasper, C.K., Brown, J.W. and Morrison, F.R. (1969). *J. Am. med. Ass.*, 208, 2045.

Weisburger, J.G., Griswold, D.P., Prejean, J.D., Casey, A.E. Wood, H.B. and Weisburger, E.K. (1975). *Recent Results in Cancer Research*, 52, 1.

Weisburger, E.K. (1977). *Cancer*, 40, 1935.

Yamada, A. (1963). *Acta Path. Jap.*, 13, 131.

10. Teratogenesis produced by drugs and related compounds

F. Beck

Introduction

Teratogenesis is difficult to define. The term is regarded as synonymous with genesis of congenital malformation, but there is an unfortunate tendency to define congenital malformation merely as physical deformity, and in order to overcome this problem, many workers now prefer to use the term congenital defect (Dudgeon, 1976). Wilson (1973) has pointed out that a quartet of *embryopathic* effects, namely foetal death, structural defect, functional defect and growth retardation should logically be considered together and there is much to be said for his point of view. He is also at pains to highlight the difficulties of producing an accurate assessment of incidence in most of these areas. Many early abortions pass undetected, while functional and even structural defects are frequently not diagnosed until well after birth and although growth retardation is perhaps the best defined, there is even here — as in two of the other categories — an arbitrary element involved in the borderline between normal variation and abnormality. A crude approximation of the estimated incidence of both structural and functional defects in liveborn infants is given in Table 10.1. Congenital defects are undoubtedly the commonest cause of death during the first year of life in all developed countries and probably account for about 20% of the incidence. Table 10.2 is an attempt at a breakdown of the causes of developmental defects in man and from it one could conclude that, given our present knowledge, only some 2-3% are due to drugs and environmental chemicals. It seems very probable, however, that many

Table 10.1. Estimated incidence of developmental defects among liveborn human infants examined under stated conditions.

Condition	Estimated %
All live births over 500g, diagnosed at birth	3-5
Born alive, diagnosed by best available means during first 2 years postnatally	5-10
Born alive but dying during first postnatal year and autopsied	18-20
Born alive but dying during first postnatal month and autopsied	25-30

From Wilson (1973), with permission.

Table 10.2.   Known causes of developmental defects in man.

Known genetic transmission	20%
Chromosomal aberration	3-5%
Environmental causes	
Radiations	<1%
Therapeutic	
Nuclear	
Infections	2-3%
Rubella virus	
Cytomegalovirus	
Herpesvirus hominis	
Toxoplasma	
Syphilis	
Maternal metabolic imbalance	1-2%
Endemic cretinism	
Diabetes	
Phenylketonuria	
Virilizing tumours	
Drugs and environmental chemicals	2-3%
Androgenic hormone	
Folic antagonists	
Thalidomide	
Organic mercury	
Some hypoglycaemics (?)	
Some anticonvulsants (?)	
Potentiative interactions	?
Unknown	65-70%

From Wilson (1973), with permission

more environmental teratogens are subsumed under the titles 'potentiative interactions' and 'unknown'.

Biology in general is largely concerned with the interaction of heredity and environment, and the study of congenital defects provides innumerable examples of this. The majority of embryopathies probably depend upon the interplay of many genetic factors and their relationship with a similar plurality of environmental influences. True, at one extreme, conditions such as achondroplasia are transmitted by dominant genes which have complete penetrance and it is difficult at this time to foresee any way in which the conditions under which development occurs might be modified to alter their expressivity. The majority of congenital defects, however, do not fall into such an extreme category and underlying genetic weaknesses can to a greater or lesser extent often be modified by the environment. At the other extreme, conditions such as rubella embryopathy and the prenatal effects of thalidomide can undoubtedly be ascribed principally to single causative agents acting during pregnancy; even then it is worth remembering that not *all* mothers who suffered from rubella or took thalidomide had deformed children, and clearly concomitant environmental and genetic factors sometimes combined to ameliorate the consequences. The genotype capable of modifying environmentally induced embryopathies is usually that of the developing conceptus, but maternal influences may also play a part, either by controlling the nature of the intrauterine environment (McLaren &

Michie, 1958) or perhaps because of extranuclear factors transmitted through the egg cytoplasm (Verrusio, Pollard & Fraser, 1968). Indeed, the general physiological status of the mother, being a combination of her environment and her phenotype (often called the 'dramatype'), is most relevant in this connection. Finally it is worth stressing that the complete elimination of embryopathy is not possible. Evolutionary drive depends upon the presence of variation within a species, which is produced by numerous factors such as mutation and genetic recombination; this will inevitably throw up extreme forms which undoubtedly merit classification as congenital 'defects'. Furthermore, phenomena such as balanced polymorphic systems in which heterozygotes are at an advantage over either homozygous genotype will often perpetrate the survival of higher levels of deleterious genes in the genetic pool than would have been possible if abnormal homozygotes were selected against in the normal way.

The analysis of variables in an embryopathic situation

Timing of the teratogenic insult

Generally speaking, the mammal passes through three broad phases of development which are relevant to abnormal development. The first precedes the formation of the primitive streak (sometimes incorrectly described as 'gastrulation' in a general sense) which occurs in the human about 16 days after fertilization. Before primitive streak formation, there is very little evidence that environmental agents are able to produce congenital defects in man or experimental animals. The reason for this is not completely known, but it is undoubtedly related to the capacity for self-regulation which the embryo is capable of before the development of the three germ layers. Thus, it is conceivable that a noxious stimulus applied before the primitive streak stage would either destroy the conceptus completely or would cause only reparable tissue damage. Even if some of the embryonic cells died, others might compensate for their absence by an alteration in their presumptive programme of differentiation and an integrated (if smaller) embryo would proceed to normal development. Thus, after environmental insults in this first stage of embryonic development there are only scattered examples of teratogenesis (Smith, 1957), though there is some evidence that litter rates may be reduced in size or indeed pregnancy terminated by death of the conceptus.

It is possible that the mode of action of certain mutagens also makes them teratogens. Germ cell mutations could in theory result in ova or sperm which, though viable, contain a sufficiently abnormal genome to result in congenital malformation. Without going into the various ways in which nucleotide sequences are altered by mutagens, it seems probable that, at their present level of use, mutagens acting on the gonads do not significantly raise the malformation rate, though they may undoubtedly lower fecundity and possibly raise the level of embryolethality. X-irradiation acting upon the somatic cells of the embryo before the formation of the primitive streak might under certain circumstances raise the incidence of non-disjunction, and the mosaicism resulting from such somatic mutation could have an effect on the level of congenital defect (Brent, 1969). The importance of these effects in the human has not been evaluated because insufficient data are available. It is unlikely to be important.

Two further points must be considered when dealing with the subject of embryopathic effects occurring before primitive streak formation. Firstly, a drug given during the pre-primitive streak stage may set off a chain of maternal events active during the second (highly susceptible) organogenetic phase of development (see below); this is clearly a special case and does not break the general rule that agents are generally speaking not teratogenic before the primitive streak develops. Secondly, a clear distinction is often not made in text books between implantation and primitive streak formation. True, they coincide in some species, e.g. rabbit and ferret, but they do not in rat (implantation 5 days, primitive streak 8.5 days) and man (implantation 7 days, primitive streak 16 days). It is important to bear in mind therefore that the early 'refractory' period relates to primitive streak formation and *not* to uterine implantation.

The developmental period at which the embryo is most susceptible to the effect of teratogens is without doubt that of major organoegenesis. This period begins quite abruptly with the development of the primitive streak and coincides with the principal processes of induction and the mass movement of cells involved in the laying down of the main organ systems. In contrast to its fairly exact beginning (about 16 days after fertilization in the human), the organogenesis period of susceptibility to teratogens tails off gradually and is somewhat arbitrarily said to end with the closure of the palate at 57 days. Within the organogenetic period, various organs and systems have their own 'critical' periods at which they are susceptible to the action of certain teratogens, while at other times they are relatively immune. There is no unitary explanation for this phenomenon, save the obvious statement that the particular morphogenetic processes affected by the teratogenic agent in question are time-limited and that in order to affect a particular structure the teratogen must 'strike' at the appropriate time. Two corollaries arise from this concept; the first is that different organs or systems differ in the timing of their critical periods to specific teratogens. In general, those involving major structural defects of the neural tube (rachischisis etc.) occur early when the neural plate folds and sinks below the surface to form a dorsal neural tube. Deformities of the palate, limbs and urogenital system, by contrast, tend to occur following teratogenic insult somewhat later during organogenesis. The second corollary arising from the 'critical time' concept is that many organ systems have more than one critical period. This follows when it is realized that most complex structures result from the sequential interaction of a large number of developmental processes. Some of these may be more susceptible to particular environmental agents than others, with the result that (often depending upon the teratogen) more than one period of high susceptibility to disordered development occurs.

Following the organogenetic period of development (sometimes popularly equated with the 'first trimester of pregnancy'), there is often an erroneous impression that the danger period is past and that environmental factors can no longer seriously harm the conceptus. However, it is precisely in the subsequent foetal period of development that, in the social sense, the most traumatic incidents can occur. The major physical malformations produced during organogenesis frequently, though by no means always, are fatal to the embryo (e.g. anencephaly) and in such cases the tragedy of a birth deformity is not permanently with the afflicted family. Following organogenesis however, the foetus undergoes a prolonged period of histogenesis and maturation of function involving most systems but in particular the central nervous system. Disturbance at this time can lead to microcephaly, gross mental defect and serious abnormalities in function of many other systems also. Indeed, the classical work of Dobbing (1970) and others has shown that even *after* birth severe malnutrition may cause irreversible mental deficit in later life. The foetal period of development therefore is classically that in which embryopathic agents cause disturbances in function and in foetal growth. The newly developing science of 'behavioural teratology' is one which is likely to become increasingly important in the toxicological evaluation of environmental agents, and the correlation of structural alteration in the CNS with behavioural modification (Rodier, Webster & Langman, 1975) will form the central theme of the research in this field.

Before leaving the general theme of a relationship between the time at which a teratogenic insult is applied and the teratogenic effect it produces, mention should be made of the extraembryonic membranes. There is no doubt that the nature of the interchange which occurs between mother and foetus in placental mammals differs not only with the species but also with stage of development of the placental system. Early embryonic nutrition is largely histiotrophic (i.e. the breakdown of macromolecules within the cells of the extraembryonic membranes for onward transmission of the products to the embryo) while later, haemotrophic nutrition (i.e. exchange of solutes between maternal and foetal circulations) supervenes to a greater or lesser extent. It is probable that various embryopathic agents will act in ways which are determined by the nature and stage of development of the 'placenta'. Thus, histiotrophic nutrition may be inhibited by chemical agents (Williams *et al.*, 1976) or access of, say, a drug to the embryo may vary with the stage of development of the placental barrier (see Beck & Lloyd 1977 for a full discussion).

The nature of the teratogenic agent

Most teratogenic agents act in ways which are not yet understood. Even when the toxicological activity of a teratogenic substance is known at a metabolic and cellular level (and this is by no means the case for the majority of teratogens), it is still usually not possible to relate this to a developmental process leading to a specific congenital defect. Nevertheless, the *specificity* of certain teratogens is beyond doubt. Thalidomide is perhaps the best known example; its principal effect is phocomelia occurring only when the mother has ingested the drug between the 27th and 40th day of gestation, although other anomalies such as defects of the external ears, facial haemangioma and atresia of the oesophagus and duodenum are also reported. Spontaneously occurring phocomelia is extremely rare in man, and this fact taken together with the observation that, among all the experimental species tested, thalidomide-induced defects can be produced only in simian primates and some strains of rabbit makes it clear that its mode of action is highly individual. We are therefore faced with a spectrum of environmental agents with examples such as thalidomide at one extreme and others such as X-irradiation at the other. The latter is a potent cytotoxin which inhibits many parameters of cell growth and division, so that providing the foetal LD_{50} is significantly lower than the maternal LD_{50}, one would expect time-dependent teratogenic activity in most species to occur at the right dose. This turns out to be the case (Brent, 1969).

Wilson (1973) has dealt with the question of teratogen specificity by enumerating nine broad basic 'causes' of congenital defect (ranging from radiation to placental failure). These in their turn, he proposes, produce nine possible reactions (e.g. mutation, mitotic interference, enzyme inhibition, etc.) which act as mechanisms inducing a pathogenic event (e.g. cell death) resulting in embryopathy. Such an attempt at classification undoubtedly provides a point of departure for constructive analysis of particular situations and as such it is of value to our thinking in the field of embryopathy. With present knowledge of normal and deranged developmental processes, however, it must be lacking both in depth and completeness and should be regarded as a general approach rather than a definitive statement.

A number of other factors require mention when the nature of teratogenic agents is discussed. The route of administration of an agent (oral, subcutaneous, intraperitoneal, intramuscular or intravenous) will clearly affect the maternal serum level it attains and the length of time at which that level will be maintained. This will usually have some effect upon the embryopathic activity of a substance, so that apparently innocuous agents administered by one route can be very dangerous when given by another. Other considerations to be borne in mind are the way in which individual agents are handled by the mother. In some cases it is conceivable that adaptive mechanisms will minimize the effects of a substance repeatedly administered during pregnancy (the development of catabolic enzymes for example), while in others cumulative toxicity will give precisely the opposite effect. For reasons such as this, a knowledge of the normal metabolism and maternotoxicity of a drug are of utmost importance in any assessment of its teratogenic potency. Other paradoxical effects are also possible; for example some agents may be embryolethal if given before primitive streak formation and this effect, when the material is administered repeatedly throughout pregnancy, may entirely mask a teratogenic effect later on. Drug interactions must also be borne in mind; an excellent example is provided by the effect of benzoic acid (which is itself not teratogenic) in maintaining the serum levels of sodium salicylate (Kimmel, Wilson & Schumacher, 1971) and enhancing the teratogenic effects of the latter.

When considering the nature of a teratogenic agent, attention must also be paid to its access or the access of its metabolites to the conceptus. Thus, the capacity for serum protein binding of a chemical is another relevant variable in the context of its embryopathic potential. So indeed is the nature of the placental system operative at the time at which the agent is acting upon the mother, for it has already been mentioned that placental systems vary between species and at various stages in gestation in an individual pregnancy. Drug access may therefore change appreciably depending upon species or time of pregnancy.

A recurrent debate in the field of teratology is whether a threshold level exists below which environmental agents are ineffective. There is probably no straightforward answer to this deceptively simple question. Generally it is assumed that a 'below threshold' level exists when the embryotoxic dose response curve is steep rather than flat, and since this is the case with most proven teratogenic agents it is felt that such substances are ineffective below the specific dose capable of interfering with the *integrated* activity of a group of cells or tissues. For all that, there is no proof that a situation might not occasionally exist (for example the induction of somatic mutation by ionizing radiation) in which a single event can produce a teratogenic result. On balance, therefore, it seems reasonable to speak of a 'no-effect dose range' in the majority of circumstances but to bear in mind that specific exceptions are possible on theoretical grounds.

Comparative teratology

The study of comparative teratology is of practical importance both in the field of environmental monitoring and in experiments designed to elucidate the specific mechanisms of action of individual teratogens. An adverse environmental agent may in theory exert its effects at one or all of three possible sites, namely the mother, the extraembryonic membranes or directly on the embryo. In an investigation of embryopathy it is therefore necessary to look at each of these three.

The many-sided toxic effects of drugs and related compounds on the adult organism are covered in other chapters. Certain special factors are operative when dealing with the toxic effects of drugs on the pregnant animal, but interspecies metabolic differences will be the major operative factor in determining variations in the extent and nature of the embryopathies produced by an action on the mother. Where the maternal toxicity of a drug is considerable, therefore, one would direct attention to the mother as perhaps the most likely site of origin of an embryopathic action. Close investigation of the comparative toxicology of a drug between adults of various species taken in conjunction with a comparison of their respective embryopathic effects will thus constitute the primary avenue of investigation when dealing with grossly maternotoxic environmental agents.

Murphy (1959) showed a great variability in the ratio of LD_{50} between mother and foetus varying from 1:1 to 530:1 for a number of teratogenic antimetabolites. Extending this concept, one is lead to speculate that where little toxicity in the mother is associated with potent embryopathic activity the agent concerned is likely to act principally (and probably directly) upon

some component of the foetoplacental unit. In such cases it is probably
most fruitful to examine the possibility of a direct action on the embryo in
the first place. Beck (1976b) has described various model systems which
help to localize the site of action of a drug to the mother, foetus or placenta.
If, indeed, a drug is acting directly upon the embryo, it is important to bear
in mind differences in the normal embryology of various common laboratory species (Nishimura & Shiota, 1977), because these may provide a clue
to the manner of action of a teratogenic agent which produces different
malformation patterns in different species or indeed appears to be teratogenic in one species and not in another.

Considerable circumstantial evidence exists for certain drugs acting upon
materno-foetal exchange mechanisms rather than directly upon the mother
or the embryo (Williams *et al.*, 1976). Fundamental variations in the
structure and function of the extraembryonic membranes between species
may therefore account for differences in the embryopathic activity of drugs
and other agents acting on them (Beck, 1976a). This explanation has been
put forward to account for the differences in the action of trypan blue on
rats and on ferrets (Beck, 1975; Beck, Swidzinska & Gulamhusein, in the
press).

The lessons to be learnt from studies in comparative teratology are of
fundamental importance in the construction of comprehensive schemes for
the testing of drugs and other potential teratogens.

The testing of drugs and related compounds for adverse effects upon reproduction

The chief practical application of studying embryopathy produced by drugs
and related compounds is to enable the rational formulation of a series of
tests to be produced with a view to protecting the unborn child from adverse
environmental agents during gestation. These tests have been extended to
cover reproductive functions in general and to insure against certain rather
special events such as transplacental carcinogenesis (Herbst, Ulfelder &
Poskanzer, 1971). Various protocols have been produced in various
countries (see Wilson (1973) and Schardein (1976) for reviews). The position
in the United Kingdom is set out in Committee on Safety of Medicines
(1974) *Notes for guidance on reproductive studies* (MAL 36) published by
the Department of Health and Social Security. However, Brent (1972) has
listed a number of factors which should be considered in establishing test
procedures and some of these are worthy of special mention here.

Because of interspecies variation, it is desirable to study as many *diverse*
species as possible. In practical terms this probably means a rodent
(popularly the rat) and at least one non-rodent species. For reasons of
phylogenetic similarity, the rabbit does not seem a good alternative to a
rodent, and a convenient laboratory animal in this respect is the ferret
(Gulamhusein & Beck, 1977). Tuchmann-Duplessis (1977) has briefly
reviewed a variety of animal species useful for teratological drug testing,
while Wilson (1971, 1972) and Poswillo, Hamilton & Sopher (1972) have led
the way in the use of non-human primates as test animals. The latter would

undoubtedly be ideal test animals if they were cheap, easy to breed and available in large enough numbers; from a practical point of view, however, the logistic difficulties are insurmountable and monkeys can only find a place in drug testing in special circumstances — they are not and can never be candidates for the *routine* screening of drugs.

Brent (1972) also considers the route, dose and timing of drug administration in routine testing. These parameters have been mentioned earlier in this chapter, and it is largely because of the inherent variables they present, together with the multiple ways in which the course and products of gestation must be examined, that the 'multi-level' reproductive tests practised by virtually all authorities have been developed (Berry & Barlow, 1976; Schardein, 1976; Wilson, 1973).

The statistical analysis of results obtained from teratological studies is still the subject of considerable controversy (Kalter, 1974; Staples & Haseman, 1974; Becher, 1974; Haseman & Hogan, 1975). The difficulty arises because in certain instances a 'within litter' effect complicates the simple addition of 'between litter' results. Put in another way, the unit of treatment is often the mother, while the unit of assessment of results is the foetus (often part of a large litter in polycotous species). No single procedure commands universal approval, but the majority of workers now seem to favour analysis which takes into account a possible litter effect (e.g. the Mann Whitney U test, even though it is a non-parametric test).

Conclusion

This chapter has considered a selection of problems associated with teratogenesis produced by drugs and related compounds. No attempt has been made to analyse the evidence that particular drugs are teratogenic in man, since present knowledge in this area is far from complete and does not illustrate any fundamental principle. Thalidomide (Lenz, 1961; McBride, 1961), some steroids (Wilkins *et al.*, 1958), anticonvulsants (see summary by Smithells, 1976) and alcohol (Jones & Smith, 1975) have little in common and there is no point in adding to the controversy which rages — often with sparse evidence — about the effects of potentially teratogenic drugs such as LSD.

I have tried to place the problem in its biological setting, isolate and analyse some of the principal factors involved in the situation and suggest why a study of comparative teratology is of value. This has been followed by a brief reference to drug testing from which I hope the reader may conclude that *rigid* adherence to a given protocol is counterproductive. The guidelines for testing drugs which have been produced in various countries should be thought of as the basic minimum requirement for safety and the research toxicologist should be turning his mind to further refining these and to the possibilities which arise when the numerous *in vitro* techniques recently introduced to mammalian embryology are adapted for use in toxicology (see for example Kochhar (1975) and Beck (1976).

References

Beck, F. (1975). In *New Approaches to the Evaluation of Abnormal Embryonic Development*, Editors: Neubert, D. and Merker, H.-J. Stuttgart: Georg Thieme.

Beck, F. (1976a). *Envir. Hlth Perspectives*, 18, 5.

Beck, F. (1976b). *Br. med. Bull.*, 32, 53.

Beck, F. (1978). *Pharm. J.*, 220, 84.

Beck, F. and Lloyd, J.B. (1977). In *Handbook of Teratology*, Editors: Wilson, J.G. and Fraser, F.C. New York, London: Plenum Press.

Beck, F., Swidzinska, P. and Gulamhusein, A. (1978). *Teratology* (in the press).

Becker, B.A. (1974). *Teratology*, 9, 261.

Berry, C.L. and Barlow, S. (1976). *Br. med. Bull.*, 32, 34.

Brent, R.L. (1969). In *Methods for Teratological Studies in Experimental Animals and Man*, Editors: Nishimura, H. and Miller, J.R., p. 223. Tokyo: Igaku Shoin.

Brent, R.L. (1972). *J. clin. Pharmac.*, 12, 61.

Dobbing, J. (1970). *Am. J. Dis. Childh.*, 120, 411.

Dudgeon, J.A. (1976). *Br. med. Bull.*, 32, 77.

Gulamhusein, A.P. and Beck, F. (1977). In *Methods in Prenatal Toxicology*, Editors: Neubert, D., Merker, H.-J. and Bedürftig, A. Stuttgart: Georg Thieme.

Herbst, A.L., Ulfelder, H. and Poskanzer, D.C. (1971). *New Engl. J. Med.*, 284, 878.

Haseman, J.K. and Hogan, M.D. (1975). *Teratology*, 12, 165.

Jones, K.L. and Smith, D.W. (1975). *Teratology*, 12, 1.

Kalter, H. (1974). *Teratology*, 9, 257.

Kimmel, C.A., Wilson, J.G. and Schumacher, H.J. (1971). *Teratology*, 4, 15.

Kochhar, D.M. (1975). *Teratology*, 11, 273.

Lenz, W. (1961). Diskussionbemerkung, Tagung der Rhein-Westfal. Kinderartztvereinigung, Düsseldorf.

McBride, W.G. (1961). *Lancet*, 2, 1358.

McLaren, A. and Michie, D. (1958). *J. Embryol. exp. Morphol.*, 6, 645.

Murphy, M.L. (1959). *Pediatrics*, 23, 231.

Nishimura, H. and Shiota, K. (1977). In *Handbook of Teratology*, Vol. 3, Editors: Wilson, J.G. and Fraser, F.C. New York and London: Plenum Press.

Poswillo, D.E., Hamilton, W.J. and Sopher, D. (1972). *Nature*, 239, 460.

Rodier, P.M., Webster, W. and Langman, J. (1975). In *Aberrant Development in Infancy: Human and Animal Studies*, Editor: Ellis, N.R. Hilsdale, New Jersey: Lawrence Erlbaum.

Schardein, J.L. (1976). *Drugs as Teratogens*. Cleveland, Ohio: C.R.C. Press Inc.

Smith, A.V. (1957). *J. Embryol. exp. Morphol.*, 5, 311.

Smithells, R.W. (1976). *Br. med. Bull.*, 32, 27.

Staples, R.E. and Haseman, J.K. (1974). *Teratology*, 9, 259.

Tuchmann-Duplessis, H. (1977). In *Methods in Prenatal Toxicology*. Editors: Neubert, D., Merker, H.-J. and Bedürftig, A. Stuttgart: Georg Thieme.

Verrusio, A.C., Pollard, D.R. and Fraser, F.C. (1968). *Science*, 160, 206.

Wilkins, L., Jones, H.W., Holman, G.H. and Stenpfel, R.S. (1958). *J. clin. Endocrin.*, 18, 559.

Williams, K.E., Roberts, G., Kidston, M.E., Beck, F. and Lloyd, J.B. (1976). *Teratology*, 14, 343.

Wilson, J.G. (1971). *Fedn Proc.*, 30, 104.

Wilson, J.G. (1972). In *Medical Primatology: Selected Papers*, Editors: Goldsmith, E.I. and Moor-Jankowski, J.K. Basel: Karger.

Wilson, J.G. (1973). *Environment and Birth Defects*. New York and London: Academic Press.

11. Unwanted dermatological responses during drug therapy

Robin H. Felix

Introduction

The dermatologist is constantly having to decide whether a patient's rash is due to a naturally occurring disease or is drug-induced, and the lack of reliable laboratory investigations to confirm that a drug is the culprit puts great emphasis on a thorough history and examination of the patient. With few exceptions it is not possible to make a confident diagnosis of a drug rash based entirely on the morphological appearance; the observation that one particular drug can produce different clinical patterns of rash emphasizes the variability of response on the skin by a drug. However, cessation of the offending drug usually leads to a prompt clearance of the rash which is not only a relief to the patient but useful confirmatory evidence to the doctor.

In addition to systemically administered drugs, the dermatologist has to be aware of the hazards encountered with countless topical preparations, the most important group being the topical steroids which have revolutionized dermatological therapy, since the advent of topical hydrocortisone over 25 years ago. Its introduction has been followed by the more potent topical steroids (alone or in combination with a topical antibiotic) which have produced their own hazards, so that knowledge of their relative potencies is essential if side effects due to continued use are to be avoided. Adverse drug reactions can be classified according to the type of mechanism which is thought to be responsible, e.g. overdose, tolerance, side effects, secondary effects, idiosyncrasy, and hypersensitivity (Rosenheim & Moulton, 1958), but in many drug reactions involving the skin the underlying mechanism is in doubt. An alternative classification (Rawlins & Thompson, 1977) which is simpler and more practical has been suggested; it divides drug reactions into two types, A and B (Table 11.1). A drug producing a type A reaction is usually an exaggerated response of a normal pharmacological action, is predictable and dose-dependent; the incidence and morbidity is high in the community whilst the mortality is low. In contrast, a drug producing a type B reaction is an atypical response, unpredictable, where the incidence and morbidity is low in the community and the mortality is high.

To understand how drugs can affect the skin, some knowledge about its anatomy is helpful. The skin is between 3 and 5 mm in thickness and is

Table 11.1.   Adverse drug reactions.

Type A		Type B	
1. Exaggerated	normal pharma-cological action	1. Atypical	
2. Predictable		2. Unpredictable	
3. Dose-dependent		3. Incidence	low in the community
4. Incidence	high in the community	4. Morbidity	
5. Morbidity		5. Mortality	high in the community
6. Mortality	low in the community		

From Rawlins & Thompson (1977).

divided into three layers (Figure 11.1); the epidermis consisting of stratified squamous epithelium, the dermis, and underneath it the subcutaneous fatty tissue layer. Cells from the basal layer (1) of the epidermis constantly divide, migrate through the epidermis to produce a protective acellular material, keratin, in the horny layer (5), which is also being constantly shed (in normal skin it takes about 28 days for cells from the basal cell layer to reach the horny layer). The dermis consists of connective tissue with a

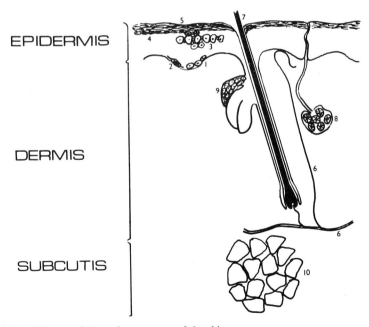

EPIDERMIS

DERMIS

SUBCUTIS

Fig. 11.1.   Digram of the main structures of the skin.
    1. Basal cell layer. 2. Melanocyte cell. 3. Prickle cell layer. 4. Granular cell layer. 5. Horny layer. 6. Blood vessel. 7. Hair follicle and shaft. 8. Sweat gland. 9. Sebaceous gland. 10. Fat cells.

network of nerve fibres and cells, blood vessels (6) and the skin appendages made up of hair follicles (7), sweat (8) and sebaceous glands (9).

The skin has many functions and among them is the ability of the horny layer to prevent the penetration of topically applied compounds. This barrier function varies according to the thickness of the horny layer; penetration of a drug across the thick palmar skin is likely to be much less than penetration across facial skin, where the horny layer is much thinner. This explains why contact dermatitis is much commoner on the face. Barrier function is also affected by hydration, dehydration and by the action of detergents and lipid solvents. In many skin diseases, the horny layer is abnormal, where barrier function is impaired allowing topical drugs to penetrate the skin more rapidly.

In general the adverse effects of topical drugs act on the epidermis producing a contact dermatitis, in which the drug behaves either as a primary irritant (type A reaction), or as an allergen (type B reaction) where an immunological mechanism is responsible. Systemically administered drugs may act either on the epidermis or against the dermis, but in some cases it is not possible to make this arbitrary distinction.

Topical steroids

The topical steroids, by their anti-inflammatory and anti-mitotic actions, are the most important class of topical drugs and since the discovery of the original active glucocorticosteroid, hydrocortisone, the natural glucocorticosteroid of the adrenal cortex, more potent steroids have been discovered. In 1960 triamcinolone acetonide, the first of the fluorinated steroids, was found to be ten times more potent than hydrocortisone. Since 1960 more have been added to the list that are available to the clinician and this has meant an increased frequency of adverse effects. The efficacy and safety of a topical steroid is dependent upon a number of factors, including whether it is in an ointment or cream base, used under polythene occlusion and the duration and amount of steroid that is applied to the skin. Certain parts of the body, particularly flexural sites such as groins or under the breasts and on the face are sites more likely to show adverse effects.

The efficacy of a steroid following continued application can be assessed by three types of test: (1) its ability to produce blanching of the skin under occlusion (vasoconstrictor test) (Mackenzie & Stoughton, 1962), and Barry & Woodford (1974, 1975) have made vasoconstrictor assays on 31 corticosteroids in ointment and cream bases; (2) fibroblast inhibition, and (3) inflammatory suppression. The last effect is used by the clinician to assess the progress of an inflammatory dermatosis, e.g. eczema, and is the method of assessment used in planning clinical trials of a new topical steroid. The relative potencies of some commonly used topical steroid preparations can be graded into four classes (Table 11.2). The complete suppression of a rash by a topical steroid in grade 1 may be achieved within a few days, in contrast to a much longer period to achieve suppression if a grade 4 steroid is used.

It has been known for over ten years that the side effects of topical steroids can either be local or systemic, but it is the local side effects which

Table 11.2. Classes of topical steroid preparations.

Active constituent	Commercial preparation
Grade 1 (very strong)	
Clobetasol propionate 0.5%	Dermovate
Fluocinolone acetonide 0.2%	Synalar Forte
Grade 2 (strong)	
Halcinonide 0.1%	Halciderm
Betamethasone valerate 0.1%	Betnovate
Fluocinolone acetonide 0.025%	Synalar
Fluocinonide 0.05%	Metosyn
Beclomethasone dipropionate 0.025%	Propaderm
Triamcinolone acetonide 0.1%	Adcortyl
Grade 3 (intermediate)	
Hydrocortisone butyrate 0.1%	Locoid
Clobetasone butyrate 0.05%	Molivate (now called Eumovate)
Betamethasone valerate 0.05%	Betnovate 50%
Grade 4 (weak)	
Hydrocortisone 1%	Efcortelan
Hydrocortisone 0.5%	

are most commonly seen today by the dermatologist in the clinic, which can be divided into five types: (1) atrophy, (2) super-infection, (3) habituation, (4) absorption and (5) contact sensitization.

Atrophy

The more potent topical steroids can produce atrophy or thinning of the dermis manifest clinically by the appearance of striae (Figure 11.2) and telangiectasia, in which the dermal vessels appear to be more prominent, features which are permanent. Striae are more commonly seen at flexural sites whereas the more gross changes of telangiectasia may develop on any area of skin which has had repeated application of a potent steroid, particularly the face. Potent steroids should not be applied for long periods under polythene occlusion or on wet areas such as the nappy area, as complete atrophy can occur. Old patients who already have an atrophic skin may notice an increased tendency to bruise more easily, particularly on the fore-arms or on the legs and repeated minor trauma may easily lead to the development of an ulcer.

Experimentally it is possible to produce epidermal atrophy (Wilson Jones, 1976) after one month's application of a potent steroid and using a radiological technique (Marks, 1976) dermal atrophy can be induced after short periods of steroid application. In this study, once the steroid was stopped, the dermal atrophy disappeared within a period of 2 months.

Super-infection

Super-infection may occur especially under occlusion, the commonest infections being either pyococcal, e.g. *Staphylococcus aureus* or due to fungi,

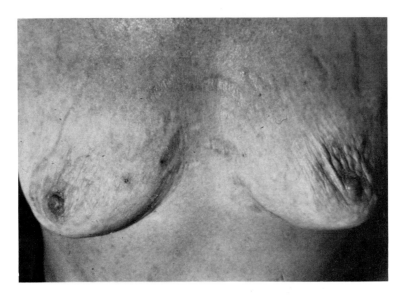

Fig. 11.2.   Presence of striae on the breasts following continued topical steroid therapy.

especially *Candida albicans*, and also the dermatophytes (ringworm species), viruses and parasites. The term tinea incognito is given (Ive & Marks, 1968) when tinea infection is masked by the application of a topical steroid resulting in a suppression of the inflammatory response, so that slight erythema and minimal scaling are the only physical signs, whilst the fungus thrives in the horny layer of the epidermis and may invade the hair follicles. Another example is unsuspected scabies infestation presenting as an eczematous eruption where the inadvertent use of a topical steroid results in a more generalized eruption.

Habituation

If a potent steroid is used continuously for long periods in patients with chronic dermatitis, it is common to observe that the steroid appears to become less effective, so that in the end it is stopped, only to be followed by the phenomenon of rebound pustulation. This observation is more liable to occur on the face (leading to rosacea and peri-oral dermatitis) and can be very troublesome in psoriasis where the development of pustular psoriasis may follow, with the risk of generalized involvement of the skin recognized as a severe form of this disease necessitating immediate admission to hospital.

Absorption

One of the more serious side effects encountered is systemic absorption which may lead to the development of Cushing's syndrome and hypothalamic-pituitary-adrenal (HPA) axis suppression by a negative feed-back mechanism. If one of the steroids in Grade 1 has been used extensively on the skin and is then stopped, adrenocortical insufficiency leading to collapse of the patient may occur, and in children can be life-threatening. Less dramatic side effects include growth retardation, steroid acne, striae, skin atrophy and purpura. Studies on the systemic effects of clobetesol propionate on normal volunteers (Carruthers, August & Staughton, 1975) showed that the HPA axis was suppressed when between 45 and 90 g was applied weekly. It was recommended that long-term administration should be restricted to less than 50 g weekly. Special care should be taken in patients with liver disease, who are at greater risk of developing side effects. An additional hazard is that topical steroids may enhance the absorption of potentially toxic compounds, e.g hexachlorophane.

Steroid rosacea and peri-oral dermatitis

Rosacea is a naturally occurring facial dermatosis most commonly seen around middle age, presenting with telangiectasia, erythema, papules and pustules. With the advent of the potent steroids it became clear that a similar picture was being produced (Sneddon, 1969), but including the more serious sign of atrophy, in patients who were applying a potent steroid to the face for long periods of time, in some cases for a number of years. Occasionally the facial skin changes can be more dramatic due to gross atrophy (Figure 11.3), the probable explanation being that the penetration of topical steroids in the head region is greater than in any other body area (Baker & Kligman, 1967). When the steroid is stopped, a rebound flare-up occurs and the patient naturally returns to using the topical steroid again. Peri-oral dermatitis is also provoked by the potent steroids (Sneddon, 1972) and is considered to be a different entity. The usual story is that the patient has borrowed a friend's steroid cream or ointment and used it on the face for a trivial complaint. Over the following months, a discrete erythematous maculo-papular rash develops at the site of application, usually around the mouth or close to the naso-labial folds (Figure 11.4). This condition is mainly seen in women and a high proportion of them are found to be taking the contraceptive pill. The role of the pill in this condition is not clear, but it may be the pill that actually provokes this eruption.

The lesson to be learnt from the recognition of these two conditions is that potent steroids should not, with few exceptions, be used on the face. It is important that the general practitioner should warn his patients about casual application.

Contact allergy

It is often overlooked that the worsening of a patient's eczema is due to a contact allergic dermatitis caused by the steroid itself rather than some ingredient in the base. In a prospective study (Alani & Alani, 1972) 6 out of 1830 patients tested were found to be allergic to hydrocortisone and one

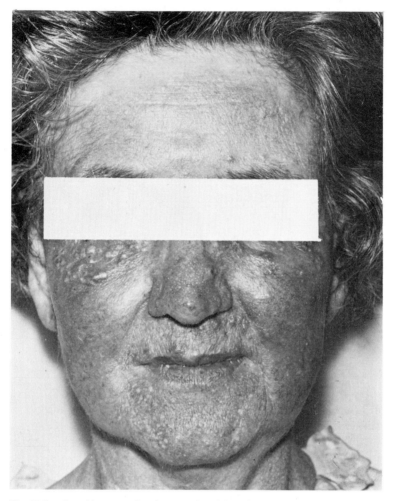

Fig. 11.3.   Steroid rosacea showing atrophy of the skin with pustules on the cheeks.

patient (Calnan, 1976) was found to be allergic following patch testing to more than one topical steroid.

Antibiotics, antifungal agents and antiseptics combined with topical steroids

Ointment and creams containing a topical antibiotic (Table 11.3) either alone or in combination with a topical steroid are commonly prescribed today to treat infected dermatoses, although both the dermatologist and bacteriologist recognize that there are dangers in using these agents, especially on a long-term basis. A drug which sensitizes the skin following topical application may produce a contact dermatitis (type B reaction) at the

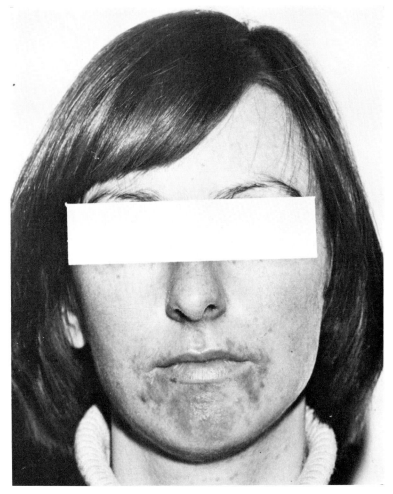

Fig. 11.4.   Peri-oral dermatitis.

site of application, and also on areas of skin, especially the face, which have
not been in contact with the sensitizing agent. If, later on, the same drug or
analogue is subsequently given by the systemic route, there is a high risk of
producing a generalized rash. Topical sensitization will therefore preclude
the use of the same drug given systemically. The aminoglycoside antibiotic
neomycin which cross-reacts with framycetin, kanamycin and gentamicin is
a well known sensitizer, particularly in eczematous conditions, and used for
chronic leg ulcers. In contrast, tetracycline is a poor topical sensitizer.

The other danger of a topical antibiotic is the emergence of resistant
strains of organisms, and the widespread use of gentamicin in a number of
centres has resulted in the isolation of gentamicin-resistant strains of
Staphylococcus aureus of epidemic proportions (Wyatt, 1977), and

Table 11.3.   Some steroid-antibiotic preparations.

Betnovate N	(Betamethasone 0.1% + neomycin 0.5%)
Betnovate A	(Betamethasone 0.1% + chlortetracycline 3%)
Synalar N	(Fluocinolone acetonide 0.025% + neomycin 0.5%)
Genticin-HC	(Gentamicin 0.3% + hydrocortisone acetate 1%)
Propaderm-A	(Beclomethasone dipropionate 0.025% + chlortetracycline 3%)
Terra-Cortril	(Oxytetracycline 3% + hydrocortisone 1%)
Aureocort	(Triamcinolone acetonide 0.1% + chlortetracycline 3%)
Fucidin H	(Sodium fusidate 2% + hydrocortisone 1%)
Tri-Adcortyl	(Triamcinolone acetonide 0.1% + nystatin + neomycin 0.25% + gramicidin 0.25%)

gentamicin-resistant strains of *Pseudomonas aeruginosa* (Chattopadhyay, 1975). Staphylococci resistant to neomycin and sodium fusidate quickly emerged after the topical use of these antibiotics in a series of infants with eczema who were followed up for twelve months (Smith, Alder & Warin, 1975). The subject of steroid antibiotic combinations has been critically reviewed by Leyden & Kligman (1977), who conclude that the risk of neomycin sensitivity is small provided that neomycin is used for short-term application, and is appropriate for use in children.

There are a number of topical antifungal agents available, including nystatin and amphotericin B, which act against the *Candida* species and the more recent imidazole derivatives, miconazole (Daktarin, Dermonistat) and clotrimazole (Canesten), which are effective against the *Candida* species and the dermatophytes. These drugs appear to be free of the hazards experienced by the aminoglycosides.

A topical antiseptic as either a cream or ointment is a useful alternative to a topical antibiotic, particularly in minor skin infections. Of the antiseptics, clioquinol (iodohydroxyquinolone, Vioform) is the ingredient of a number of topical steroid preparations (Table 11.4), but like the topical antibiotics it has the reputation of provoking a contact dermatitis.

Table 11.4.   Topical steroids + clioquinol.

Vioform-HC	(Clioquinol 3% + hydrocortisone 1%)
Betnovate-C	(Betamethasone 0.1% + clioquinol 3%)
Synalar-C	(Fluocinolone acetonide 0.025% + clioquinol)
Nystaform HC	(Nystatin, clioquinol 3% + hydrocortisone 1%)
Propaderm-C	(Beclomethasone dipropionate 0.025% + clioquinol 3%)

Topical antihistamines and anaesthetic agents

Itch, also referred to as pruritus, a cardinal symptom of many dermatoses, is extremely variable in its severity and attempts at relief can be achieved with drugs either applied topically or given systemically. The antihistamines and phenothiazines are a class of drugs which are effective anti-pruritic agents, but unfortunately they readily sensitize the skin following topical use, leading to the development of an acute contact allergic dermatitis (Figure 11.5). The eruption will be made worse if the same drug or analogue is given systemically and as the patient will be complaining of much

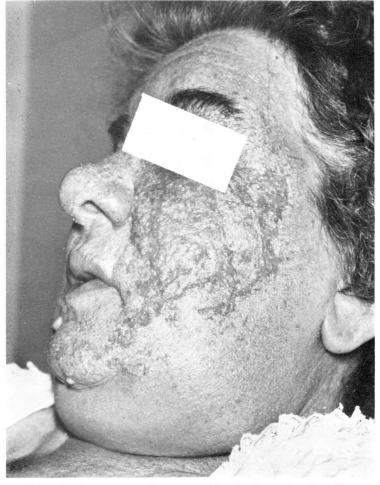

Fig. 11.5.   Acute contact allergic dermatitis following sensitization with a
topical antihistamine.

discomfort, including pruritus, the addition of the drug systemically will
merely aggravate the symptoms rather than relieve them. Although derma-
tologists no longer use these drugs topically, they are still widely bought
over the counter, the usual need being for insect bites. Equally topical
anaesthetic agents, derivatives of *p*-aminobenzoic acid, such as benzocaine,
amethocaine, procaine and dibucaine are strong sensitizers and are prescribed for a variety of conditions where pruritus is a prominent symptom.

Vehicles — bases

It is sometimes overlooked that the cause of either a contact irritant or
allergic dermatitis may be due to the cream or ointment base rather than

the active agent, so that knowledge of the individual constituents is essential for elucidating the cause. Individual constituents may be added as preservatives to the base; chlorocresol is found in 1% hydrocortisone cream B.P.C. as a preservative and might explain why some patients experience stinging or discomfort immediately after application.

Parabens (*p*-hydroxybenzoate esters), another preservative in many creams, is a known sensitizer as well as lanolin (wool alcohols), which is used as the ointment base in a number of steroid preparations as well as numerous cosmetic agents. Confirmation of suspected parabens and lanolin sensitivity can be achieved by appropriate patch tests (*vide* patch testing). Examples of creams containing parabens are Adcortyl cream, Adcortyl lotion, Betnovate lotion, Cidomycin cream, Genticin cream and Genticin ointment. Examples containing lanolin are Aureomycin ointment, calamine lotion oily B.P.C., 1% hydrocortisone ointment, E.45 cream, Golden Eye ointment, Hewlett's antiseptic cream, Germolene and Nivea cream.

Exposure to ethylenediamine, an antihistamine, may occur in the industrial preparation of dyes, fungicides, insecticides and is a potent sensitizer. One group particularly at risk from exposure are pharmacists and nurses who handle aminophylline suppositories (theophylline and ethylenediamine). White, Douglas & Main (1978), who investigated 159 consecutive patients with a clinical diagnosis of contact dermatitis, found 20 patients to be allergic to ethylenediamine and all had previously used Tri-Adcortyl cream (Tri-Adcortyl ointment does not contain ethylenediamine). Ethylene diamine is a constituent of aminophylline suppositories, Mycelog cream (USA) and Tri-Adcortyl cream, as well as being the parent substance of certain antihistamines such as Phenergan cream.

Drugs by the systemic route

While it must be admitted that the mechanism for adverse reactions in this group is ill-understood, the majority can be classed as a type B reaction, and in general are more severe than type A reactions. Prompt admission of the patient to hospital as a dermatological emergency may be indicated in a minority of cases, where the whole skin is involved, e.g. exfoliative dermatitis. Skin rashes account for most of the reactions, but the skin appendages, including hair and nails, may be affected either alone or in combination with a rash. It is convenient to discuss the variety of drug reactions in this group according to the type of reaction produced, since certain groups of drugs are more likely to produce particular types of rashes, e.g. the thiazide diuretics in light sensitive dermatoses.

Exanthematous

This is probably the commonest group encountered with different clinical features in which the cause may be other than drug such as the childhood infectious diseases.

Toxic erythema. This eruption is typically erythematous, and often measles-like, it develops on one part of the body, later becoming generalized, and is extremely itchy. This type of reaction is seen with the penicillin group, but there must be many patients labelled as being 'allergic to penicillin' where the evidence is extremely tenuous. Ampicillin is known to produce a similar kind of rash in almost all patients with glandular fever, but once the patient has recovered, re-exposure to ampicillin no longer produces a rash. The risk of an ampicillin rash is also high in patients with lymphatic leukaemia (Cameron & Richmond, 1971).

Erythema multiforme. This eruption presents as circular, red raised lesion, which are most prominent on the limbs. In more severe cases, blisters may develop within the lesions associated with mucosal involvement, where the patient can be extremely ill, and before the use of systemic steroids, this disease carried a 10% mortality.

Drugs that can produce erythema multiforme are barbiturates, phenylbutazone and the long-acting sulphonamides; also drugs chemically related to the sulphonamides, chlorpropamide, thiazide diuretics and the sulphones. The hydantoins (phenytoin) and succinimide group can produce severe bullous erythema multiforme (Levantine & Almeyda, 1972) in addition to aspirin, codeine, tetracyclines, and penicillin.

Vasculitis. This refers to an acute inflammatory reaction involving the walls of the blood vessels within the dermis, and there are different types depending upon the size of the blood vessels involved. In one variety known as an allergic vasculitis, lesions start as discrete circular erythematous spots which later may become vesicular and pustular through necrosis (Figure 11.6). The site of involvement is the small upper dermal blood vessels. Implicating a drug is often circumstantial since there are other causes including infections, but the evidence is strongly in favour of an immunological mechanism in which circulating immunoglobulins can be identified by immunofluorescent techniques in and around capillaries in the upper dermis. The author has seen three patients with an allergic vasculitis which developed soon after frusemide was started and cleared once this diuretic was stopped. Three patients developed a severe form of vasculitis while taking alcofenac (Billings *et al.*, 1974), and more recently an identical picture has been reported in two patients who were being treated with the immuno-stimulant drug levamisole. In both patients, the eruption promptly cleared once the drug had been stopped (MacFarlane & Bacon, 1978; Scheinberg *et al.*, 1978). Inflammation of the medium-sized arteries produces a slightly different clinical picture in which small dermal or subcutaneous nodules occur along the course of a superficial artery. This form of vasculitis is referred to as cutaneous polyarteritis nodosa — a rare disease — and numerous drugs have been incriminated including the sulphonamides, iodides, penicillin, chloramphenicol and streptomycin.

Drug-induced lupus erythematosus. The naturally occurring disease systemic lupus erythematosus (S.L.E.) is a multi-system disorder which can be fatal and is controlled by the use of systemic steroids with immunosuppressive agents. The skin signs consist of dusky red plaques which are most prominent on light-exposed areas on the face, neck and dorsa of the hands. Certain laboratory investigations help to confirm the diagnosis, in particular the presence of L.E. cells which are white cells of the

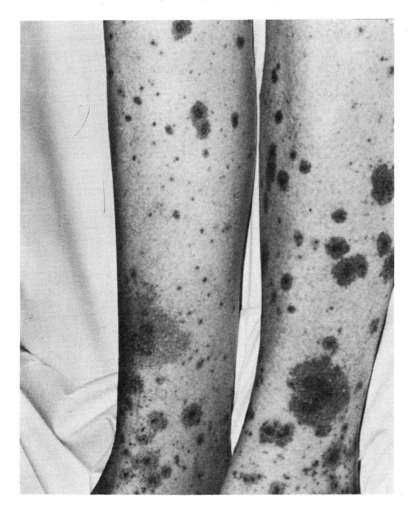

Fig. 11.6. Allergic vasculitis involving the legs.

polymorphonuclear series with ingested white cell nuclei producing a characteristic appearance. In addition circulating antibodies against cell nuclei are found and the presence of anti-DNA antibodies is specific and indicates activity of this disease. Drugs also can produce an almost identical disease with an identical rash and over 27 drugs have been reported (Harpey, 1973), the most important being procainamide, hydrallazine, isoniazid and phenytoin. More recently practolol has been shown to produce the lupus syndrome (Raftery & Denman, 1973). The prognosis in the drug-induced lupus syndrome is more benign compared with the naturally occurring disease but it may take several months for the patient to make a full recovery. The absence of anti-DNA antibodies is confirmatory evidence in support of the drug-induced disease.

Toxic epidermal necrolysis. This condition aptly described as the 'scalded skin syndrome' is a rare and sometimes lethal disease, in which part or whole of the epidermis separates from the underlying skin, leaving red weeping areas which look typically like a burn (Figure 11.7). It can occur in infants where it is caused by a staphylococcal infection, but it is seen in adults where drugs are more likely to be the cause and where the mortality is higher. In one series (Lyell, 1967) of drug-induced cases, the mortality was over 20%.

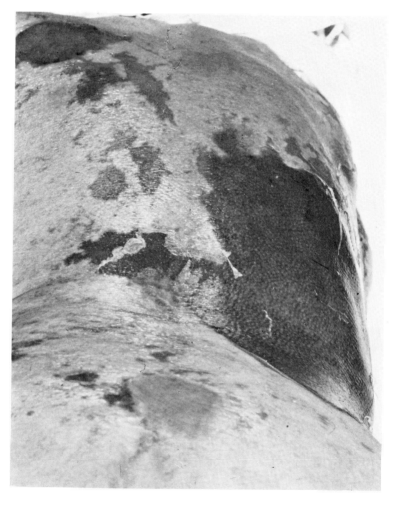

Fig. 11.7.   Toxic epidermal necrolysis of the back showing denuded areas of skin.

Fixed drug eruption. The usual story in this curious eruption is the development of a circular, red, raised lesion which may ultimately develop a blister (Figure 11.8) usually affecting the limbs. After the first episode, the

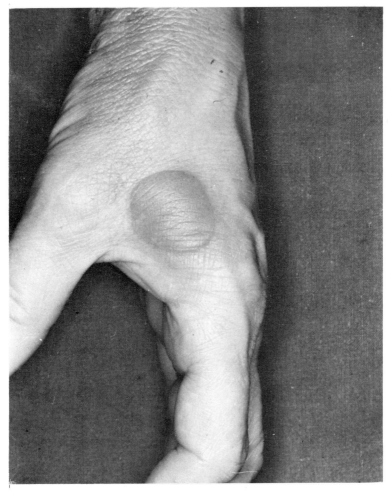

Fig. 11.8.   Fixed drug eruption — early phase with blister formation.
By courtesy of Dr. A. Levantine.

lesion resolves after a few days leaving some scaling and a brown stain due
to melanin pigmentation. At a later date, the same site erupts again and may
be associated with other lesions developing on the skin and including the
mucous membranes, the mouth or the genital region. If the patient is seen at
a time when the physical signs have settled down, there may be some
difficulty in making the diagnosis, but the clinician should be alerted to this
diagnosis, where the history highlights a fixed site. Fixed drug eruptions can
be caused by barbiturates, quinine, tetracyclines and sulphonamides, and
one of the commonest offenders is phenolphthalein, an ingredient in a
number of laxatives. A thorough history is essential and once the suspected
drug has been identified, the patient can be challenged with the drug orally.
Reappearance of the eruption within a few hours of ingestion confirms the

diagnosis. It is difficult to explain why certain areas of skin should repeatedly be involved, although injection of the patient's serum intradermally into a previously involved area of skin produces an inflammatory response (Wyatt, Greaves & Sondergaard, 1972), evidence in favour of a blood-borne mediator.

Purpura

This refers to the leakage of red cells into the skin, which may be due to a blood disorder, but in dermatological practice, the probable cause is damage to the blood vessel wall. Among the drugs that can cause purpura are gold, chlorothiazide, oestrogens, mercurials, antimetabolites, oxytetracycline, salicylates, quinidine, streptomycin, sulphonamides, tolbutamide and troxidone (Wintrobe, 1967; Whitby & Britton, 1969). Carbromal, also found in Carbrital, a hypnotic, can produce a very distinct purpuric eruption on the extremities which fades once the drug is discontinued.

Lichen planus-like, lichenoid

Lichen planus, a disease of unknown aetiology, is characterized by the appearance of discrete flat-topped papules typically on the wrist, back and legs. Certain drugs can produce a similar and in some cases identical eruption. Of the modern drugs, the phenothiazines (Groth, 1961), thiazide diuretics (Harber, Lashinsky & Baey, 1959) and methyldopa (Stevenson, 1971; Almeyda & Levantine, 1973; Holt & Navaratnam, 1974) are occasionally responsible.

Eczematous eruptions and exfoliative dermatitis

Eczematous rashes from systemically administered drugs are uncommon unless the patient has previously been sensitized following topical application. If the drug is not stopped in time, there is a risk of a generalized eruption with redness and scaling developing, referred to as exfoliative dermatitis (erythroderma) which will necessitate hospital treatment.

While exfoliative dermatitis can complicate such conditions as eczema and psoriasis, the importance of suspecting a drug is underlined by the observation that the rash will clear swiftly once the drug has been stopped. The one exception is gold, the likely explanation being the very slow clearance of gold from the body. Other drugs responsible for producing exfoliative dermatitis are organic arsenicals, phenylbutazone, streptomycin, sulphonamides, sulphonylureas and practolol.

Church (1973) has described a number of patients with a seborrhoeic-like eczema, who were taking methyldopa, which cleared once methyldopa was stopped.

Blistering eruptions (vesicular or bullous)

These eruptions may be seen in the more severe forms of other cutaneous reaction, e.g. erythema multiforme or fixed drug eruption. The blister develops following splitting between the epidermis and dermis and may be haemorrhagic. Drugs commonly involved are the barbiturates, typically seen in patients who have taken an overdose (Beveridge & Lawson, 1965). A severe haemorrhagic bullous eruption is rarely seen with the coumarin group of anticoagulant drugs (Nalbandian *et al.*, 1965).

Urticaria

The presence of large itchy weals, like a nettle rash, which may last for a few hours to be followed by fresh lesions is called urticaria; it is produced by the release of certain blood-borne mediators, including histamine, resulting in swelling within the dermis. Drugs may be involved in the acute variety but are seldom responsible in chronic urticaria, which can persist for many months. Penicillin, codeine, salicylates, indomethacin are common offenders, although it is known that these drugs can release histamine into the skin by a direct pharmacological effect (type A reaction), so that patients with chronic urticaria should avoid these drugs. Unfortunately tartrazine and other azo-dyes, used to colour some drug tablets and many foods, are known to enhance the urticarial reaction.

Light-sensitive reactions

Sunlight, especially its ultra-violet component, is responsible for provoking light-sensitive eruptions and can provoke rashes on exposed areas of skin in combination with a number of drugs. The time relationship between exposure to ultra-violet light and the onset of the rash may vary depending upon whether the reaction is a photo-toxic eruption (type A reaction), or a photo-allergic eruption (type B reaction) in which an immunological mechanism is involved. With a photo-toxic eruption, the rash, similar to a sun-burn, may appear within a few hours, in contrast with a photo-allergic eruption, where there is a delayed onset. The morphology of the rash may vary between an eczematous, lichenoid or bullous eruption.

The most common group of drugs known to be photo-sensitizers are the tetracycline antibiotics, particularly demethylchlortetracycline, phenothiazines, antihistamines, thiazide diuretics and sulphonylureas. The oestrogen component of the contraceptive pill is also a photo-sensitizer (Erickson & Peterka, 1968), and can precipitate the development of blisters on light-exposed skin in patients suffering from a metabolic blood disease called porphyria. Nalidixic acid can cause a photo-toxic bullous eruption (Birkett, Garretts & Stevenson, 1969).

A rare photo-sensitive reaction of demethylchlortetracycline (Bethell, 1977) is the development of onycholysis which refers to the separation of the nail from the nail bed. Although this phenomenon has been recognized for a number of years in countries where there is more sunlight, this is the first report in the UK, and arose during the hot summer of 1976.

Disorders of pigmentation

The pigment melanin produced by the melanocyte cell (Figure 11.1) is responsible for the pigmenting effect of the skin, and many disorders of pigmentation, either increased or decreased, can be produced by drugs, but the mechanism in many cases is uncertain. A distinct patchy hyperpigmentation, known as chloasma, is quite often seen in women taking the contraceptive pill and the pigmentation is accentuated by exposure to sunlight. Other drugs producing hyperpigmentation are the phenothiazines, phenytoin, chloroquin, mepacrin, cytotoxic drugs (Figure 11.9), corticotrophin and oxprenolol (Harrower & Strong, 1977). Leukoderma — decreased areas of pigmentation — is rare and can be produced by hydrochlorothiazide.

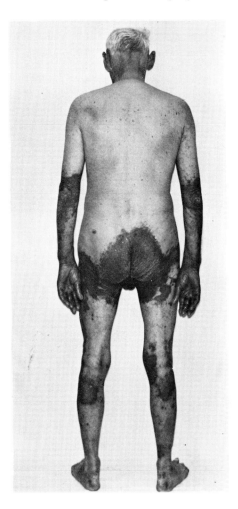

Fig. 11.9.   Hyper-pigmentation occurring in patches following cytotoxic therapy.

Acne-like eruptions

Acne is a common complaint of adolescence in which there is an increased sebum production, but in an atypical case the role of a drug should be suspected. The corticosteroids, corticotrophin, barbiturates and the anticonvulsant drugs, hydantoins and troxidone are acnegenic. Isoniazid treatment can produce an acne-like eruption (Cohen, George & Smith, 1974) with pellagra (deficiency of nicotinic acid-niacin) and in one patient topical niacinamide 1% in cetomacragol cream produced an improvement in the skin (Comaish, Felix & McGrath, 1976). Acneiform lesions have also been reported in African patients treated with rifampicin (Nwokolo, 1974).

Itch (pruritus)

Many drugs can produce irritation of the skin without any signs, and it is often the first confirmatory piece of evidence in support of a drug eruption following oral challenge.

Disorders of hairgrowth

Some loss of hair may develop after the contraceptive pill is stopped, but a toxic effect on the dividing cells of the hair follicle resulting in alopecia is observed with the cytotoxic drugs, heparin and coumarin group of drugs. Increased hair growth — hypertrichosis — can occur with diazoxide (Burton *et al.*, 1975) and phenytoin, glucocorticosteroids and psoralens.

Super-infection

Systemic steroids, like topical steroids, and immunosuppressive agents predispose to skin infections and even scabies infestation (Patterson, Allen & Beveridge, 1973). A course of antibiotics may be followed by the emergence of candida in the gut leading to infection around the anal margin spreading to the groins and genital sites if left untreated.

β-Adrenergic-blocking drugs

In the early 1970s, isolated reports of adverse effects seen with practolol, a very effective β-blocker, were published (Wiseman, 1971; Rowland & Stevenson, 1972; Raftery & Denman, 1973). In 1974, Felix, Ive & Dahl reported 21 patients who presented with a variety of rashes, amongst which was one with a characteristic psoriasiform (psoriasis-like) appearance (Figure 11.10). In addition patients noticed a gradual thickening and scaling of the palms and soles (Figure 11.11) which was insidious in onset, and unlike most drug eruptions, the different rashes in most patients took up to four and a half months to develop. Since then, more serious side

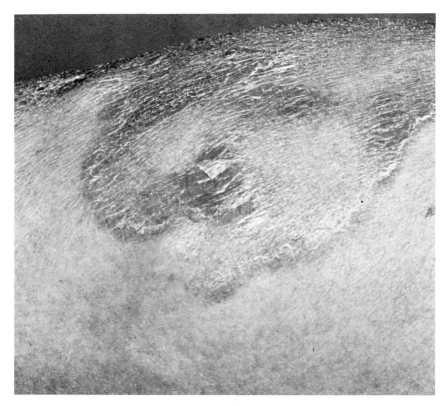

Fig. 11.10.   Practolol therapy producing psoriasiform lesion.

effects have been reported including damage to the eye, ear, gastro-
intestinal tract and lungs, culminating with the withdrawal of practolol
apart from short-term use in hospital. These side effects were thought
originally to be peculiar to practolol, but atypical rashes, some psoriasiform, have been reported with other β-blockers, oxprenolol (Holt &
Waddington, 1975) and propranolol (Aerenlund *et al.*, 1976). It is interesting that although propranolol was the first β-blocker to be introduced in
1964, it is only recently that psoriasiform rashes have been reported.

   The mechanism behind the 'practolol syndrome' remains obscure; a
likely hypothesis concerns the role of cyclic adenosine monophosphate
(cAMP) on epidermal cell turnover. High levels of cAMP depress mitotic
activity, and blockade of epidermal β-receptors may lead to reduced levels
of cAMP. This mechanism would explain why some patients with psoriasis
experienced a deterioration of their rash following practolol therapy, as it is
generally accepted that the skin in patients with psoriasis, a common skin
disease, is already low in cAMP.

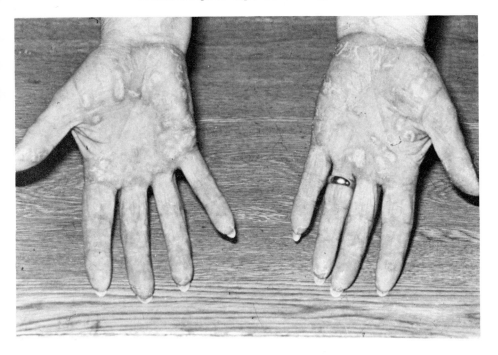

Fig. 11.11.   Hyperkeratosis of palms observed in patient taking practolol.

Penicillamine

Penicillamine (dimethylcysteine), a chelating agent used in Wilson's disease to remove copper, is increasingly being used in the treatment of rheumatoid arthritis. Exanthematous and urticarial eruptions are the usual types of rashes seen within the first ten days of treatment, but rheumatologists are familiar with a 'late eruption' which occurs after about six months' treatment; the onset is slow with few lesions appearing on the upper trunk scalp and face, but may extend to cover the whole body with the formation of small blisters, later turning into crusts (Figure 11.12). The hall-mark of this late-onset eruption is the development of blisters which appear within the epidermis, where the normal cohesion between the epidermal cells is lost, identical to a group of blistering diseases referred to as pemphigus.

The unusual feature about this pemphigus-like rash is that it takes many weeks to clear and in one series (Marsden *et al.*, 1976), the rash persisted for over twelve months after penicillamine was stopped. The cause is likely to be immunological in origin, since circulating antibodies to the epidermal cells are found, typical of the pemphigus group, and in one patient circulating antibodies to penicillamine (Sparrow, 1978) were present. Other drugs that produce a pemphigus-like rash are rifampicin and phenylbutazone.

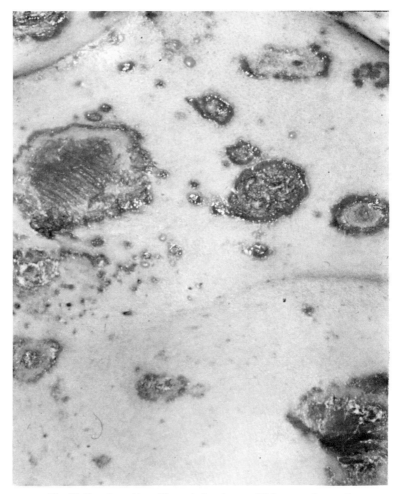

Fig. 11.12.　Pemphigus-like rash showing small blisters and crusts in
patient taking penicillamine.

Investigating adverse drug reactions

To decide whether a rash is drug-induced or due to some other cause is not
helped by the lack of reliable *in vivo* and *in vitro* tests. Oral challenge is the
simplest method of identifying the suspected drug but this method is
hazardous and can be fatal if anaphylaxis with circulatory collapse occurs.
With other types such as a fixed drug eruption, the diagnosis can with safety
easily be confirmed by oral challenge. With reactions following systemic
administration, skin testing in the form of patch, prick and intradermal
tests can be useful under certain circumstances (Felix & Comaish, 1974) and
should be performed in this sequence, since even these tests, particularly
prick and intradermal are potentially hazardous. With medicaments

applied topically and producing a contact dermatitis, the established method of investigation is patch testing.

Patch testing

The procedure is to apply the test compound or drug made up in a suitable base, e.g. soft paraffin or propylene glycol, on a piece of filter paper placed on an impermeable sheet and secured to the skin with some adhesive tape. The patch test is removed after an interval of 48-72 hours and the presence of an inflammatory response indicates a positive reaction, producing either a primary irritant effect or clinically more significant an allergic reaction, aptly described as delayed-type hypersensitivity (Figure 11.13). With the

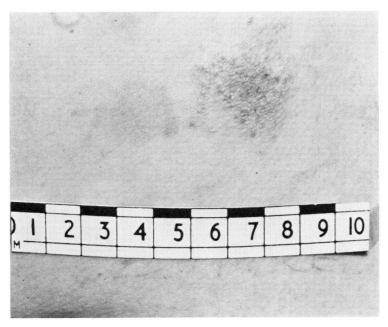

Fig. 11.13.   Patch test: allergic reaction.

introduction of a standardized battery of patch tests, the frequency of false positive or negative results is much less; where a new compound or drug is being patch tested, the result of a positive reaction is only significant provided that a negative result is obtained in a number of control subjects. Unfortunately the results of patch testing in eruptions produced by drugs given systemically is extremely variable; probably a metabolized derivative of the drug rather than the drug itself is the antigen, which would explain why the results of testing are so often negative, and why there are no established *in vitro* tests. Knowledge of the type of eruption is important; an eczematous reaction is an epidermal event and under these circumstances the drug on subsequent patch testing is more likely to produce a positive result compared with other types of reactions.

Prick and intradermal tests

These tests involve minute quantities of the drug in a soluble form being introduced into the skin, and the presence of a weal and flare after 15-20 minutes indicates a positive response, typical of immediate-type hypersensitivity. Allergy to penicillin may be confirmed by this technique in which penicilloyl-polylysine, a conjugated form of the penicilloyl group, is considered to be one of the antigenic determinants.

Presented with an unusual rash, the differential diagnosis must always include iatrogenic skin disease, and it is a sobering thought that drugs are the commonest cause of iatrogenic diseases today especially in the elderly, where drug clearance by the kidneys is impaired and where the practice of polypharmacy is commonplace. The late Richard Asher (1972), Physician and Essayist, once wrote: 'It is a wise physician who knows as much about the dangers of the drugs he uses as he does about their good effect.'

References

Aerenlund, H., Jensen, H.I., Mikkelson, S., Wadskov, S. and Sondergaard, J. (1976). *Acta med. Scand.*, 199, 363.
Alani, M.D. and Alani, S.D. (1972). *Ann. Allergy*, 30, 181.
Almeyda, J. and Levantine, A. (1973). *Br. J. Derm.*, 88, 313.
Asher, R. (1972). *Richard Asher Talking Sense,* Editor: Avery Jones, Sir Francis. London: Pitman.
Baker, H. and Kligman, A.M. (1967). *Arch. Derm.*, 96, 441.
Barry, B.W. and Woodford, R. (1974). *Br. J. Derm.*, 91, 323.
Barry, B.W. and Woodford, R. (1975). *Br. J. Derm.*, 93, 563.
Bethell, H.J.N. (1977). *Br. med. J.*, 3, 96.
Beveridge, G.W. and Lawson, A.A.H. (1965). *Br. med. J.*, 1, 835.
Billings, R.A., Burry, H.C., Emslie, F.S. and Kerr, G.D. (1974). *Br. med. J.*, 4, 263.
Birkett, D.A., Garretts, M. and Stevenson, C.J. (1969). *Br. Med. J.*, 81, 342.
Burton, J.L., Schutt, W.H. and Caldwell, I.W. (1975). *Br. J. Derm.*, 93, 707.
Calnan, C.D. (1976). *Dermatologica*, 152 (Suppl. 1), 247.
Cameron, S.J. and Richmond, J. (1971). *Scottish med. J.*, 16, 425.
Carruthers, J.A., August, P.J. and Staughton, R.C.D. (1975). *Br. med. J.*, 4, 203.
Chattopadhyay, B. (1975). *Lancet*, ii, 934.
Church, R.E. (1973). *Br. J. Derm.*, 89 (Suppl. No. 9), 10.
Cohen, L.K., George, W. and Smith, R. (1974). *Arch. Derm.*, 109, 377.
Comaish, J.S., Felix, R.H. and McGrath, H. (1976). *Arch. Derm.*, 112, 70.
Erickson, L.R. and Peterka, E.S. (1968). *J. Am. med. Ass.*, 203, 980.
Felix, R.H. and Comaish, J.S. (1974). *Lancet*, i, 1017.
Felix, R.H., Ive, F.A. and Dahl, M.G.C. (1974). *Br. med. J.*, 321.
Groth, O. (1961). *Acta derm-venereol.* (Stockholm), 41, 168.
Harber, L.C., Lashinsky, A.M. and Baey, R.L. (1959). *J. Invest. Derm.*, 33, 83.
Harpey, J.P. (1973). *Adv. Drug Reaction Bull.*, 43, 140.
Harrower, A.D.B. and Strong, J.A. (1977). *Br. med. J.*, 3, 296.
Holt, P.J.A. and Navaratnam, A. (1974). *Br. med. J.*, 3, 234.
Holt, P.J.A. and Waddington, E. (1975). *Br. med. J.*, 2, 539.
Ive, F.A. and Marks, R. (1968). *Br. med. J.*, 3, 149.
Levantine, A. and Almeyda, J. (1972). *Br. J. Derm.*, 87, 246.
Leyden, J.J. and Kligman, A.M. (1977). *Br. J. Derm.*, 96, 179.
Lyell, A. (1967). *Br. J. Derm.*, 79, 662.
MacFarlane, D.G. and Bacon, P.A. (1978). *Br. med. J.*, 1, 407.
Mackenzie, A.W. and Stoughton, R.B. (1962). *Arch. Derm.*, 86, 608.
Marks, R. (1976). *Dermatologica*, 152 (Suppl.), 117.

Marsden, R.A., Vanhegan, R.I., Walse, M., Hill, H. and Mowatt, A.G. (1976). *Br. med. J.*, 4, 1423.
Nalbandian, R.M., Mader, I.J., Barrett, J.L., Pearce, J.F. and Rupp, E.C. (1965). *J. Am. med. Ass.*, 192, 603.
Nwokolo, U. (1974). *Br. med. J.*, 3, 473.
Patterson, W.D., Allen, B.R. and Beveridge, G.W. (1973). *Br. med. J.*, 4, 211.
Raftery, E.B. and Denman, A.M. (1973). *Br. med. J.*, 2, 242.
Rawlins, M.D. and Thompson, J.W. (1977). *Textbook of Adverse Drug Reactions,* Editor: Davies, D.M. Oxford University Press.
Rosenheim, M.L. and Moulton, R. (1958). *Sensitivity Reactions to Drugs*: Symposium, Oxford.
Rowland, M.G.M. and Stevenson, C.J. (1972). *Lancet*, i, 1130.
Scheinberg, M.A., Bezerra, J.B.G., Almeida, F.A. and Silveira, L.A. (1978). *Br. med. J.*, 1, 408.
Smith, R.J., Alder, V.G. and Warin, R.P. (1975). *Br. med. J.*, 3, 199.
Sneddon, I. (1969). *Br. med. J.*, 1, 671.
Sneddon, I. (1972). *Br. J. Derm.*, 87, 430.
Sparrow, G.P., (1978). *Br. J. Derm.*, 98, 103.
Stevenson, C.J. (1971). *Br. J. Derm.*, 86, 246.
White, M.I., Douglas, W.S. and Main, R.A. (1978). *Br. med. J.*, 1, 415.
Whitby, L.G. and Britton, C.J.C. (1969). *Disorders of the Blood*, 10th edition. London: Churchill Ltd.
Wilson Jones, E. (1976). *Dermatologica*, 152 (Suppl. 1), 107.
Wintrobe, M.W. (1967). *Clinical Haematology*, 6th Edition. London: Henry Kimpton.
Wiseman, R.A. (1971). *Postgrad. med. J.* (Suppl. 2), p. 68.
Wyatt, E., Greaves, M.W.G. and Sondergaard, J. (1972). *Arch. Derm.*, 106, 671.
Wyatt, T.D. (1977). *J. Antimicrobial Chemotherapy*, 3, 1.

12. The effects of drugs and their metabolites on blood and blood-forming organs

Ronald H. Girdwood

The alert clinician is likely to be worried about the possible adverse effects of drugs on the blood and blood-forming organs. Most doctors are aware of the fact that there is a hazard of this type for some individuals when certain preparations, particularly non-narcotic analgesics, are taken, but, when any completely new product is marketed, there must be concern as to whether the drug will be yet another to add to the list of over a thousand that may have such effects. In general, there is no way of predicting this, no real knowledge of the mechanism by which it is caused, and no test to identify those who will develop this type of adverse effect as a consequence of treatment. In some instances, despite active attempts to remedy the situation, the result will be death, and in a paper based on reports to the UK Committee on Safety of Medicines (Girdwood, 1974), the commonest alleged cause of death was a thrombotic episode caused by the contraceptive pill, closely followed by blood dyscrasias after the taking of non-narcotic analgesics. However, the Register of Adverse Reactions (which is supplied to hospitals and Medical Schools by this Committee) cannot be regarded as a scientific document because of gross under-reporting of adverse reactions by doctors, together with the difficulty of deciding which drug caused a blood dyscrasia when several have been given simultaneously. In some instances the problem results from drug interactions.

A list of types of drug-induced blood disorders is given in Table 12.1.

Pancytopenia

Few patients are more distressing to see than those whose bone marrows have been ablated because of drug therapy. With certain preparations, such as those used in cancer therapy, the risk has to be taken, but, in most instances, it is a patient suffering from a non-fatal illness who is one of the unfortunate few to react in an abnormal way to treatment, and who has lost the precursors of erythrocytes, leucocytes and platelets. Before 1948, pancytopenia was commonly thought to be idiopathic unless it followed the taking of one of a few drugs, such as amidopyrine, which had been identified as causative agents, but it is likely that in many instances a full drug history had not been taken. From 1948 onwards it became obvious

Table 12.1.   Types of drug-induced blood disorder.

Pancytopenia (usually named aplastic anaemia)
Reversible erythroid suppression
Agranulocytosis or granulocytopenia
Thrombocytopenia
Haemolytic anaemia
    Immune type
    Autoimmune type
    Red cell destruction
        – in normal persons
        – in association with deficiency of glucose-6-phosphate dehydrogenase
        – in association with other enzyme deficiencies
        – in association with unstable haemoglobins
Coagulation problems
    Anticoagulants
    Plasminogen activators
    Prostaglandin inhibitors
Thrombosis
Megaloblastic anaemia
    Folate reductase inhibition
    Uncertain mechanism
    Interference with DNA synthesis
    Malabsorption of vitamin B_{12}
Sideroblastic anaemia
Leukaemia induced by drugs
Anaemia from drug-induced gastro-intestinal bleeding
Methaemoglobinaemia and sulphaemoglobinaemia
Drug-induced porphyrias

Glossary

Pancytopenia	Deficiency of red cells, white cells and platelets in the circulating blood because of marrow depression.
Aplastic anaemia	Lack of red cells from marrow depression.
Agranulocytosis	Absence of neutrophil polymorphs in peripheral blood.
Granulocytopenia	Less severe deficiency of neutrophil polymorphs in peripheral blood.
Thrombocytopenia	Deficiency of platelets in peripheral blood.
Haemolytic anaemia	Anaemia due to excessive destruction of red cells.
Megaloblastic anaemia	Anaemia with large red cells in peripheral blood and large abnormal red cell precursors in the bone marrow. Caused by deficiency of folic acid or of vitamin B_{12}.
Sideroblastic anaemia	Anaemia with abnormal red cell precursors containing a perinuclear ring of iron-staining granules in their cytoplasm. These are in the marrow.

that the symptoms appeared in a small proportion of patients receiving chloramphenicol (perhaps about 1 in 50 000). The mechanism has never been explained (Yunis, 1973), but it may be that chloramphenicol can have such an effect because it contains a nitrobenzene moiety in its structure. More commonly, this antibiotic causes reversible and dose-related erythroid suppression. In this type of anaemia there is inhibition of protein synthesis by mitochondria, and the enzyme *haem synthetase* is suppressed. Accordingly, the last step in haem synthesis is blocked. There is no true understanding of the way in which the more serious aplasia of the marrow is produced.

Non-narcotic analgesics

Amidopyrine is no longer used in the United Kingdom because it may cause agranulocytosis or marrow aplasia. Phenylbutazone and oxyphenbutazone are used extensively despite the fact that in the Register of the Committee on Safety of Medicines, covering the period from July 1963 to June 1976, the former drug was reported to have caused marrow depression on 272 occasions, with 172 deaths, while oxyphenbutazone was reported in relation to 102 instances of marrow depression, with 64 deaths. The figures for numbers of prescriptions suggest, however, that oxyphenbutazone may have a greater tendency to cause marrow depression than does phenylbutazone. It is not possible to suggest an incidence of adverse reactions solely from consulting this or any other available British Register. However, Inman (1977) has studied deaths from blood dyscrasias where a drug had not been mentioned as a factor, and has also obtained data about the prescribing by general practitioners of phenylbutazone and oxyphenbutazone. He calculates that the mortality from the former drug, as a result of aplastic anaemia or agranulocytosis, is 2.2 per 100 000 and from the latter it is 3.8 per 100 000. Those chiefly at risk appeared to be women over the age of 65. He concludes that 'When compared with other anti-inflammatory drugs prescribed to a similar extent, phenylbutazone and oxyphenbutazone clearly account for a disproportionately large number of fatal blood dyscrasias — probably over one third of all drug-induced blood dyscrasias in the United Kingdom (excluding cancer chemotherapy)'. This is in accord with the findings of Böttiger & Westerholm of Stockholm (1972, 1973), whose mortality figures were almost identical (Böttiger, 1977).

Many firms have attempted to produce a 'safe' non-narcotic analgesic. Evidence of safety in the animal model is not a sufficient safeguard, and it may be some time before the first incident of marrow depression is noticed after marketing. This adverse effect has been reported frequently after indomethacin but very seldom with ibuprofen, ketoprofen, naproxen, flufenamic acid, mefenamic acid, fenoprofen, ibufenac and aloxiprin. On the other hand, it has also been reported after paracetamol or aspirin, but it is likely that these had been given together with one or more of the drugs referred to above. The Register does not give this information.

It is essential for us to have non-habit-forming analgesics and difficult to know how best to advise an uninformed patient. Perhaps a survey of what is taken by knowledgeable physicians themselves, suffering from active rheumatoid arthritis, would be of interest. Certainly in some instances indomethacin or ibuprofen has been chosen by them, but the former may cause mental confusion.

Other drugs believed to cause marrow depression

A list of these has been published elsewhere (Girdwood, 1976), and a useful North American list is published by the American Medical Association Department of Drugs in their *AMA Drug Evaluations Manual* (1977). Attention should perhaps be drawn to sulphonamides and to sodium aurothiomalate as occasional causes of marrow depression. The mistake of attempting to attribute scientific accuracy to the data received by the Committee on Safety of Medicines in relation to gold injections has been commented on by Gumpel (1978). The much rarer pure red cell aplasia after this form of treatment, fortunately with recovery, has been reported by Reid & Patterson (1977).

Agranulocytosis

A low granulocyte count may be caused by a variety of drugs in those who have developed an abnormal response. Seventy-four such drugs are listed elsewhere (Girdwood, 1976) and again the non-narcotic analgesics are high on the list. Inman (1977) suggested that co-trimoxazole was an important cause of fatal agranulocytosis, but Lawson & Henry (1977) point out that there has been no increase of deaths from agranulocytosis since co-trimoxazole was first marketed as an antibacterial drug.

It has been suggested that there is an 'amidopyrine type' of agranulocytosis which is immunological, in that the offending drug alters the leucocytes to form a complex with them, making them antigenic (Moeschlin & Wagner, 1952). In contrast, there is said to be a 'chlorpromazine type' which comes on after a drug has been in use for several weeks or months. This seems to be a dose-related toxic effect that occurs in susceptible subjects (Pisciotta, 1969). Antibody studies are fruitless, and the administration of small doses of chlorpromazine, after recovery has occurred, does not necessarily cause a relapse.

It is not, however, possible to divide the offending drugs neatly into two categories with different modes of causation of this adverse reaction. In many instances the patients may have some inborn or developed abnormality of drug-metabolizing power.

Thrombocytopenia

More drugs have been alleged to cause thrombocytopenia than to be responsible for aplastic anaemia or agranulocytosis. In one publication (Girdwood, 1976) 85 of these are listed, the commonest reported being phenylbutazone, co-trimoxazole, oxyphenbutazone, indomethacin and frusemide. Occasionally, paracetamol (acetaminophen) may be the causative agent, and the clinician must remember this when he is faced with apparent idiopathic thrombocytopenic purpura. Sometimes a patient may have forgotten that she has taken this drug, and apparent spontaneous recovery may be the adverse results of this medicament wearing off.

No doubt with some drugs there is a central toxic effect on megakaryocytes and in others there is an immunological disorder operating along the lines suggested by Ackroyd (1949) in relation to apronal, which he thought to combine with circulating platelets to form antigens which then provoked antibodies.

Haemolytic anaemia

Immune type

Here there are immune antibodies which can only be detected if the drug is also present, and it is then that they react with normal red cells. Commonly the direct antiglobulin (Coombs) test is positive, but not invariably (Worlledge, 1969). However, in the presence of the drug, the *indirect* antiglobulin test is positive, and the serum antibodies are of the IgM or IgG type. These antibodies are fairly specific, but there may be cross-reaction with related drugs.

The agents that have been reported are shown in Table 12.2.

Table 12.2.   Drugs reported as having caused the 'immune type' of haemolytic anaemia.

Amidopyrine	Insulin	Quinine
Antazoline	Isoniazid	Rifampicin
Cephalosporins	*p*-Aminosalicylic acid	Sulphasalazine
Chlorpromazine	Penicillin	Stibophen
Dipyrone	Phenacetin	Sulphonamides
Insecticides	Quinidine	Sulphonylurea

Penicillin is a very rare cause of haemolysis; when this occurs, the penicillin is bound strongly to the red cell and cannot be removed by washing. A very large dose of penicillin has usually been administered.

Haemolytic anaemia may be caused by cephalosporins. A positive direct antiglobulin test without haemolysis is commonly found when cephalothin has been given, particularly if there is renal failure. There is thought to be a non-immune binding of a cephalothin-protein complex to the surface of the erythrocyte (Kosaki & Miyakawa, 1970). New cephalosporins being developed could show similar effects.

Autoimmune haemolytic anaemia

This is now the most commonly encountered form of haemolytic anaemia, the causative agent usually being methyldopa. The condition is serologically similar to idiopathic autoimmune haemolytic anaemia. Autoantibodies that react with normal red cells are present and the direct antiglobulin test is positive. The abnormality usually does not occur until after three months or more of treatment with methyldopa. However, the direct antiglobulin test does not become negative again until a month or more after the taking of the drug ceases. Haemolysis occurs in less than 1% of patients taking methyldopa, but the extent to which the serological test becomes positive is much greater. The indirect antiglobulin test is usually positive as well as the direct one, indicating that autoantibody is free in the serum. The antibodies are of the IgG type. To enhance recovery it may be necessary to treat with corticosteroids.

Other drugs which may cause this type of anaemia include mefenamic acid, *l*-dopa, chlorpromazine, hydantoins and methysergide (Worlledge, 1973).

Red cell destruction in normal persons

Certain drugs or other agents may cause destruction of the erythrocytes in anyone exposed to them in sufficient concentration, no immunological action being necessary. Dapsone is an oxidant drug which may do this, and sulphasalazine may also act in this way. Other agents that may do so are acetanilide, arsine, lead, methyl chloride, naphthalene, nitrobenzene, and phenacetin in large amounts.

Red cell destruction in those with glucose-6-phosphate dehydrogenase deficiency

The erythrocyte requires energy which is obtained from the breakdown of glucose. The main path of breakdown is to pyruvate or lactate, but about 10 to 15 per cent is by a shunt mechanism. From glucose is formed glucose-6-phosphate, and it is here, by the shunt, that a proportion is acted on by the red cell enzyme glucose-6-phosphate dehydrogenase. A series of steps from this point lead back to pyruvate, but on the way to this there is a need for the reduction of nicotinamide adenine dinucleotide phosphate (NADP). In turn, NADPH is an essential coenzyme in the reduction of oxidized glutathione to reduced glutathione. The latter is required for the protection of sulphydryl groups within the red cell against oxidation (Kosower, Keum-Ryul Song & Kosower, 1969). The shunt mechanism seems to be the only source of NADPH in the red cell. If the glucose-6-phosphate dehydrogenase (G6PD) is not acting normally, NADPH formation is impaired, and the red cell is not properly protected against oxidant damage, hence it is destroyed prematurely. Oxidant drugs appear to form hydrogen peroxide and an oxidized disulphide form of glutathione may be attached to haemoglobin, giving a mixed disulphide-glutathione-haemoglobin complex that is unstable. Precipitated denatured haemoglobin appears in the red cells as Heinz bodies (see Chapter 1).

There are over 70 variants of the normal G6PD, and, of these, it is said that 20 are associated with potential hereditary haemolytic anaemia occurring primarily in white subjects, whereas the more common variants occur in black subjects or persons from the Mediterranean littoral (Miller & Wollman, 1974). About 100 million persons are thought to carry the trait for a G6PD variant (Carson & Frischer, 1966). There may be no obvious clinical abnormality or, rarely, chronic hereditary haemolytic anaemia may occur. More commonly, haemolysis becomes evident only if an oxidant drug is given or if stress, particularly an infection, occurs. Sometimes both the drug and an infection are needed. Since a number of variants of G6PD are involved, there may be racial and geographical variations in the drugs that may lead to haemolysis. For instance, chloramphenicol, quinine and quinidine are said not to cause haemolysis in Negroes, but, occasionally, to do so in susceptible subjects of Mediterranean racial extraction. Other causative agents are listed in Table 12.3.

Table 12.3.   Drugs believed to cause haemolysis in subjects with glucose-6-phosphate
dehydrogenase abnormalities.

Acetanilide	Methylene blue	Phenacetin
Aspirin	Naphthalene	Primaquine
Chloroquine	Neoarsphenamine	Probenecid
Dapsone	Nitrofurantoin	Sulphonamides
Dimercaprol	Nitrofurazone	Sulphoxone
Furaltadone	Pamaquin	Thiazosulphone
Furazolidine	p-Aminosalicylic acid	Vitamin K (water-soluble analogues)
Mepacrine	Pentaquine	

The infections that may trigger off haemolysis include acute viral
hepatitis, influenza, pneumonia and typhoid fever. In some, the taking of
the fava bean, *Vicia fava*, will act as a precipitating factor.

Red cell destruction in those with other enzyme deficiencies

Other abnormalities are rare, but there can be deficiency of glutathione
synthetase, glutathione reductase or glutathione peroxidase. In these, drugs
may very rarely cause haemolysis.

Unstable haemoglobins

Unstable haemoglobins have an amino acid substitution that gives a haemoglobin that is less stable than normal. In some, such as Hb_{Zurich}, a
haemolytic event may be precipitated by a drug such as a sulphonamide.

Coagulation problems

Anticoagulants

Anticoagulants given by injection (e.g. heparin) or by mouth (e.g. warfarin)
are administered with the intention of making the blood less readily
coagulable. Occasionally a patient may have an apparent bleeding disorder
through having taken an overdose of an anticoagulant. In one such case, a
16-year-old girl was admitted to hospital literally bleeding to death. She
denied having taken any drugs, but responded rapidly to treatment with
phytomenadione. Her blood warfarin level was found to be very high and,
although she still denied having taken the drug, it was discovered that the
same day she had unwillingly signed adoption papers in relation to her
illegitimate baby. There was no question of anyone else having given her
warfarin.

One important aspect of therapy with oral anticoagulants is the danger of
interactions with an increasing number of drugs. For instance, amylobarbitone is one that induces the activity in the liver of microsomal enzymes that
metabolize warfarin. Accordingly, if a patient has been receiving both drugs
and the amylobarbitone is then stopped, it will be necessary to reduce the
dose of warfarin. On the other hand, phenylbutazone and related drugs

displace warfarin from binding sites on plasma albumin. A serious bleeding problem was seen in a patient with mitral stenosis and atrial fibrillation who had been given warfarin on a long-term basis to prevent embolism, and, simultaneously, amylobarbitone as a hypnotic. She developed joint pains and was seen by a consultant who continued the warfarin in the same dosage, stopped the amylobarbitone and prescribed phenylbutazone. The bleeding episode that resulted was particularly severe.

Plasminogen activators

In the body, blood clots are removed by a process in which plasminogen is activated to plasmin and this latter substance causes degradation of fibrin. Streptokinase is a fibrinolytic agent which activates plasminogen and it can be used as a therapeutic agent if given with care. If an overdose is given, an antidote is aminocaproic acid, which inhibits, competitively, the activation of plasminogen to plasmin.

Prostaglandin inhibitors

The substances thromboxane, prostaglandin and prostacyclin are derived from arachidonic acid. Thromboxane A_2 produces platelet aggregation and vasoconstriction, whereas prostacyclin inhibits platelet aggregation and relaxes vascular smooth muscle (Vane, 1978). Aspirin-like drugs inhibit prostaglandin synthesis, and it seems likely that the release of thromboxane A_2 in platelets is inhibited by aspirin-like drugs. The use of aspirin as an anticoagulant drug is being investigated but so far has had no dramatic results (Verstraete, 1976).

Thrombosis

The main interest here concerns the possible dangers of thrombosis in a small number of women who have taken the combined oestrogen/progestogen type of contraceptive pill. Two articles, published in 1977 (Beral & Kay, 1977a; Vessey, McPherson & Johnson, 1977) aroused much interest and led to considerable correspondence about the degree of risk (Kuenssberg & Dewhurst, 1977; Fowler & Burch, 1977; May, 1977; Turner, 1977; Lloyd, 1977; Marchant, 1977; Russell, 1977; Beral & Kay, 1977b; Simons, Gibson & Jones, 1977).

Soon after the introduction of the combined contraceptive pill it became apparent that women who took it had a slight but increased risk of having a thrombotic episode, which could be venous or arterial, and that death could occur. The reasons for this are complex and little understood (Girdwood, 1976), but it was found that there was some relationship to the oestrogen content of the pill, and hence in most preparations this concentration was reduced to 50 μg or less. In a survey, published in 1973, the Boston Collaborative Drug Surveillance team had considered the risk of venous thromboembolism in women aged 20 to 44 who did not use oral contraceptives to be about 6 per 100 000 per annum, whereas it was 66 per 100 000 in those who did; moreover, this referred particularly to the taking of low oestrogen dose preparations. There is, therefore, a risk, but there is also a certain danger in being pregnant. The pill transfers a slight risk from one cause to a lower risk from another, but in a different individual. The paper by Beral & Kay (1977a), based on a large prospective study by general practitioners, appeared to show the death rate from diseases of the circulatory system in women who had used oral contraceptives to be five times that of controls who had never used them, and the death rate in those who had taken the pill continuously for five years or more to be ten times that of controls. Those particularly at risk were women over the age of 35, and a variety of vascular accidents occurred. The reported difference in death rate from diseases of the circulatory system between ever-users of oral contraceptives and controls was 20 per 100 000 women per year. It was suggested that women over 35 years should reconsider their method of contraception (Kuenssberg & Dewhurst, 1977). The conclusions were criticized by various contributors. Thus, Lloyd (1977) concluded: 'The R.C.G.P. study may have identified that women, who smoke more heavily and become older, have a higher risk of death due to arterial disease. Any direct connection with oral contraceptives is very far from substantiated'. This was not accepted by Beral & Kay (1977b), who make the important point that, in the R.C.G.P. study, 79% of the women-years of observation in the takers related to pills containing 50 μg oestrogen or less and a large majority of these related to the 50 μg dosage.

Megaloblastic anaemia

Drugs used to treat epilepsy

In studies of megaloblastic anaemias throughout a 15-year period in Britain, war-time India and, later, the United States, I was able to explain for the causation of the condition in each of several hundreds of patients, except in one lady who had been receiving primidone. Megaloblastic anaemia after the taking of hydantoins had just been reported (Mannheimer *et al.*, 1952), but the formula of primidone is different, being more closely related to that of phenobarbitone. Since then it has readily been accepted that phenytoin or primidone may cause megaloblastic anaemia when given over long periods, and that this is due to folate depletion. The mechanism is not known, but the theories have been summarized elsewhere (Girdwood, 1973).

Folate antagonists

Unlike most blood disorders induced by drugs, the occurrence of megaloblastic anaemia after the taking of folate antagonists is predictable. In the diet, folates are present as a variety of complex substances derived from pteroylglutamic acid. In the alimentary tract these are converted by γ-glutamyl carboxypeptidase (folate conjugase) to simpler forms which are absorbed by the small intestine.

It is possible that this action occurs in the epithelial cells of the villi, and perhaps it is here, too, that the next stage occurs. Monoglutamates are reduced to the dihydro- and then tetrahydro- forms by an enzyme known as dihydrofolate reductase (sometimes called folate reductase). In the liver there is stored a 5-methyltetrahydropteroylglutamate complex, and in both the red cells and the plasma, the main form is 5-methyltetrahydropteroyl-glutamate. The important feature in relation to the present consideration is that the active forms of folate in the body are reduced ones and that any-thing that interferes with the dihydrofolate reductase step is likely to cause megaloblastic anaemia. It was discovered at a very early stage that aminopterin (4-aminopteroylglutamic acid) not only could not be used to treat megaloblastic anaemia, but, in fact, could be lethal in that condition. This was because it is a folate antagonist, as is methotrexate. Others which are less active in this respect in man are pyrimethamine and trimethoprim. The latter, a constituent of co-trimoxazole, is 50 000 times more active against bacterial folate reductase than it is against that of man. In fact, it does not cause folate depletion unless the patient already has another cause for this deficiency. Even then, it is possible to give folic acid together with co-trimoxazole since preformed folic acid is not available to bacteria.

Other drugs that may cause folate depletion

Some drugs produce megaloblastic anaemia by interfering with DNA formation: these include cytarabine, hydroxyurea, cyclophosphamide, fluorouracil, mercaptopurine, azathioprine and thioguanine.

Reports that oral contraceptives may cause megaloblastic anaemia have been made by Paton (1969), Strieff (1970) and a few others. Wood, Goldstone & Allan (1972) reported three patients who developed megalo-blastic anaemia when taking oral contraceptives, but one had a poor nutritional state, another had a diet with a rather low folate content, while the third had gluten enteropathy. However, at an International Workshop on Human Folate Requirements held in Washington, D.C. in 1975, not one of the 37 investigators in this field had encountered a patient who had developed folate deficiency or megaloblastic anaemia from taking contra-ceptive pills. If it does occur, the reason is not clear, and perhaps another cause of folate depletion, such as malnutrition or malabsorption, must also be operating.

Related to this is the question of whether oral contraceptives, if they fail to be effective, can cause foetal abnormalities. This is unlikely, but the same question arises, possibly with more reason, in relation to pregnancy in epileptic women receiving phenytoin or primidone. Several workers have suggested that folate depletion may cause foetal deformities (*Lancet*, 1977).

Alcoholics may develop folate deficiency and this may merely indicate malnutrition. On the other hand, it has been claimed that macrocytosis and megaloblastic change may occur in alcoholism in the absence of folate deficiency, and suggested that this may be a direct toxic action of alcohol on the erythroblast (Chanarin & Perry, 1977).

Drug-induced vitamin B$_{12}$ deficiency

It seems that the hypoglycaemic agent, metformin, may cause malabsorption of vitamin B$_{12}$ (Berchtold *et al.*, 1969; Tomkin *et al.*, 1971). It has been suggested that metformin may either inhibit vitamin B$_{12}$ absorption competitively in the distal ileum or inactivate the enzyme system involved in the normal absorption of vitamin B$_{12}$.

Sideroblastic anaemia

This is a condition in which some of the red cell precursors contain a perinuclear ring of iron-staining granules in the cytoplasm. These are called sideroblasts. Occasionally, the condition is a familial disorder, there being an enzyme deficiency affecting the synthesis of haem. More commonly, sideroblastic anaemia is a complication of another disorder such as megaloblastic anaemia, hypothyroidism or metastatic carcinoma. Various drugs may cause it, again by interfering in some way with haem synthesis. Drugs that may do this include isoniazid, cycloserine, pyrazinamide, chloramphenicol and lead.

Leukaemia induced by drugs

There have been some reports of the occurrence of myeloblastic leukaemia after a patient has developed aplastic anaemia which itself may have been induced by chloramphenicol.

There have also been reports that leukaemia may follow the taking of phenylbutazone (Bean, 1960; Dimitrov, Faix & Ellegaard, 1973), but it has not been satisfactorily established that this is a true cause and effect. Certainly some patients may have joint pains in association with leukaemia and take phenylbutazone or a related drug to relieve this pain. It may then be thought that the drug caused the leukaemia.

Drug-induced gastro-intestinal bleeding

Aspirin is absorbed as such, but much is fairly rapidly hydrolysed to salicylic acid in the gastro-intestinal mucosa. Aspirin in any form is potentially irritant and it is perhaps not surprising that so many of those who become anaemic from alimentary bleeding have been taking aspirin in one form or another. Phenylbutazone, oxyphenbutazone and most of the newer non-narcotic analgesics can cause alimentary bleeding in a small number of patients who take the drug.

Methaemoglobinaemia and sulphaemoglobinaemia

Methaemoglobinaemia is usually caused by the taking of drugs which preferentially oxidize haemoglobin, and, in sufficient quantities, they may overcome the normal reducing mechanisms of red cells. Causative agents include acetanilide, phenacetin, potassium chlorate and certain sulphonamides, such as sulphanilamide, sulphathiazole and sulphapyridine.

Sulphaemoglobinaemia is due to the presence of a haemoglobin derivative not normally found in red cells. It is almost always produced by drugs, particularly phenacetin and acetanilide.

Porphyria

The porphyrias are a group of metabolic abnormalities characterized by the excretion in abnormal quantities of substances that are either precursors or by-products in the metabolic pathways leading to the formation of haem. The complexities of the enzyme deficiencies involved have been discussed recently (Kramer, Becker & Viljoen, 1977). Acute intermittent porphyria may be precipitated by a variety of agents, including barbiturates, sulphonamides, methyldopa, griseofulvin and contraceptive pills. General anaesthesia with thiopentone may be lethal in this condition.

With regard to any information quoted from the Register of Adverse Reactions of the Committee on Safety of Medicines, any interpretation placed upon the figures is that of the author and not that of the Committee.

References

Ackroyd, J.F. (1949). *Clin. Sci.*, 7, 249.
AMA Drug Evaluations (1977). 3rd Ed. Prepared by the A.M.A. Department of Drugs. Littleton, Massachusetts: Publishing Sciences Group Inc.
Bean, R.H.D. (1960). *Br. med. J.*, 2, 1552.
Beral, V. and Kay, C.R. (1977a). *Lancet*, 2, 727.
Beral, V. and Kay, C.R. (1977b). *Lancet*, 2, 1276.
Berchtold, P., Bolli, P., Arbenz, U. and Keiser, G. (1969). *Diabetologia*, 5, 405.
Boston Collaborative Drug Surveillance Programme (1973). *Lancet*, 1, 1399.
Böttiger, L.E. (1977). *Br. med. J.*, 2, 265.
Böttiger, L.E. and Westerholm, B. (1972). *Acta med. scand.*, 192, 315.
Böttiger, L.E. and Westerholm, B. (1973). *Br. med. J.*, 3, 339.
Carson, P.E. and Frischer, H. (1966). *Am. J. Med.*, 41, 744.
Chanarin, I. and Perry, J. (1977). In *Folic Acid, Biochemistry and Physiology in Relation to the Human Nutrition Requirement*. Editors: Broquist, H.P., Butterworth, C.E. and Wagner, C., p. 156. Washington, D.C.: National Academy of Sciences.
Dimitrov, N.V., Faix, J.D. and Ellegaard, J. (1973). In *Drugs and Haematologic Reactions*. Editors: Dimitrov, N.V. and Nodine, J.H., p. 223. New York: Grune & Stratton.
Fowler, P.B.S. and Burch, P.R.J. (1977). *Lancet*, 2, 879.
Girdwood, R.H. (1973). In *Blood Disorders Due to Drugs and Other Agents*. Editor: Girdwood, R.H., p. 49. Amsterdam: Excerpta Medica.
Girdwood, R.H. (1974). *Br. med. J.*, 1, 501.
Girdwood, R.H. (1976). In *Haematological Aspects of Systemic Disease*. Editors: Israels, M.C.G. and Delamore, I.W., p. 495. London: W.B. Saunders Co.
Gumpel, J.M. (1978). *Br. med. J.*, 1, 215.
Inman, W.H.W. (1977). *Br. med. J.*, 1, 1500.
Kosakai, N. and Miyakawa, D. (1970). *Postgrad. med. J.* (Suppl.), 46, 107.
Kosower, N.S., Keum-Ryul Song and Kosower, E.M. (1969). *Biochim. biophys. Acta*, 192, 23.
Kramer, S., Becker, D.M. and Viljoen, J.D. (1977). *Br. J. Haemat.*, 37, 439.
Kuenssberg, E.V. and Dewhurst, J. (1977). *Lancet*, 2, 757.
Lancet (1977). Leading article, 1, 462.
Lawson, D.H. and Henry, D.A. (1977). *Br. med. J.*, 2, 316.
Lloyd, G. (1977). *Lancet*, 2, 921.

Mannheimer, E., Pakesch, F., Reimer, E.E. and Vetter, H. (1952). *Med. Klin.*, 47, 1397.
Marchant, J. (1977). *Lancet*, 2, 922.
May, D. (1977). *Lancet*, 2, 921.
Miller, D.R. and Wollman, M.R. (1974). *Blood*, 44, 323.
Moeschlin, S. and Wagner, K. (1952). *Acta Haemat. (Basel)*, 8, 29.
Paton, A. (1969). *Lancet*, 1, 418.
Pisciotta, A.V. (1969). *J. Am. med. Ass.*, 208, 1862.
Reid, G. and Patterson, A.C. (1977). *Br. med. J.*, 2, 1457.
Russell, H. (1977). *Lancet,* 2, 922.
Simons, L.A., Gibson, J.C. and Jones, A.S. (1977). *Lancet*, 2, 1277.
Strieff, R.R. (1970). *J. Am. med. Ass.*, 214, 105.
Tomkin, G.H., Hadden, D.R., Weaver, J.A. and Montgomery, D.A.D. (1971). *Br. med. J.*, 2, 685.
Turner, R.W.D. (1977). *Lancet*, 2, 921.
Vane, J.R. (1978) (Personal communication).
Verstraete, M. (1976). *Am. J. Med.*, 61, 897.
Vessey, M.P., McPherson, K. and Johnson, B. (1977). *Lancet*, 2, 731.
Wood, J.K., Goldstone, A.H. and Allan, N.C. (1972). *Scand. J. Haemat.*, 9, 539.
Worlledge, S.M. (1969). *Semin. Hemat.*, 6, 181.
Worlledge, S.M. (1973). In *Blood Disorders Due to Drugs and Other Agents*. Editor: Girdwood, R.H., p. 11. Amsterdam: Excerpta Medica.
Yunis, A.A. (1973). In *Blood Disorders Due to Drugs and Other Agents*. Editor: Girdwood, R.H., p. 107. Amsterdam: Excerpta Medica.

13. Mechanisms of ocular toxicity

A. J. Bron

Introduction

The eye is as subject to adverse reactions as other parts of the body and almost every part of the eye, its adnexal organs and the neuromuscular systems responsible for coordinating the movements of the eyes, has been involved in toxic reactions of one form or other.

In many instances the ocular changes may be of incidental interest, apparently neither harming the eye nor indicating more widespread systemic toxicity; the keratopathy of indomethacin is of this nature. In other instances, the toxic reactions may be bilateral, and may threaten sight, as with the cataracts of corticosteroid therapy, the retinopathy of chloroquine therapy and the optic neuropathy of ethambutol therapy. Ocular toxicity may also be part of a more widespread toxic reaction, as in the mucocutaneous syndrome caused by practolol. However, in certain cases, it may be possible to make use of mild toxic reactions on the visual system as an indicator of more serious systemic toxicity, permitting adjustment of dosage. This is being attempted in the case of digitalis overdose.

The advent of a toxic reaction is often delayed because it is dose dependent. This is the case with phenothiazine and chloroquine retinopathy. The delay in onset of clinical signs may be such that their features do not become apparent until after therapy has ceased. The cataract caused by the tricyclic compound Triparanol appeared only after a latent period and rarely while the patient was on therapy. In chloroquine and phenothiazine therapy, the toxic effect may persist after withdrawal of the drug, resulting in continued deterioration of vision.

Many of the drugs having toxic ocular effects are used for life-saving therapy, as with corticosteroids used in the management of collagen vascular disease, immunosuppressive therapy for renal transplant patients, and the treatment of bronchial asthma. Though the ophthalmologist may guide the physician in the safe ocular dose, it may be necessary to exceed these levels and accept an adverse reaction, such as cataract, which is remediable by surgery. But where continued therapy will cause irreversible blindness, as with ethambutol or practolol toxicity, it is imperative to find an alternative form of therapy for the primary condition.

This chapter touches briefly on the toxic implications of topical ocular therapy and deals mainly with the ocular toxicity of systemic drugs and certain other substances. I shall discuss the incidence of toxicity, clinical features, onset, reversibility, and sequelae. The known toxic daily and total dose and presumed safe dose are mentioned where appropriate and the site of action and mechanism of toxicity where known. Finally, where it is possible to modify dosage to within safe limits, the techniques of monitoring are noted.

Ocular anatomy and physiology

The outer corneo-scleral envelope of the eye houses the dioptric system of the eye, which focuses an image of the outside world on the light-sensitive retina. Change in focus from distance to near is effected by change in shape of the lens, through the action of the ciliary muscle. Accommodation for near is accompanied by pupil constriction through the action of the iris sphincter. The ciliary muscle and iris sphincter are under parasympathetic control. The pupil dilator muscle is under adrenergic control.

The integrity of the corneal epithelium, and that of conjunctival mucous membrane which lines the lids and globe, is achieved by a constant bathing of these surfaces by the tears. The aqueous component is secreted by the lacrimal gland and auxilliary lacrimal tissue in the conjunctival sac. The lacrimal gland is innervated by the parasympathetic system, but tear production may also be stimulated by beta-adrenergic agonists.

The lens is made up of an outer collagenous capsule, a concentric arrangement of spindle-shaped fibres, the outer of which are nucleated, and an anterior epithelial sheet, sandwiched between the capsule and the fibre zone. Division of equatorial epithelium gives rise to fresh lens fibres as the human lens grows throughout life. The lens respiration is predominantly anaerobic. The small amount of aerobic metabolism (Hockwin *et al.*, 1971) (accounting for about 3% of the glucose metabolized) takes place in the epithelium. Although this is capable of supplying about 20% of lens ATP, it appears that the lens can survive in entirely anaerobic conditions. Disturbance of the ionic environment of the lens fibres and of their normal hydration disturbs their regular packing and optical homogeneity, and results in less of transparency or cataract.

Ocular pressure averages around 16 mmHg with an upper limit of 21 mmHg. This is a result of the homeostatic balance between inflow of aqueous humour, secreted by the ciliary gland, and outflow through the trabecular meshwork and Schlemm's canal. Aqueous secretion is under autonomic control, but the physiologic regulation of outflow resistance has not been clarified.

In pre-disposed eyes, with shallow angles, dilation of the pupil may cause the peripheral iris to abruptly shut off the outflow of aqueous. With continued secretion of aqueous, a rapid rise in ocular pressure results in acute angle closure glaucoma.

The rods and cones contain visual pigment and are the light-sensitive elements of the retina. The cones are concentrated at the fovea and macula, and are in lesser density elsewhere in the retina. They are responsible for colour vision and daylight vision. The high resolution achieved at the macula accounts for the excellence of visual acuity at the fixation point. The rods are sensitive to dim illumination, and distributed outside the macula and are responsible for night vision. The retinal pigment epithelium lies outside the photoreceptors and is intimately concerned with their metabolic requirements, which are supplied through the outer vascular coat, the choroid.

Stimulation of the photoreceptors generates nervous impulses in the intermediate cells of the retina, the bipolar cells, and the impulse is transmitted thence to the retinal ganglion cells. Their axons make up the fibres of the optic nerve. The electrical activity of the retina is detected clinically by electroretinography (ERG), where the characteristic waveform in response to a light flash indicates, in a general way, the integrity of the retinal elements. The early receptor potential (ERP) is generated at the outer portion of the rods and cones. The later receptor potential is the a-wave which is a small negative deflection arising from the inner portion of the rods and cones. The well-defined positive potential, the b-wave, arises at the bipolar cells. The secondary slow positive wave is called the c-wave, and is generated at the level of the resting potential of the eye, i.e. in the pigment epithelium and the outer tips of the rods and cones. The functions of the rods and cones can be distinguished by eliciting the ERG with coloured flashes (the cones are more red-sensitive, the rods more blue-sensitive) or with different frequencies of flickering flash (since the cones have a much higher temporal resolution than the rods) (Galloway, 1975). The drug furaltadone has been associated with an acquired cone degeneration with day blindness and nystagmus (Siegel & Smith, 1967). Damage to the ganglion cells or optic nerve alone or the higher visual pathways will produce a normal ERG. Damage to the photoreceptor and pigment epithelial layer will affect the a- and c-waves, while damage to the bipolar layer (such as will be caused by retinal artery occlusion) results in depression of the b-wave.

The resting potential of the eye is low in the dark and rises with increasing illumination. Changes in the size of this potential reflect events occurring in the pigment epithelium and the retinal receptors. This potential change is recorded as the electro-oculogram (EOG). Disease affecting the pathway from bipolar cells to the visual cortex does not affect the EOG, which reflects only pre-synaptic retinal function. Various drug induced retinopathies affect the EOG (Ikeda, 1976).

Acquired defects in colour vision may arise from damage to the retina or optic nerve. Severe damage to either may result in uniform affection of hue discrimination. Less severe damage tends to affect either red/green discrimination or blue/yellow discrimination preferentially. Koellner (1912) suggested that post-synaptic lesions from the bipolar cells to lateral geniculate body preferentially affect the red/green discrimination (as in many toxic neuropathies), while lesions of the neurosensory retina are associated with a disturbance of blue/yellow discrimination. However, there are many exceptions to this rule (Foulds, 1976).

The Ishihara pseudo-isochromatic plates detect red/green colour defects, while the American Optical Harvey-Rand-Rittler (HRR) plates detect both groups of defects. The City University colour vision test also detects both forms of colour defect, as does the more complex but highly sensitive Farnsworth Munsell 100 Hue Test.

Further information about macular (cone) function can be derived from the macular threshold and photostress tests, and about rod function from measurement of dark adaptation.

Table 13.1 summarizes a comprehensive assessment of ocular functions in monitoring for ocular toxicity. Table 13.2 cites the multiplicity of forms in which ocular toxicity may be expressed.

Table 13.1.   Monitoring for ocular toxicity.

Biomicroscopy
Schirmer's Test
Ocular Pressure
Visual Acuity: Near and distance
Visual Fields: Central and Peripheral
Electrodiagnosis: E.R.G., E.O.G., E.N.G.
Colour Vision
Dark Adaption
Macular Thresholds
Photo Stress Test
Fluorescein Angiography

Table 13.2.   Modes of toxic ocular response.

Disturbed Vision	Oculo-motor Disturbance	Other Changes
Corneal deposits	Convergence weakness	Pigmentations and deposits
Accommodative paresis	Paralytic squint	Dry eye
Cataract	Nystagmus	Lacrymation
Glaucoma	Oculo-gyric crises	Teratogenicity
Retinal damage		
Optic nerve and other visual pathway damage		

Local toxicity of topical drugs

A vast number of local adverse reactions are encountered which result from topical therapy. The most common are allergic reactions to antibiotics, anaesthetics, mydriatics (Theodore, 1953) and adrenaline (Grant, 1974) in addition to constituents in the vehicle of drops or ointments.

Table 13.3 specifies other forms of toxic reaction.

Anticholinesterases

Anticholinesterases such as phospholine iodide are used in the management of accommodative squint in children. Dilute drops (0.06%) may induce epithelial cysts at the pupil margin, which in the presence of intense miosis,

Table 13.3.   Local toxicity of topical drugs.

Class	Drug	Toxic effect
Anticholinesterase	Phospholine iodide	Iris cysts; cataract; retinal detachment
Antiviral	I.D.U.; Ara-A	Ptosis; conjunctivitis; keratitis; dry eye; punctual stenosis
Corticosteroid	Prednisone	Glaucoma; cataract; ptosis; mydriasis
Mydriatic	Atropine	Angle-closure glaucoma
Preservatives	B.Z.K.	Epithelial keratitis
	P.M.N.	Band-keratopathy; mercuria lentis
Sympathomimetic	Adrenalin	Aphakic macular oedema

may interfere with vision. The mechanism is not known, but the effect may be mechanical, since it may be prevented by combining the drug with the mydriatic phenylephrine.

Retinal detachment may also be induced by strong anticholinesterases particularly in aphakics, presumably by the transmission of the pull created by the intense contraction of the ciliary muscle to the peripheral retina.

Anticholinesterases were in the past used extensively in the management of chronic glaucoma. The ability of anticholinesterases, particularly the irreversible cholinesterases, echothiophate iodide (phospholine iodide), diethyl-*p*-nitrophenyl phosphate (Mintacol) and di-isopropylfluorophosphate (DFP) to cause cataract was first suspected in 1954, by Kreibig, who reported its development in a patient receiving treatment with DFP over a period of several weeks. These observations have been confirmed by several retrospective (Axelsson, 1969a; Axelsson & Holmberg, 1966; De Roetth, 1966; Shaffer & Hetherington, 1966; Tarkkanen & Karjalainen, 1966) and prospective studies (Morton, Drance & Fairclough, 1969).

The cataract affects the anterior subcapsular zone of the lens, starting with minute vacuoles which later aggregate into larger configurations associated with 'mossy' patches and streaks. The effect on vision is severe, because the pupil is intensely miosed by such drugs.

The incidence of cataract due to phospholine iodide in strengths ranging from 0.06-0.25% is cited between 33-62% after treatment for six months or more (Patterson, 1971).

The effect is said to be dose-related, accelerated by increasing age and static or progressive after cessation of therapy (Drance, 1969; Axelsson, 1969b). Harrison (1960) observed complete reversal in three weeks of a cataract which developed after three months' treatment of a child, with DFP.

Mechanism of anticholinesterase cataract

No convincing model of anticholinesterase cataract exists, but biochemical changes have been produced *in vitro*.

Michon & Kinoshita (1968) demonstrated a depression of oxidative metabolism in the lens, differing in degree with different miotics. Since aerobic metabolism does not appear essential for lens transparency, the significance of this finding is not clear. However, they demonstrated increased permeability and altered sodium and potassium content, albeit at high levels of the drugs.

De Roetth (1966) demonstrated reduced lens anticholinesterase activity and Laties (1969) demonstrated localization of DFP at the anterior lens surface. It has been suggested that cholinesterase may be involved with ion transport.

Antiviral agents such as IDU or ARA-A produce a distinctive form of follicular conjunctivitis with ptosis, pain and punctal occlusion and epithelial keratitis. The reaction develops after weeks or months of therapy and the reaction is accelerated over a newly grafted cornea. For this reason, antivirals should be avoided in the immediate post-graft period except at low dosage.

Corticosteroids given topically for inflammatory conditions of the eye may raise the ocular pressure and produce glaucoma. The pressure rise is due to an increase in outflow resistance in the absence of an increase in flow. It has been suggested that the effect is due to an increased hydration of mucopolysaccharide in the trabecular meshwork (Oppelt, White & Halpert, 1969).

Topical Dexamethazone 0.1% q.d.s. will produce a pressure rise after 4-6 weeks in one third of the general population. This may be intermediate (6-16 mmHg) or high (16 or more). Armaly (1967) suggested that the high response occurred in subjects homozygous for the chronic simple glaucoma gene. (An increased proportion of responders is met in myopes over 5.0 diopters (Podos, Becker & Marten, 1966), angle recession and with pigmented angles (Becker & Hahn, 1964; Armaly *et al.*, 1968).

Certain other steroids, which retain an anti-inflammatory action, have a lower tendency to induce a pressure rise, for example hydroxymethyl-progesterone (Bedrossian & Eriksen 1969), fluomethalone, and clobetazone butyrate. Topical steroids have produced cataract (Becker, 1964; Streiff, 1964; Valerio, Carones & De Poli, 1965) and the mechanism will be discussed further under systemic toxicity.

The ability of mydriatic drops to precipitate angle closure glaucoma, is well known, and will not be discussed further.

Preservatives, such as benzalkonium chloride, may occasionally cause a punctate keratitis. This possibility is increased when they are used in the presence of a hydrophilic contact lens, which may concentrate the agent over a period of time.

Phenyl mercuric nitrate, for a long time used as a preservative in miotics and other drops used chronically in the treatment of glaucoma, is able to induce a band-shaped keratopathy in the cornea and a deposit of heavy metal in the anterior lens capsule, where it appears as a brown discolouration in the pupil zone — mercuria lentis (Abrams & Majzoub, 1970).

Kolker & Becker (1968) found that 20-30% of aphakic patients on adrenalin therapy for glaucoma developed a reversible oedema of the macula, associated with blurring, distortion and decreased acuity. The mechanism is not known, but the interesting implication is that removal of the lens leads to a breakdown of the so-called vitreous barrier, which obstructs the diffusion of drugs in the aqueous from the posterior chamber into the vitreous space in the intact eye.

Systemic toxicity of topical drugs (Table 13.4)

Drugs are readily absorbed from the conjunctival sac and nasopharynx after topical application to the eye, and may cause systemic toxicity either directly or through interaction with other agents.

Table 13.4. Systemic toxicity of topical drugs.

Class	Drug	Toxic effect
Anticholinesterase	Phospholine iodide	Systemic toxicity Succinylcholine apnoea Hyperreactivity in mongols Rhinorrhoea in children
Antimuscarinic Mydriatic	Atropine	Fatalities in mongols
Sympathomimetics	Phenylephrine	Hypertension in neonates Hypertension with M.A.O.I.?
	Adrenalin	Arrhythmias with digitalis, halothane? Hypertension with tricyclics
	Isoprenaline	Arrhythmias

(See Davidson, 1974)

Phospholine iodide, used chronically in the treatment of glaucoma, has a deserved reputation for producing symptoms of systemic toxicity on the gastro-intestinal, respiratory, cardiovascular and other systems. It may produce prolonged apnoea after use of the muscle-relaxant succinylcholine and rhinorrhoea in children. A syndrome of hyperreactivity is described in mongols.

Mongols too are more sensitive to the local and systemic action of atropine, and fatalities have been described. Various sympathomimetics given topically or subconjunctivally may theoretically or actually cause hypertension or cardiac arrhythmias by their direct action or through interaction with monoamine oxidase inhibitors, cardiac glycosides, anaesthetic agents or tricyclic antidepressants (Davidson, 1974).

The ocular toxicity of systemic drugs

What makes the eye a target organ for so many drugs? Perhaps this is more apparent than real. Certainly patients who develop optic atrophy from isoniazid may also exhibit a peripheral neuropathy, presumably through a similar mechanism of pyridoxine deficiency. Triparanol cataract was associated with and always preceded by severe changes in the skin and hair. The neuropathy of tobacco amblyopia appears to be confined to the optic nerve, but the related toxic amblyopia associated with consumption of cassava plant may be accompanied by a peripheral neuropathy; both are regarded by some workers as secondary to chronic cyanide intoxication. On the other hand, the affinity of chloroquine and the phenothiazines for ocular melanin may well dictate the severity of their local ocular manifestations. The occurrence of fresh forms of adverse reaction in the eye is a constant challenge to the ophthalmologist confronted for the first time with an unusual ocular disorder.

Practolol

Practolol is a potent cardioselective beta-adrenergic receptor agent which was used in the treatment of angina, cardiac dysrhythmia and systemic hypertension.

In 1974, Felix, Ive & Dahl noted a peculiar skin rash in patients receiving practolol for periods ranging from two to twenty-six weeks and on doses from 100-600 mg daily. The rash was psoriasiform and erythematous, and showed a hyperkeratosis affecting the plantar, palmar and digital surfaces. They noted three patients with eye signs, two of whom had 'dry eyes' and one of whom underwent corneal grafting.

Wright (1974, 1975) described similar changes in association with kerato conjunctivitis sicca, as part of a mucocutaneous syndrome in which dry eyes and rashes might occur in conjunction with mucosal ulceration, a sclerosing peritonitis (Brown *et al.*, 1974), pleurisy and conduction deafness due to secretory otitis media.

The incidence of eye lesions was almost as high as the skin changes. The eye lesions are most marked on the lid and conjunctiva and consist of:
1. Conjunctival hyperaemia with papillary changes and a disorderly vessel pattern.
2. A reduction of tears and fall in tear lysozyme and secretory IgA (indices of lacrimal gland function).
3. Subsequent development of subconjunctival fibrosis, leading to tarsal scarring, shrinkage of the fornix and symblepharon.

A severe dry eye may result, with a staining pattern with Bengal Rose dye, not only of the exposed interpalpebral epithelium of the cornea and bulbar conjunctiva, but also in the upper and lower fornices, associated with metaplasia and keratinization. Corneal perforation and blindness may occur. The doses employed were 200-1200 mg/day over periods 6-48 months before the onset of eye symptoms.

Immunological mechanisms may be involved in the disorder, and circulating and fixed antibodies against an intercellular component of epithelium have been identified as well as circulating and fixed antinuclear antibody and autoantibody against smooth muscle (Amos, Brigden & McKerron, 1975; Rahi & Garner, 1976). Though antibody against intercellular component is also found in pemphigus (Sams & Jordan 1971), the component in pemphigus is not trypsin-sensitive, whereas in practolol toxicity it is.

Histology shows chronic inflammatory changes in the conjunctiva, with loss of goblet cells and where lacrimal gland has been examined, no functioning tissue has been identified (Rahi *et al.*, 1976). Both factors may contribute to the corneal and conjunctival xerosis, but it is thought that the sub-epithelial fibrosis probably represents a primary lesion caused in some way by practolol, though the mechanism is unclear. IgG and Cl_3 component of complement have been localized between epithelial cells and the antinuclear antibody is of IgM class.

The incidence of the disorder is low, and could represent some genetically determined idiosyncratic immunological disturbance.

The symptoms are in part relieved by artificial tears and other measures designed to conserve tears. However, the tear deficiency usually persists.

Other beta-blocking agents may be used in practolol toxicity patients without reactivating the skin disorder, though re-introduction of practolol does so within a short time.

Although patients present with reduced tears, while on other beta-blockers such as propranolol, or oxprenolol (Holt & Waddington, 1975; Clayden, 1975), there is not yet evidence of a similar mucocutaneous syndrome caused by other blocking agents. It is possible that reduced tear production may be a pharmacological action of these drugs.

Corticosteroids

Long-term systemic glucocorticoid therapy may reduce resistance to infection (especially herpes simplex and fungal infection), may delay corneal wound healing (for instance after corneal graft) and produce changes such as lid swelling, ptosis, mydriasis, exophthalmos, papilloedema (associated with raised intra-cranial pressure) and also open angle glaucoma and cataract (Slansky, Kolbert & Gartner, 1967).

Glaucoma is an uncommon occurrence after systemic corticosteroid therapy in genetically predisposed subjects compared to the ease with which it may be induced with topical therapy (Bernstein & Schwarz, 1962; Kalina, 1969). This contrasts with the rarity of cataract after topical therapy though cataract may be produced consistently in patients on long-term high-dose systemic therapy.

This presumably implies that different concentrations reach the target organs according to the mode of delivery, and that the trabecular meshwork is more accessible to topical therapy, the lens to systemic therapy.

The cataract of corticosteroid toxicity was first described by Black *et al* (1960) and Oglesby *et al.* (1961a, b) in patients on long-term therapy for rheumatoid arthritis. The subject has been reviewed by Spaeth & von Sallmann (1966) and Leopold & Barnert (1967). Clinically, the opacities resemble those due to radiation, and are initially composed of a discoid cluster of posterior subcapsular vacuoles which gradually increase in size with time. The effect on vision is great and is accentuated in bright light, when the pupil is small. Patients experience blurring, dazzle, difficulty reading and reduced acuity.

The incidence of posterior subcapsular cataract in patients (rheumatoid arthritis, asthma and others) on steroids was 21% in the report of Spaeth & von Sallmann (1966) compared to 0.2% in the general population and 0.4% in a rheumatoid population.

Steroid cataract has been reported in children as well as adults (Havre, 1965; Schwenk, 1967; Bihari & Grossman, 1968; Dikshit & Avashti, 1965), shows a dose response (Black *et al.*, 1960; Giles *et al.*, 1962; Crewes, 1963) and rarely is reversible (Frandsen (1965) described disappearance over three years). The cataract may progress or regress after withdrawal of therapy.

On a dose of less than 10 mg/day of prednisone, no cataract developed in the studies of Giles *et al.* (1962) and Crewes (1963), while on 16 mg/day 75% of recipients developed changes. Spaeth & von Sallmann (1966) suggested a safe total dose of 3.5 g at a rate of 10 mg/day over one year.

An experimental steroid cataract has been difficult to produce, but this has been achieved, e.g. in the rabbit (Wood *et al.*, 1967) with topical steroids. No potentiation of experimental 2,4-DNP cataract (chicken) radiation, xylose or triparanol cataract (rat) was found by Cotlier & Becker (1965), but whereas phenylbutazone alone produced no cataract, prednisolone plus phenylbutazone produced cataract in 33% of treated rats.

The mechanism by which corticosteroids produce cataract is not certain. The permeability of the posterior lens surface to fluorescein is increased by topical steroids in rabbits (Maurice, 1963; Oshima, 1968) and steroids increase the permeability of the lens *in vitro* to ^{86}Rb and ^{22}Na, resulting in a cation and water imbalance.

Lenses lost potassium and gained sodium and water when incubated with prednisolone but not dexamethazone or triamcinolone. All these steroids prevented the rewarmed lens from re-establishing normal cation levels after cooling (Becker & Cotlier, 1965). Harris (1966) showed that ^{22}Na exchangeability of the lens *in vitro* is increased on incubation of the lens with prednisolone or 9-L-fluorohydrocortisone.

Patterson (1971) suggests that the posterior location of the lens opacity may be best explained as follows: the lens fibre permeability is affected equally at the front and back of the lens, but the anterior lens surface has the additional capacity to correct the ionic shift anteriorly by reason of its active cation transport.

Two other cataractogenic drugs may now be mentioned whose mode of action is known and which shed some light on the cataractogenic process.

2,4-Dinitrophenol (2,4-DNP)

2,4-DNP was found to be cataractogenic in women taking the drug for weight reduction (Horner, 1942). Approximately 0.1-1.0% of users developed cataract (Grant, 1974). The drug has since been withdrawn. Clinically, cataracts developed in subjects taking about 300 mg/day, several months after onset of therapy. They started in the anterior cortex with fine grey cloudy opacities and a lustreless capsule, and progressed to involve the posterior cortex with golden granular polychromatic opacities. The lens later became swollen and mature cataracts resulted (Grant, 1974).

Species differences were noted in the ability to induce cataracts in animals. Cataract is induced in the duck and chicken (within a few hours of feeding), in obese mice and in the newborn rabbit, but not in the mature rabbit and only in the scorbutic guinea-pig. Gehring & Buerge (1969) showed that 2,4-DNP was capable of inducing cataract in the mature rabbit lens *in vitro* and showed further that penetration of the drug into the aqueous of the intact animal after systemic administration was better in the duckling than mature rabbit. They postulated that susceptibility depended on differences in permeability of the blood aqueous barrier.

2,4-DNP is an uncoupler of oxidative phosphorylation, and it has been suggested that cataract is produced in this way, but since lens metabolism does not rely on oxygen, such a mechanism is not fully accepted, though it might explain the initial opacification of the anterior cortex. DNP produced opaque lenses at a molar concentration of 10^{-3}-10^{-5}; at the former concentration DNP does inhibit the temperature-reversible cation shift of the lens. However, this may be higher than that achieved by DNP *in vivo* (Harris, 1966).

Many compounds related to DNP are capable of inducing cataract (e.g. 2,4-dinitro-6-aminophenol and 2-butyl-4,6-dinitrophenol) and have in common a phenolic hydroxyl and at least one nitro group, preferably in the *para*-position.

Triparanol (MER/29)

Triparanol was introduced in the 1950s, as a drug to reduce blood cholesterol in patients with hypercholesterolaemia. It acts by blocking the enzymic reduction of 2,4-dehydrocholesterol to cholesterol. It was withdrawn in April 1962 because of ocular and dermatological side effects.

A posterior subcapsular lens opacity with mild anterior subcapsular changes was reported in 1961. Altogether 25 patients were reported out of many thousands of users. In the majority a delay between use of the drug and development of cataract occurred (Kirby, 1967).

The drug was used in a dose of 250 mg or more daily. Von Sallmann, Grimes & Collins (1963) were able to induce cataracts in rats which resembled the human cataract, on a diet of 0.1% triparanol over 3 to 4 months. They identified a sudanophilic material within normal or swollen lens fibres, which they assumed to contain desmosterol, among other lipids, such as phospholipid, cholesterol and cholesterol esters.

It is thought that changes in the lens cell membranes may have been responsible for causing permeability changes. Kirby (1967) and Harris & Gruber (1969) showed increased sodium and water content and reduced potassium content in experimental cataractous lenses due to triparanol. The latter authors were able to produce a reversible cataract.

Lüllmann *et al.* (1975) have suggested that certain cationic, amphiphilic drugs (possessing both hydrophobic and hydrophilic moieties) are capable of producing a generalized lipidosis in experimental animals by reason of their ability to form tight complexes with phospholipid (Seydel & Wasserman, 1973). It is suggested that these complexes are poorly digestible by acid lipases and accumulate within lysosomes as membranes lamellar and crystalloid inclusions.

The amphiphilic compounds chloroquine (anti-malarial and anti-rheumatic drug) chlorphentermine (appetite suppressant) and iprindole (tricyclic antidepressant) each produce a similar form of cataract in rats, exhibiting

1. a diffuse anterior and faint posterior sub-capsular opacity, and
2. anterior sutural opacities.

The former were due to the presence of numerous vacuoles and lamellar inclusions of a size order (100-600 nm) thought to be capable of scattering light (Benedek, 1971).

Phenothiazines

The phenothiazines are widely used as tranquillizers and anti-emetics. Three categories of phenothiazine exist according to the substitution of side-chains in the 2 and 10 positions of the parent molecule. These are:

1. The piperidines, such as thioridazine (Melleril) NP-207, and KS-24;
2. The dimethylamines such as chlorpromazine, promazine and promethazine;
3. The piperazines such as prochlorperazine, perphenazine and trifluoperazine.

In the high doses required for psychotropic action, certain piperidines have been responsible for retinotoxicity, the dimethylamine chlorpromazine has been responsible for pigmentation of the skin, conjunctiva, cornea and lens and at lower dosages, certain piperazines have been responsible for transient myopia and oculo gyric crises (Table 13.5).

Table 13.5.   Toxic effects of phenothiazine drugs.

Derivative:	Phenothiazines		
	Piperidines	Dimethylamines	Piperazines
Examples:	Thioridazine NP-207 KS-24	Chlorpromazine	Prochlorperazine Perphenazine Trifluoperazine
Toxic effects on:			
Skin	–	+	–
Conjunctiva	–	+	–
Cornea	–	+	–
Lens	–	+	–
Retina	+	rare?	–

Piperidines. Thioridazine (Melleril) and NP-207 (piperidylchlorophenothiazine) have caused a pigmentary degeneration of the retina leading to impaired vision in dim light, reduced acuity, visual field constriction and a scattered fine pigmentary change through the fundus, which becomes coarse with time (Burian & Fletcher, 1958; Scott, 1963).

The dark adaption is impaired and the ERG (b-wave) amplitude is depressed. There is some uncertainty as to whether the piperidines produce skin, corneal and lens changes (Grant, 1974).

NP-207 was withdrawn soon after its introduction in 1954. Effects on vision were noted at doses of 0.4-0.8 g per day over 2-3 months, whereas doses below this did not cause problems over the same period (Table 13.6).

Table 13.6.   Toxic effects of NP-207.

Impaired vision in dim light
Reduced acuity
Field constriction
Macular and peripheral retinal pigmentation
Reduced dark adaptation
Depressed E.R.G.

Thioridazine produces retinotoxicity at massive daily doses usually over 1000 mg per day. Toxicity has been reported at below 700 mg per day. Toxic daily doses have ranged from about 700 mg per day to 2900 mg per day and have caused damage in periods ranging from 15 days to 3 years. Total doses range from 40 g to 1045 g (Grant, 1974).

Grant (1974) suggests that doses up to 600 mg per day are safe and that the range 600-800 mg per day is probably so. With doses of over 800 mg/day, periodic eye examination with inspection for pigmentary change and a fall in acuity should be made. The pigmentary change may precede the effect on vision, but in acute cases with large initial dosage, blurred vision may precede pigmentary change, though retinal oedema has been noted. In thioridazine toxicity, unlike chloroquine, there is no bull's-eye pigmentation and no ring scotoma.

The mechanism of retino-toxicity of NP-207 has been fully studied by Meier-Ruge (1969), who showed binding of the drug to choroidal melanin in the cat, similar to that shown by chloroquine and other phenothiazines (Potts, 1962). They found a toxic action on the rod ellipsoids accompanied by inhibition of ATP-ase and lactic dehydrogenase, and disruption of the outer segments, whose products were taken up into the retinal pigment epithelium. Another factor may be inhibition of oxidative phosphorylation secondary to blocking of flavine nucleotides.

Chlorpromazine in high dosage produces skin, cornea, lens and sometimes retino toxicity. A daily dose of 300 mg per day for a total dose of at least 500 g appears to be the minimum dose to produce ocular effects. (A dose of 160 mg daily for 9-12 years to total doses exceeding 500 g did not produce ocular toxicity in one group of patients (Sarin, Leopold & Winkelman, 1966), suggesting that both daily and total dose are important).

The incidence of skin and conjunctival pigmentation is probably similar (0.1-1%) and occurs only at the high dose level, a minimum of 800 mg per day for 20-24 months. The incidence of corneal and lens changes is higher, e.g. 20-35% of patients receiving over 500 mg daily over three years. The skin change darkens from a blue-grey to a purple hue over the exposed areas of face, neck and hands. The conjunctival grey-brown pigmentation is also in the exposed, interpalpebral conjunctiva (Bernstein, 1970).

Corneal deposits are interpalpebral, and biomicroscopically appear as central fine brownish-yellow or yellowish-white granules in deeper layers of the stroma, in Decemets membrane, and in and around endothelial cells (Goldstein, 1971). These changes may be associated with symptoms of haloes round lights, watering and photophobia (editorial, *British Medical Journal*, 1969). Corneal deposits appear at a total dose of between 500-1000 g (Goldstein, 1971).

The lens opacities precede the corneal changes and develop from a brown anterior capsular dusting in the pupillary zone, to a large stellate opacity and finally anterior polar cataract (Bernstein, 1970).

Chlorpromazine is a well-known photosensitizing agent. Absorption of light energy by the drug leads to the formation of highly reactive free radicals. This may be concerned in phototoxic damage to the lens or cornea, though this is still unproven. Binding to melanin may involve transfer of an electron from the chlorpromazine to the melanin polymer, to form a charge-transfer complex. Lüllmann *et al.* (1975) have suggested that chlorpromazine is another of those drugs capable of binding to phospholipid and producing intra-lysosomal storage of polar lipid.

Chloroquine

Chloroquine is a 4-aminoquinoline used in the treatment and prophyllaxis of malaria, and since the early 1950s used also in daily doses of 100-250 mg per day in the long-term treatment of such diseases as rheumatoid arthritis, discoid and systemic lupus and other conditions.

The chief features of chloroquine toxicity are keratopathy, retinopathy, and possibly effects on the lens (a flake-like posterior subcapsular lens opacity) and ciliary body (difficulty with accommodation) (Bernstein, 1970) (Table 13.7).

Table 13.7.   Ocular toxicity of chloroquine.

Clinical features of toxicity	
Keratopathy	
Retinopathy	Bull's-Eye Macular Pigmentation
	Late : optic atrophy
	vessel attenuation
	peripheral pigmentation
	Field defects
	central, pericentral, ring and
	bitemporal
	Colour vision defect: Late
	Disturbed E.R.G. and E.O.G.: Late
Lens opacities?	
Accommodative weakness?	

Monitoring for toxicity
Fundoscopy
Visual fields, especially to red targets
Photostress test
Retinal threshold test
Fluorescein angiography
E.R.G.; E.O.G.; colour vision

The keratopathy is not clearly dose-related. It may appear within two weeks of therapy and in less than 50% of patients are there any visual complaints. It consists of a vortex pattern in the corneal epithelium and a number of other drugs are capable of producing an identical pattern. The keratopathy disappears rapidly on withdrawing therapy.

The opacification of the epithelium may be another example of the toxic lipidosis proposed by Lüllman *et al.* (1975). Membranous lamellar inclusions have been observed in the corneal epithelium of patients treated with chloroquine and it is of interest that the same sort of vortex pattern is encountered in the corneae of patients with the genetically determined glycolipid storage disorder, Fabry's disease. It has been suggested that the tiny posterior lens opacities observed in 20-40% of patients on chloroquine are the human counterpart of the experimental chloroquine cataract in which myeloid bodies are also found.

Retinopathy may occur at a dose of 250 mg/day for a period of one year (100 g) but the incidence rises with increase in daily and total dose and duration of therapy. The majority of cases occur after 2-3 years of treatment but may occur as soon as seven months after the start of therapy, or as late as ten years. Incidence has ranged in various series, between 0.1 and 50%, according to dosage regimes and definition of retinopathy.

Like the phenothiazines, chloroquine shows a strong affinity for ocular melanin and is concentrated in the choroid and retinal pigment epithelium. This produces a gradual retinal degeneration which starts in the outer retinal layers. The earliest sign of retinal toxicity is increased macular pigmentation, leading to a classical 'bull's-eye' or target lesion. This is associated with visual disturbance and a central, pericentral or ring scotoma which may be detected in the earliest stages with a red field target.

The binding of chloroquine to melanin leads to an extremely slow release of the drug from the eye. This is thought to explain the continued development of the retinopathy and field loss after withdrawal of the drug, and onset of toxicity as late as five years after stopping the drug. Advanced toxicity can lead to total blindness.

Monitoring of objective and subjective features of retinal function is imperative to prevent severe and irreversible toxicity. The most sensitive tests are:
1. Identification of early macular pigmentation;
2. Visual field to the red target;
3. Retinal threshold tests;
4. Photostress test;
5. Electrodiagnosis.

Although a fall in EOG was thought to be an early sign of involvement of the retinal pigment epithelium (Kolb, 1965; Arden & Fogas, 1962) the EOG may on occasion be normal despite severe toxicity. The relationship of the ERG to the level of retinal toxicity is also erratic. The visual acuity, dark adaptation response and colour vision are not early indicators of toxicity. It has been suggested that fluorescein angiography may permit early detection of the macular disturbance.

Bernstein (1970) suggests a safe daily level of 250 mg per day in adults with periodic assessments every 3-6 months after the first year of therapy.

Chloroquine binding in tissues involves nucleic acid and nucleoprotein, as well as melanin. The binding to melanin may be a means by which a high concentration of chloroquine is maintained in the retina for a prolonged period. It is possible that the retinotoxic effects result in an inhibition of the capacity of melanin to inactivate potentially toxic photochemically induced free radicals in, say, the retinal pigment epithelium. Chloroquine is capable of inhibiting many intracellular enzymes, such as DNA polymerase, NADH-cytochrome reductase, and NADH-monodehydroascorbic acid transhydrogenase (Cohen & Yielding, 1963; Henkind, Carr & Rothfield, 1966).

Since melanin acts as a cationic exchange resin, binding of chloroquine is reduced at lowered pH. Although chloroquine excretion has been increased in animals receiving ammonium chloride, this therapy does not reduce chloroquine in the ocular tissues.

Clioquinol (5,7-dichloro-8-hydroxyquinoline)

In recent years attention has been drawn to the remarkable number of cases in Japan of subacute myelo-optico neuropathy (SMON), characterized by damage to the optic nerves, spinal tracts and peripheral nerves after taking unusually large amounts of the chlorinated hydroxyquinoline, clioquinol (Enterovioform) (Cavanagh, 1973).

The drug was used for treatment of chronic diarrhoea of bacterial or parasitic origin in larger doses and for longer periods in Japan than in other countries. Visual impairment occurs in about 40% of cases and ranges from complete blindness to a transient blurring (Tsubaki, Honma & Hoshi, 1971). It is estimated that some 10 000 cases of this illness occurred in recent years in patients taking doses ranging from 0.6 to 1.6 g daily. Neurological effects are shown when such quantities are taken for more than 14 days.

When the sale of clioquinol in Japan was banned in 1970, there was a dramatic cessation of new cases. Although there does not seem to be a satisfactory animal model for this intoxication, and there have been suggestions that the condition is due to a viral infection (Inoue, Nishibe & Nakamura, 1971), it appears more likely that SMON is a toxic disorder, possibly modified by other environmental factors.

Digitalis

The toxic action of digitalis on the eye is probably at the level of the photoreceptors rather than the ganglion cells of the retina.

Up to 10-25% of patients on digitalis may experience visual symptoms of toxicity, which may develop after weeks or years of therapy. Though the ocular aspects are not serious, this has become of increasing interest in parallel with the interest in systemic toxicity of digitalis and bioavailability of digitalis preparations.

Typical disturbance of colour perception comprises a tinging of perceived objects with a green or yellowish hue. Objects may appear to be glittering or frosted, and there may be flashing lights (photopsiae), scintillating scotomata (teichopsiae), or photophobia. There may be blurred vision, difficulty with reading and diminished acuity. These complaints may diminish towards the end of the day (Henkes, 1972).

Although small central scotomata have been recorded with digitalis intoxication, Robertson, Hollenhorst & Callahan (1966) have recorded an elevation of dark adaptation in an area 5° from fixation, and believe that toxicity is at the level of the photoreceptors, with cone function affected more than rod function. These were reversible asymptomatic changes, developing after 2 to 4 weeks of therapy.

In a recent instance of digitalis/digitoxin overdose, affecting 179 patients, 95% of patients suffered visual symptoms and where colour vision was examined nearly all subjects showed disturbed colour perception (dyschromatopsia) of protan type, by the Farnsworth Munsell test (Lely & van Enter 1970). At the MRC Unit of Pharmacology at Oxford, the value of colour vision testing in monitoring for toxicity is being explored and preliminary studies suggest that the degree of defect may parallel other indices of systemic intoxication, such as plasma digitalis levels, red cell digoxin binding, intra-erythrocyte sodium concentration, and ^{86}Rb transport (Aronson & Ford, 1978).

Toxic amblyopia

A number of drugs are capable of damaging the optic nerve or pre-geniculate visual pathways, or have their effect on the ganglion cells of the retina so that optic atrophy may finally supervene. They are described under the general term of toxic amblyopia. These toxic optic neuropathies commonly present with visual disturbances or alteration of the visual fields without fundus abnormality, in chronic intoxications, and may be reversible to some extent on withdrawing therapy. This is referred to as retrobulbar neuritis though the inflammatory element may be small, or conjectural.

The field defect may comprise a central scotoma, as with chlorpropamide, clomiphene and disulfiram toxicity or peripheral constriction of the field, as with organic arsenical, isoniazid and quinine. With chloramphenicol and pheniprazine, a mixed picture may occur (Table 13.8).

Some toxic amblyopias may be associated with disc swelling (unrelated to raised intracranial pressure), and may be diagnosed as papillitis.

The toxic amblyopias may show a dyschromatopsia with a defect to red; the ERG is generally normal.

In the majority of cases the incidence of toxic amblyopia with a given drug is low, but with, for instance, Ethambutol, the incidence was high enough to make monitoring of therapy mandatory, and to establish schemes of safe dosage.

Ethambutol

Ethambutol is a drug of choice in the treatment of pulmonary tuberculosis.

Drug toxicity

Table 13.8. Optic nerve damage — selected systemic drugs.

Drug	Disc* swelling	Retro-bulbar neuritis	Scotoma Central	Scotoma Peripheral	Optic atrophy
Arsenicals–organic				+	+
Broxyquinoline					+
Chloramphenicol		+	+	+	+
Chlorpropamide		+	+		
Clomiphene			+		+
Disulfiram		+	+		
Emetine	(+)		+	+	
Ethambutol	(+)	+	+	+	+
Ethyl alcohol			+		
Ethyl hydrocupreine				+	+
Hexamethonium					+
Isoniazid	(+)	+		+	+
Octamoxin		+	+		+
Pheniprazine		+	+	+	+
Piperidylchlorophenothiazine	(+)			+	
Plasmocid			+		+
Quinine				+	+
Streptomycin			+		+
Sulphonamides			+		

*Excluding benign intracranial hypertension

(Grant 1974)

Early experience with the racemic mixture demonstrated ocular toxicity in 44% of patients on a regime of 40-100 mg/kg/day (Carr & Henkind, 1962). The dextro-rotatory isomer is regarded as less toxic and is the form in current use.

Leibold (1966) found toxicity in 18.6% of patients receiving 35 mg/kg/day, and 2.25% in a group receiving 25 mg/kg/day. The delay in onset of toxic signs has varied from 139 days to 2 years at this level.

The field defect may be axial (with involvement of the papillo-macular bundle and a dyschromatopsia involving the sense to green more than red) or it may be periaxial, when no dyschromatopsia may occur. The former is more common at higher dose levels. Sometimes a bitemporal defect suggests chiasmal involvement.

Recovery of visual function after withdrawing therapy may take two to four months, or as long as two years, but vision may initially deteriorate after stopping therapy and recovery may not be complete in a small proportion (Leibold, 1971; Bronte-Stewart, Pettigrew & Foulds, 1976).

Demyelination of optic nerve, chiasm and tract has been produced in experimental studies in monkeys (Schmidt, 1966) and in chiasm and optic nerve in the rat (Lessell, 1976).

The recommended safe dose is 15 mg/kg/day and it is recommended that patients be assessed at two month intervals. Bronte-Stewart *et al.* (1976) found five patients with toxicity on the standard regime of 25 mg/kg/day for two months, followed by 15 mg/kg/day.

Ethambutol is highly retino-toxic in dogs, possibly by reason of an ability to chelate zinc, which is in high concentration in the dog tapetum, but no such mechanism has been incriminated as a cause of toxic amblyopia in man.

Isoniazid

Another antituberculous agent, isoniazid, may produce toxic amblyopia in addition to the more frequently observed peripheral polyneuritis. Toxicity is more common in malnourished individuals and alcoholics (see Chapter 4). A variety of field defects have been encountered, in doses ranging from 200 to 900 mg/day with onset from 10 days to 2 months after start of therapy.

Isoniazid is detoxicated in the liver by acetylation, and the inactive conjugates so produced are rapidly excreted in the urine. It has been shown that the ability to inactivate isoniazid is genetically determined (Boone & Woodward, 1953) and that only the 'slow' inactivators develop the polyneuritis, due to the fact that the drug persists in the body at higher levels for a longer period (see Chapter 3).

The neuropathy is thought to be due to interference with vitamin B_6 metabolism and the administration of pyridoxal or pyridoxamine has a clear-cut protective effect in animals and man against neuropathy (Biehl & Vilter, 1954).

Isoniazid forms a hydrazone by condensing with pyridoxal phosphate and interferes with the enzyme (pyridoxal phosphate kinase), which phosphorylates pyridoxal, both directly and through the action of the hydrazone. This deprives affected tissues of the cofactor required for a variety of decarboxylation and transamination reactions.

It is possible that *L*-penicillamine, which can occasionally cause optic atrophy, may work through a similar mechanism (Holz & Palm, 1964) and that the optic neuropathy associated with monoamine oxidase inhibitors is also dependent on pyridoxine deficiency.

Disulfiram

Methanol toxic amblyopia is abrupt in onset and characterized by retinal and disc oedema in the acute stage and later, optic atrophy. The patient is totally blind, and later shows a variable degree of recovery. Ingestion of as little as 8 ml methanol may cause blindness, while as little as 30 ml may be lethal. Retinal damage is due to a toxic effect on the ganglion cells of the retina, probably resulting from the accumulation of oxidation products of methanol, such as formaldehyde (Potts, 1962). Experimentally and clinically, treatment with ethanol may have a protective effect (Roe, 1969).

A reversible retrobulbar neuritis is described in patients taking disulfiram and peripheral neuropathy also occurs in patients taking this drug.

This has been attributed to the effects of accumulated acetaldehyde, whose breakdown is inhibited by disulfiram which acts on alcohol dehydrogenase in the liver. However, it may have a direct toxic action on nerve through its degradation products diethyldithiocarbamide and carbon disulphide. It has been suggested that these compounds may chelate polyvalent metal ions, copper and zinc, or reduce the availability of pyridoxal (Thorne & Ludwig, 1962; Vasák & Kopecky, 1967).

Tobacco-amblyopia

In certain toxic amblyopias there is a focal depression of the central and caeco-central areas of the visual field due to an involvement of those nerve fibres arising from the macular region and the zone between macula and disc, the papillo-macular bundle.

The optic neuropathy associated with smoking, tobacco amblyopia, is of this variety.

Tobacco amblyopia is usually associated with the smoking of heavy pipe tobaccos, but may follow heavy cigarette smoking. Its occurrence is in part related to the amount of tobacco smoked.

Foulds uses the following strict criteria of tobacco amblyopia:
1.   Bilateral reduction of central vision;
2.   Centro-caecal field defect most marked for red and green targets;
3.   An acquired red/green colour defect;
4.   No fundus pathology to explain the defect.
(Bronte-Stewart *et al.*, 1976), though it is evident that lesser degrees of amblyopia exist. Temporal pallor of the discs may be observed, and rarely overt atrophy.

Boerhaabe first described, in 1749, the association between smoking and amblyopia, Caroll (1944) showed that visual improvement would occur despite persistent smoking with an adequate intake of the B group vitamins, but that B_1 alone was not sufficient. Leishman (1951) drew attention to an association between pernicious anaemia and tobacco amblyopia. Heaton (1958) showed a statistically lower level of serum B_{12} in thirteen patients with tobacco amblyopia, suggesting a role for vitamin B_{12} in protecting against this toxic neuropathy.

Wokes (1958) advanced the view that the toxic agent in tobacco is cyanide, which is present in high concentrations in tobacco smoke. Smith (1968) suggested that hydroxycobalamine detoxifies cyanide and is converted into cyanocobalamine in the process.

It appears that cyanide is also detoxicated in the liver by conjugation with sulphur-containing amino acids to produce thiocyanate, its main detoxifying product which is found in both serum and urine (Stoa, 1957). One liver pathway to produce thiocyanate involves the enzyme rhodanase. This enzyme may well be inactivated by alcohol.

Vitamin B_{12} appears to be required (as well as folate) for the interconversion of the sulphur-containing amino acids. This may be a regulatory factor influencing the availability of sulphur donors involved in cyanide detoxication. Vitamin B_{12} may also be required to maintain sulphydryl compounds in the reduced state (Dubnoff, 1950a, b, 1951). In vitamin B_{12} deficiency, a decrease in the activity of the enzyme glutathione reductase (Biswas & Johnson, 1964) results in lowered concentrations of reduced glutathione in the blood. These levels are restored by treatment with vitamin B_{12} (Register, 1954).

In smokers without amblyopia, the levels of thiocyanate in blood and urine are higher than in age-matched non-smokers. In tobacco amblyopia these thiocyanate levels are reduced. This has suggested a failure to detoxicate cyanide. Levels of red cell glutathione are also reduced (Pettigrew, Fell & Chisholm, 1972) as are levels of sulphur amino acids (Bronte-Stewart *et al.*, 1976).

Tobacco amblyopia can be effectively treated by stopping smoking, by intra-muscular or oral hydroxycobalamine with or without stopping smoking, or by adding sulphur-containing amino acids to the diet (such as cystine and perhaps methionine). These measures result in improved visual acuity, and colour vision and resolution of the field defect. Resolution is associated with a rise in levels of thiocyanate in serum and urine, and a rise in red-cell glutathione.

It is therefore postulated, particularly by the Glasgow group, that tobacco amblyopia results from the conjunction of two events: an increased cyanide intake from tobacco smoke, and a shortage of sulphur donors involved in cyanide detoxication. The latter could arise in a number of ways:

1. Dietary deficiency of protein (30% of tobacco amblyopia patients (Bronte-Stewart *et al.*, 1976). These patients tend to be undernourished, and from the lower end of the social scale;
2. Deficiency of vitamin B_{12} affecting interconversion of sulphur amino acids and availability of sulphydryl radicals. (This may arise by malabsorption or dietary deficiency).

Despite the excellent studies demonstrating the relationship between cyanide metabolism, detoxification and tobacco amblyopia, it is still not clear what the cause of the optic neuropathy is.

There is no evidence of raised serum cyanide levels in tobacco amblyopia patients, despite the lowered thiocyanate levels. Animal experiments have only produced optic nerve demyelination at near-lethal doses of cyanide (Smith & Duckett, 1965; Lessell, 1976) and a primate model of cyanide intoxication simulating tobacco amblyopia, has not yet been produced.

It has been suggested that the existence of a faulty thiocyanate detoxication mechanism results in a greater proportion of cyanide being converted into other, potentially toxic products through different metabolic pathways. 2-Amino-4-thiazolidine carboxylic acid is such a compound, and it is possible that this may interfere with myelination and myelin turnover through its action on choline synthesis (Foulds, Chisholm & Pettigrew, 1974).

Implications of the cyanide hypothesis. The cyanide toxicity hypothesis implies that other factors which increase intake of cyanide or disturb detoxication should be capable of simulating the neuropathy of tobacco amblyopia. A similar mechanism probably explains the amblyopia associated with the eating of cassava in parts of Africa. The delivery of cyanide is dependent on the manner in which the fruit is cooked. Although the association between high tobacco consumption and high alcohol intake with so-called 'tobacco-alcohol' amblyopia is unclear, it is noteworthy that there is a high cyanide content in beer.

Occasional patients with tobacco amblyopia show low folate levels. It may be that the requirement of folate for interconversion of sulphur amino acids plays a role here and it could explain the occurrence of optic neuropathy resulting from the use of folate antagonists such as Epanutin or cytotoxic drugs (Bronte-Stewart *et al.*, 1976). Pyridoxal phosphate is also involved in the interconversion of sulphur amino acids, which may explain some successes claimed for B vitamins other than B_{12} in treating tobacco amblyopia.

Tobacco-alcohol amblyopia. The association of tobacco amblyopia with alcohol intake is unclear. Certainly the neuropathy may occur in non-drinkers (about 50% of tobacco amblyopia patients in the studies by Foulds *et al.* (1969, 1970) were drinkers; see also Sedan & Farnarier (1965)).

Harrington (1962) suggests that there is no such thing as a toxic alcohol (ethyl) amblyopia, but that the amblyopia associated with chronic alcoholism is a nutritional amblyopia.

Table 13.9.   Ocular toxicity of systemic drugs. Guidelines for monitoring.

Agent	Toxicity	Safe dose		Potentially toxic dose	
		Daily	Total	Daily	Total
Chloramphenicol	Optic neuritis		19.5g[1]		100g
Chlorpromazine	Cataract + corneal pigmentation		500g	300mg to a total of:	500g[2]
Chloroquine sulphate phosphate	Retinopathy			200mg[3] 250mg[3]	100-300g[4]
Corticosteroid Prednisolone	Cataract	10mg[5]			3.5g
Ethambutol		15mg/kg[6]		25mg/kg	
Thioridazine		600mg		600-800mg[4]	40-1045g[4]

As the toxic manifestations of drugs are often dependent upon the duration of treatment as well as daily or total dosage and other factors, the above dose levels represent opinions selected from the literature and where not expressed in terms of body weight, should be taken to reflect adult regimes.

Notes

1. One report of toxicity at this dosage; usually rare under 100g total (see Grant, 1974).
2. Bernstein (1971).
3. Toxicity is rare at this dosage and may take years to develop (Grant, 1974).
4. Bernstein (1971).
5. Spaeth & von Sallmann (1966).
6. But see Bronte-Stewart *et al.* (1976). Five patients developed toxicity while receiving 15mg/kg *after* an initial dose of 25mg/kg/day for two months.

Conclusions

The occurrence of toxic reactions in the eye may depend on the delivery of the drug in toxic concentrations to a vulnerable tissue site.

This in turn will depend on dosage and the idiosyncrasies of systemic and local detoxication of the drug, and on the existence of penetration barriers to entry into the tissue. Further determinants of a toxic effect may be the nutritional state of the patient, and peculiarities of metabolism of specific tissues. In many instances the biochemical pathways involved in toxic action are well known, but their application to the specific situation of ocular toxicity may be unclear. In other instances the mechanism of toxicity may be merely conjectural.

Experience has taught us when to eliminate potentially toxic drugs from our therapeutic armamentarium, when to modify the use of other drugs and how to monitor for toxic effects where this is feasible (Tables 13.1 and 13.9). It has also taught us to be watchful for adverse reactions at all times.

References

Abrams, D. and Majzoub, U. (1970). *Br. J. Ophthal.*, 54, 59.
Amos, H.E., Brigden, W.D. and McKerron, R.A. (1975). *Br. med. J.*, 1, 589.
Arden, G. and Fojas, M. (1962). *Arch. Ophthal.*, 68, 369.
Armaly, M.F. (1967). *Arch. Ophthal.*, 77, 747.
Armaly, M.F., Montavicius, B.F. and Saygeh, R.E. (1968). *Arch. Ophthal.*, 80, 354.
Aronson, J.K. and Ford, A.P. 7th International Congress of Pharmacology, Paris. 1978. Abstract 2894.
Axelsson, U. (1969a). *Acta Ophthal.*, 47, (Suppl.) 102.
Axelsson, U. (1969b). *Acta Ophthal.*, 47, 1049.
Axelsson, U. and Holmberg, A. (1966). *Acta Ophthal.*, 44, 421.
Becker, B. (1964). *Am. J. Ophthal.*, 58, 872.
Becker, B. and Hahn, K.A. (1964). *Am. J. Ophthal.*, 57, 543.
Becker, B. and Cotlier, E. (1965). *Invest. Ophthal.*, 4, 117.
Bedrossian, R.H. and Eriksen, S.P. (1969). *Arch. Ophthal.*, 81, 184.
Benedek, G.B. (1971). *Appl. Optics*, 10, 459.
Bernstein, H.N. (1970). *Int. Ophthal.*, 10, 553.
Bernstein, H.N. and Schwartz, B. (1962). *Arch. Ophthal.*, 68, 742.
Biehl, J.P. and Vilter, R.W. (1954). *Proc. Soc. exp. Biol. Med.*, 85, 389.
Bihari, M. and Grossman, B.J. (1968). *Am. J. Dis. Childh.*, 116, 604.
Biswas, D.K. and Connor Johnson, B. (1964). *Arch. Biochem. Biophys.*, 104. 375.
Black, R.L., Oglesby, R.B., von Sallmann, L. and Bunim, J.J. (1960). *J. Am. med. Ass.*, 174, 166.
Boerhaabe, A. (1749). *Les Maladies des Yeux*. Paris: Huartet Moreaux Fils.
Boone, I.U. and Woodward, K.T. (1953). *Proc. Soc. exp. Biol. Med.*, 85, 389.
Bronte-Stewart, J., Pettigrew, A.R. and Foulds, W.S. (1976). *Trans. Ophthal. Soc. U.K.*, 96, 355.
Brown, P., Baddeley, H., Read, A.E., Davies, J.D. and McGarry, J. (1974). *Lancet*, 2, 1477.
Burian, H. and Fletcher, M. (1958). *Arch. Ophthal.*, 60, 612.
Cavanagh, J.B. (1973). *Critical Rev. Toxicol.*, 2, 365.
Carroll, F.D. (1944). *Am. J. Ophthal.*, 27, 847.
Carr, R.E. and Hendkind, P. (1962). *Arch. Ophthal.*, 67, 566.
Clayden, J.R. (1975). *Br. med. J.*, 2, 557.
Crews, S.J. (1963). *Br. med. J.*, 1, 1644.
Cohen, S. and Yielding, Y. (1963). *Am. Rheum. Ass.*, Dec. 6-7.
Cotlier, E. and Becker, B. (1965). *Invest. Ophthal.*, 4, 806.
Davidson, S.I. (1974). *Trans. Ophthal. Soc. U.K.*, 94, 487.

De Roetth, A. (1966). *Am. J. Ophthal.*, 62, 619.

Dikshit, S.K. and Avasthi, P.N. (1965). *Indian J. Pediat.*, 32, 93.

Drance, S.M. (1969). *Symposium on Ocular Therapy*, 4.

Dubnoff, J.W. (1950a). *Fedn Proc.*, 9, 166.

Dubnoff, J.W. (1950b). *Arch. Biochem.*, 27, 466.

Dubnoff, J.W. (1951). *Fedn Proc.*, 10, 178.

Felix, R.H., Ive, F.A. and Dahl, M.G.C. (1974). *Br. med. J.*, 4, 321.

Foulds, W.S. (1969). *Trans. Ophthal. Soc. U.K.*, 89, 125.

Foulds, W.S., Chisholm, I.A. and Pettigrew, A.R. (1974). *Br. J. Ophthal.*, 58, 386.

Foulds, W.S. (1976). In *Medical Ophthalmology*, Editor: Rose, C. London: Chapman & Hall.

Foulds, W.S., Chisholm, I.A., Bronte-Stewart, J. and Reid, H.C.R. (1970). *Trans Ophthal. Soc. U.K.*, 90, 739.

Frandsen, E. (1965). *Acta Ophthal.*, 43, 605.

Galloway, N.R. (1975). In *Ophthalmic Electrodiagnosis*. Editor: Saunders, W.B. London.

Gehring, P.J. and Buerge, J.F. (1969). *Toxic. appl. Pharmac.*, 15, 574.

Giles, C.L., Mason, G.L., Duff, I.F. and McLean, J.A. (1962). *J. Am. med. Ass.*, 182, 719.

Goldstein, J.H. (1971). *Int. Ophthal. Clin.*, 2, 2.

Grant, W.M. (1974). *Toxicology of the Eye*, 2nd Ed. Springfield, Ill., Charles Thomas.

Harrington, D.O. (1962). *Am. J. Ophthal.*, 53, 967.

Harris, J.E. and Gruber, L. (1969). *Docum. Ophthal.*, 26, 324.

Harris, J.E. (1966). *Trans. Am. Ophthal. Soc.*, 64, 675.

Harris, J.E. and Becker, B. (1965). *Invest. Ophthal.*, 4, 709.

Harrison, R. (1960). *Am. J. Ophthal.*, 50, 153.

Havre, D.C. (1965). *Arch. Ophthal.*, 73, 818.

Heaton, J.M. (1958). *Lancet*, 2, 286.

Henkes, H.E. (1972). *Drug Induced Diseases*, Vol. 4, p. 524. Editors: Meyler, L. and Peck, H.M. Amsterdam Excerpta Medica.

Henkind, P., Carr, R. and Rothfield, N. (1966). Reported at *Annual Meeting of Rheumatism Association*. Cincinatti, Ohio.

Hockwin, O., Blum, G., Korte, I., Murata, T., Radetzki, W. and Rast, F. (1971). *Ophthal. Res.*, 2, 143.

Holt, P.J.H., and Waddington, E. (1975). *Br. med. J.*, 2, 539.

Holz, P. and Palm, D. (1964). *Pharmac. Rev.*, 16, 113.

Horner, W.D. (1942). *Arch. Ophthal.*, 27, 1097.

Ikeda, H. (1976). In *Medical Ophthalmology*, Editor: Rose, C. London: Chapman & Hall.

Inoue, Y.K., Nishibe, G. and Nakamura, Y. (1971). *Lancet*, 1, 853.

Kalina, R.E. (1969). *Arch. Ophthal.*, 81, 788.

Kirby, T.J. (1967). *Trans. Am. Ophthal. Soc.*, 65, 493.

Koellner, H. (1912). *Die Storungen des Farbensinnes, ihre Klinische Bedeutung und ihre Diagnose*. Berlin: Karger.

Kolb, H. (1965). *Br. J. Ophthal.*, 49, 573.

Kolker, A.E. and Becker, B. (1968). *Arch. Ophthal.*, 79 (5), 552.

Kreibig, W. (1954). *Klin. Mbl. Augenheilk*, 125, 39.

Laties, A.M. (1969). *Amer. J. Ophthal.*, 68, 848.

Leibold, J.E. (1966). *Ann. N.Y. Acad. Sci.*, 135, 904.

Leibold, J.E. (1971). In *Side Effects of Drugs in Ophthalmology*. International Ophthalmology Clinics, Vol. 11, No. 2. Boston: Little Brown.

Lely, A.H. and van Enter, C.H.J. (1970). *Br. med. J.*, 3, 737.

Leopold, I.H. and Barnert, A.H. (1967). *Adv. Ophthal.*, 18, 1.

Lessell, S. (1976). *Invest. Ophthal.*, 15, 765.

Lüllmann, H., Lüllmann-Rauch, R. and Wassermann, O. (1975). *Critical Rev. Toxicol.*, 4, 185.

Maurice, D.M. (1963). *Exp. Eye Res.*, 2, 33.

Meier-Ruge, W. (1969). *Ophthalmologica Addit. Ad.*, 158, 561.

Michon, J. and Kinoshita, J.H. (1968). *Arch. Ophthal.*, 79, 611.

Morton, W.R., Drance, S.M. and Fairclough, M. (1969). *Am. J. Ophthal.*, 68, 1003.

Oglesby, R.B., Black, R.L., von Sallmann, L. and Bunim, J.J. (1961). *Arch. Ophthal.*, 66, 519.

Oglesby, R.B., Black, R.L., von Sallmann, L. and Bunim, J.J. (1961). *Arch. Ophthal.*, 66, 625.

Oppelt, W.W., White, E.D. and Halpert, E.S. (1969). *Invest. Ophthal.*, 8, 535.
Oshima, T. (1968). *Acta Soc. Ophthal. Jap.*, 72, 1753.
Patterson, C.A. (1971). In *Side Effects of Drugs in Ophthalmology*. International Ophthal-mology, Vol. 11, No. 2. Boston: Little Brown.
Pettigrew, A.R., Fell, G.S. and Chisholm, I.A. (1972). *Exp. Eye Res.*, 14, 87.
Podos, S.M., Becker, B. and Morton, W.R. (1966). *Am. J. Ophthal.*, 62, 1039.
Potts, A.M. (1962). *Invest. Ophthal.*, 1, 290.
Rahi, A.H.S. and Garner, A. (1976). *Br. J. Ophthal.*, 60, 684.
Rahi, A.H.S., Chapman, C.M., Garner, A. and Wright, P. (1976). *Br. J. Ophthal.*, 60, 312.
Register, U.D. (1954). *J. biol. Chem.*, 206, 705.
Robertson, D.M., Hollenhorst, R.W. and Callahan, J.A. (1966). *Arch. Ophthal.*, 76, 640, 852.
Roe, O. (1969). *Trans. Ophthal. Soc. U.K.*, 89, 235.
Sams, W.M. and Jordan, R.E. (1971). *Br. J. Derm.*, 84, 7.
Sarin, L., Leopold, I. and Winkelman, N. (1966). *J. Am. med. Ass.*, 198. 789.
Schmidt, I.G. (1966). *Ann. N.Y. Acad. Sci.*, 135, 759.
Schwenk, V.D. (1967). *Z. Rheumaforsch.*, 26, 153.
Scott, A.W. (1963). *Arch. Ophthal.*, 70, 775.
Sedan, J. and Farnarier, G. (1965). *Arch. Ophthal. (Paris)*, 25 (1), 53.
Seydel, J.K. and Wasserman, O. (1973). *Chim. Ther.*, p. 427.
Shaffer, R.N. and Hetherington, J., Jr. (1966). *Am. J. Ophthal.*, 62, 613.
Siegel, I.M. and Smith, B.F. (1967). *Arch. Ophthal.*, 77, 8.
Slansky, H.H., Kolbert, G. and Gartner, S. (1967). *Arch. Ophthal.*, 77, 579.
Smith, E.L. (1968). *Pl. Fds. Hum. Nutr.*, 1, 7.
Smith, A.D.M. and Duckett, S. (1965). *Br. J. exp. Path.*, 46, 612.
Spaeth, G.L. and von Sallmann, L. (1966). *Int. Ophthal. Clin.*, 6, 915.
Stoa, K.F. (1957). Medisinsk rekke no. 2 University of Bergen Arbok 1957.
Streiff, E.B. (1964). *Ophthalmologica*, 147, 143.
Tarkkanen, A. and Karjalainen, K. (1966). *Acta Ophthal.*, 44, 932.
Theodore, F.H. (1953). *J. Am. med. Ass.*, 151, 25.
Thorne, G.D. and Ludwig, R.A. (1962). *The Dithiocarbamates and Related Compounds*. Amsterdam: Excerpta Medica Foundation, Elsevier.
Tsubaki, T., Honma, Y. and Hoshi, M. (1971). *Lancet*, 1, 696.
Valerio, M., Carones, A.V. and De Poli, A. (1965). *Boll. Oculist*, 44, 127.
Vasák, V. and Kopecky, J. (1967). In *Toxicology of Carbon Disulphide*, Editors: Brieger, H. and Teisinger, J. Amsterdam: Excerpta Medica Foundation, Elsevier.
Von Sallmann, L., Grimes, P. and Collins, E. (1963). *Arch. Ophthal.*, 70, 522.
Wokes, F. (1958). *Lancet*, 2, 526.
Wood, D.C., Sweet, D., Smith, J.C. and van Dolah, J. (1967). *Ann. N.Y. Acad. Sci.*, 141, 346.
Wright, P. (1974). *Br. med. J.*, 2, 560.
Wright, P. (1975). *Br. med. J.*, 1, 595.

14. Toxic effects of compounds on the pulmonary system

M. L'Estrange Orme

Introduction

The pulmonary system may be damaged by a variety of compounds and is especially vulnerable to damage by compounds inhaled in the air. Similar principles apply to the adverse effects of drugs and to the damage produced by other compounds. In this chapter, therefore, the effects of both drugs and non-drugs on the pulmonary system will be considered.

Adverse reactions due to drugs

Recent concern over the possible harmful effects of drugs has led to a much closer examination of the way in which such reports are collected. No longer is it satisfactory to rely on a patient reporting a toxic effect without prompting. Most studies now rely on direct questioning of patients to identify all possible adverse effects. The Boston collaborative drug surveillance programme was started to study this problem and a typical programme is shown in Table 14.1. Patients in an Israeli hospital (1239) were compared with 11 891 patients in a number of hospitals in Boston, USA. Adverse reactions were seen in 28% of patients and in 9% of drug exposures in Israel; similar figures for the Boston sample were 27% and 5% respectively.

Table 14.1. Incidence of adverse drug reactions in hospitals in Israel and the USA.

	Israel		USA
Average number of drug exposures per patients	6.3		8.8
Adverse reactions per patient per drug exposure	28% 9%		27% 5%
Drug-attributed deaths		0.44%	
Hospitalization due to drugs	5.9%		6.7%

Deaths attributed to drugs occurred in 0.44% of patients, while in about 6% of patients, hospital admission had been the direct result of an adverse drug reaction (Levy *et al.*, 1973). These and similar results show that adverse reactions to drugs do contribute significantly to the amount of illness in society, although this is more related to the extensive use of drugs than to their intrinsic toxic potential (Jick, 1974).

Drug-induced lung disease has been the subject of a number of recent reviews and as a result a number of useful classifications have been suggested (Davies, 1976; Lippman, 1977). One of the most useful is that put forward by Brewis (1977) and shown in Table 14.2.

Table 14.2. Compounds causing damage to pulmonary systems.

Industrial and occupational exposure
Air pollution
Poisons – e.g. Paraquat
Drugs – effect on bronchi and airways
    Pulmonary vasculature
    Lung parenchyma
    Pleural space
    Mediastinum
    Respiratory muscles and control

Adverse drug effects on bronchi and airways

The most common type of adverse drug reaction on the airways is that of obstruction of the airways, resulting in the development of asthma. The pharmacological control of bronchial smooth muscle tone is illustrated in Figure 14.1. The mediators involved include histamine, S.R.S. A, brady-kinin and prostaglandins. Drug-induced asthma may arise from a wide variety of drugs, by five possible mechanisms: (1) drugs that are themselves antigens, (2) drugs that cause release of mediators, (3) drugs that are themselves mediators, (4) drugs that affect autonomic receptors, and (5) drugs that affect the metabolism or action of other drugs used in asthma.

1. Drugs that are antigenic. Some substances used in medicine are directly antigenic and may result in either immediate or delayed broncho-constriction due to either type I or type III hypersensitivity. Intradermal injection of suspected allergens, used in the diagnosis of extrinsic asthma, may provoke severe asthma, as may the nasal insufflation of pituitary snuff for the treatment of diabetes insipidus. Penicillins, in particular, may cause drug-induced anaphylaxis, and asthma and laryngeal oedema are life-threatening components of this reaction. Most patients showing this reaction have previously been exposed to penicillin, and the antigen appears to be an impurity in the injected penicillin preparation (Garrod, Lambert & O'Grady, 1973). Penicillin should not be given to patients who have had even slight reactions in the past. Similar reactions may occur with other antibiotics such as cephalosporins.

2. Drugs that may release mediators. All aerosols may trigger a reflex, vagally mediated bronchoconstriction which can usually be blocked by

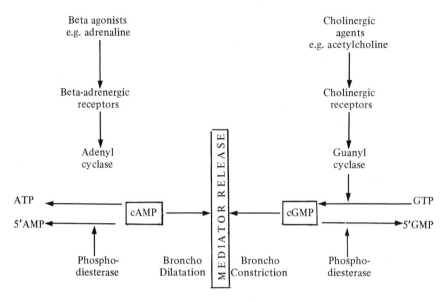

Fig. 14.1.   Model of pharmacological mediation of bronchodilation and bronchoconstriction (cAMP is cyclic adenosine monophosphate, and cGMP is cyclic guanosine monophosphate.)

atropine. Iodine-containing contrast media used in X-ray examinations, or iodine-containing drugs, may induce a syndrome known as iodism, in which obstruction of the airways, together with collapse, purpura and rhinorrhoea, may occur. It is thought to be due to the release of histamine.

Asthma may develop in sensitive individuals about half an hour after the ingestion of acetylsalicylic acid (aspirin) and is accompanied by flushing and rhinorrhoea. The attacks may be mild or severe and appear to be associated with late onset asthma in individuals with nasal polyposis (Samter & Beers, 1967). Such patients may be sensitive to other analgesics such as indomethacin and pentazocine but not usually to sodium salicylate. The mechanism of this adverse effect is unknown, but appears to be associated with drugs that have anti-inflammatory properties, thought to be due to inhibition of prostaglandin synthetase activity. The lung contains a bronchodilator prostaglandin (E_1 and E_2) and a bronchoconstrictor prostaglandin (F_{2a}) and it may be that the balance between these prostaglandins is disturbed by aspirin. Exercise-induced asthma may be improved by therapy with aspirin (*British Medical Journal*, 1973).

3. *Drugs that are mediators themselves.* This group of drugs comprises only histamine, which may be given in tests of gastric acidity, and prostaglandins, which have a number of therapeutic uses in the obstetric field.

4. *Drugs that affect autonomic receptors.* These drugs, like those in group 3, can be expected to produce airways obstruction to a greater or lesser extent in all patients given the drug, unlike drugs in groups 1 and 2. Cholinergic drugs may provoke asthma, especially in patients with labile asthma, such agents include carbachol, given to promote bladder contractility, and neostigmine, used in the treatment of myasthenia gravis. Asthma

is more commonly seen with the use of beta-adrenoreceptor-blocking drugs, because these drugs interfere with the bronchodilation produced by adrenalin. Propranolol, a non-selective beta-blocking drug, will produce an increase in airways resistance in all patients, but this is of clinical importance only in patients with a previous history of airways obstruction. Selective beta-blocking drugs (e.g. atenolol or metoprolol) and non-selective beta-blocking drugs with intrinsic sympathomimetic activity (e.g. oxprenolol, pindolol) are perhaps less likely to produce this effect, but all beta-blocking drugs should be used with caution in patients with a history of asthma or chronic bronchitis.

Isoprenaline is a pure beta-adrenergic agonist used in the treatment of patients with asthma. However, after prolonged use, resistance to the effects of isoprenaline may be noted with rebound bronchoconstriction (Paterson *et al.*, 1968; Conolly *et al.*, 1971). Between 1959 and 1966 there was a dramatic increase in the death rate from asthma in the UK (Speizer, Doll & Heaf, 1968) and analysis of the figures led to the suggestion that the use of pressurized aerosols (usually containing a higher than normal dose of isoprenaline) might be responsible. The mechanisms behind these adverse effects are probably complex. Overdosage of isoprenaline may have led to cardiac arrhythmias, particularly if resistance to the bronchodilatory action of isoprenaline occurred and the fluorocarbons in the aerosols may have sensitized the myocardium to the arrhythmic effects of isoprenaline.

5. *Drug interactions.* The regular use of phenobarbitone may reduce the therapeutic effects of corticosteroid drugs used to control asthma. This is due to the enzyme-inducing effect of phenobarbitone, which results in a lowering of the plasma concentration of the corticosteroid (Brooks *et al.*, 1972).

Adverse drug effects on pulmonary vasculature

Pulmonary thromboembolism. Venous thrombosis is known to be associated with the use of the combined oral contraceptive steroid preparations. The risk of venous thrombosis is increased some five- or six-fold in women taking oral contraceptives and is likely to occur in one in every 2000 women taking these drugs (Vessey & Doll, 1969; Royal College of General Practitioners, 1974). The risk of venous thrombosis with the subsequent development of pulmonary embolism is related to the dose of oestrogen used, and since 1970 all oral contraceptive steroid preparations have had the equivalent of 50 μg or less of ethinyloestradiol per tablet. The cause appears to be, in part, a rise in the concentration of certain clotting factors in the blood, notably factors II, VII, VIII and X (*British Medical Journal*, 1972). Recently the risks of thromboembolic disease have been shown to be associated with increasing age and smoking in women taking oral contraceptives (Royal College of General Practitioners, 1977). A woman of 35 or over who smokes would be wise to consider alternative forms of contraception.

Pulmonary hypertension. An epidemic of pulmonary hypertension was noted in Europe between 1967 and 1969, where some clinics reported a 20%

increase in incidence (Follath, Burkart & Schweizer, 1971). The disease was characterized by progressive breathlessness, effort syncope and heart failure, and most patients had been taking the drug aminorex fumarate to assist weight loss. In the UK, where the drug was not marketed, no cases were noted. The exact mechanism is in doubt in this case, since animal studies have failed to reproduce the effect seen in man (Kay, 1974).

Pulmonary oedema. Pulmonary oedema may occur after over-zealous infusion of intravenous fluids, especially sodium chloride solutions. Pulmonary oedema is sometimes seen in heroin and morphine addicts, apparently due to the injection of excessive dosages, perhaps resulting in the release of histamine. Pulmonary oedema in heroin addicts may be severe and prolonged and does not necessarily respond to the injection of the antidote naloxone (Frand, Shim & Williams, 1972). Pulmonary oedema has been reported following the use of phenylbutazone and carbenoxolone, both of which may cause sodium retention. A typical chest radiograph of pulmonary oedema is shown in Figure 14.2.

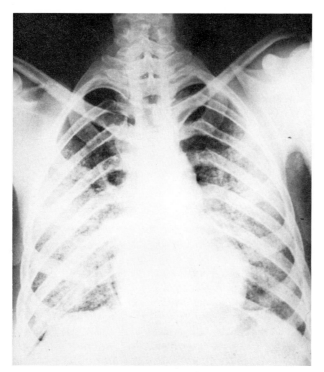

Fig. 14.2. Chest radiograph showing acute pulmonary oedema in a 45-year-old man following inhalation of smoke fumes containing nitrogen dioxide.

Drug-induced disease of lung parenchyma

It is often difficult to be certain that a drug is responsible for causing damage to the lung parenchyma. Acute reactions are often manifest as pulmonary oedema, which has a number of other causes, and chronic reactions such as pulmonary fibrosis may be considerably delayed after the initial exposure to the drug. Inhalation of a number of compounds may produce a pneumonia through irritation or osmotic effects. Thus the use of liquid paraffin or oily nose drops may lead to an inhalation type of lipoid pneumonia. Lung infections may occur more commonly as a result of drug therapy. Such opportunistic infections often involve relatively non-pathogenic organisms and occur in people taking drugs that suppress the immune response. Such drugs include corticosteroids, azathioprine and a variety of antineoplastic drugs such as methotrexate, vinblastine and cyclophosphamide. The infecting organism may be a fungus such as *Candida albicans* or *Nocardia asteroides*, a virus such as cytomegalovirus or protozoal such as *Pneumocystis carinii*.

Drug-induced disseminated lupus erythematosus (D.L.E.). A diffuse pneumonitis may occur as a result of D.L.E. induced by drug therapy (Harpey, 1973). Such patients usually present with cough, shortness of breath and pleural pain. The drugs which may produce this condition are shown in Table 14.3. The syndrome of drug-induced D.L.E. has most

Table 14.3. Drugs reported as causing disseminated lupus erythematosus.

Definite	Probable
Hydrallazine	Penicillin
Procainamide	*p*-Aminosalicylic acid
Isoniazid	Streptomycin
Phenytoin	Phenylbutazone
Primidone	Carbamazepine
	Practolol
	Reserpine
	Oral contraceptives

commonly been reported following the use of hydrallazine, procainamide and isoniazid. These three drugs are all metabolized by acetylation, and patients vary in the rate at which they acetylate drugs (see Chapter 3). In Caucasians, slow acetylators predominate, but in the Japanese and Eskimos, fast acetylators are more common (Evans, 1971). The acetylation of drugs shows genetic polymorphism.

In general, slow acetylators are more likely to develop the D.L.E. syndrome than fast acetylators (Perry, 1973). In the use of hydrallazine, the dose should be kept under 200 mg/day in slow acetylators and under 300 mg/day in fast acetylators to avoid drug-induced D.L.E. Symptoms of drug-induced D.L.E. may occur at any time, but usually between 1 and 35 weeks after the start of treatment (Byrd & Schanzer, 1969). Recovery usually occurs on stopping the drug and corticosteroids are often useful in suppressing symptoms of the condition.

Diffuse pneumonitis. Pneumonitis may occur with a variety of different drugs and often produces an appearance in the chest radiograph very similar to that seen with pulmonary oedema (see Figure 14.2). In some cases the condition is reversible, but in other cases it progresses to pulmonary fibrosis. Pneumonitis is usually accompanied by eosinophilia and is known as Loeffler's Syndrome. The eosinophil count in the blood may be very high and many eosinophils may be seen in the pulmonary exudate that fills the alveolar spaces. The pulmonary response is probably due to a hypersensitivity reaction occurring in the alveolar walls. Symptoms are usually limited to a mild cough but can, on occasion, be quite severe. Drugs that may cause pulmonary eosinophilia include nitrofurantoin, sulphonamides, aspirin, methotrexate, *p*-aminosalicylic acid, penicillin, sulphasalazine and imipramine. Nitrofurantoin and sulphonamides are probably the best known drugs capable of producing this reaction (Israel & Diamond, 1962; Fiegenberg, Weiss & Krishnan, 1967; Jones & Malone, 1972). Methotrexate may also produce a similar type of lesion in patients who have been on treatment for several weeks (Whitcomb, Schwarz & Tormey, 1972). Radiological changes may persist for some time after the clinical features have disappeared, but recovery is usually uncomplicated, unlike the disease that may follow the use of other antineoplastic agents.

Diffuse pneumonitis and fibrosis. Pulmonary fibrosis following drug therapy was first reported after the administration of ganglion-blocking drugs. Doniach, Morrison & Steiner (1954) reported shortness of breath and shadowing on the chest X-ray in three patients who had been treated with hexamethonium for hypertension. The pathological changes were those of widespread fibrosis with destruction of the alveoli (Heard, 1962). Mecamylamine and pentolinium have also been shown to be associated with the development of pulmonary fibrosis (Hildeen, Krogsgaard & Vimtrup, 1958) but these drugs are now rarely used in the treatment of hypertension. More commonly used drugs that may cause pulmonary fibrosis include nitrofurantoin, bleomycin, azathioprin, busulphan, chlorambucil, methotrexate, melphalan and gold salts. Nitrofurantoin, as well as producing pulmonary eosinophilia, may produce a more chronic form of lung damage. The two types of lung damage appear to be fundamentally different; they are not seen together and one form does not usually lead to the other (Hailey, Glascock & Hewitt, 1969). The features of the two types are shown in Table 14.4. The chronic type is usually insidious in onset and although symptoms may improve when the nitrofurantoin is stopped, permanent pulmonary fibrosis may result (Israel *et al.*, 1973). Figure 14.3 is a typical chest radiograph of diffuse pulmonary fibrosis.

Table 14.4. Features of nitrofurantoin-induced lung damage.

	Acute	Chronic
Symptoms	Fever prominent Chills, cyanosis, dyspnoea	Low grade fever increasing dyspnoea
Course	2 hours to 10 days	6 months to 6 years
X-Ray	Pleural effusion Diffuse pneumonitis	Basal fibrosis
Laboratory	Eosinophilia	Increased lactic dehydrogenase
Outcome	Good	Poor

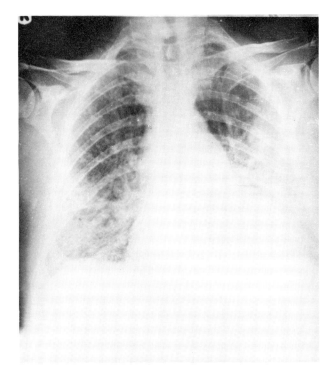

Fig. 14.3.   Chest radiograph showing diffuse pulmonary fibrosis in a 60-year-old man.

Pulmonary fibrosis may also occur after therapy with a number of cytotoxic drugs. This is most commonly associated with busulphan, but may occur with other anti-neoplastic drugs such as bleomycin and chlorambucil. The condition is not common (Littler & Ogilvie, 1970) and treatment may have been in progress for many months or even years before the onset of symptoms. Fever is commonly present, accompanied by cough and shortness of breath. The pathological changes are those of a fibrinous alveolar exudate with institial fibrosis and, in severe cases, honeycombing of the lung (Heard & Cooke, 1968). These changes, once established, are usually irreversible and often lead to death, but corticosteroid therapy may be beneficial in some patients (Boyles, 1969).

Drugs causing pleural damage

Pleural fibrosis has been reported following the use of both methysergide and practolol. Methysergide, used in some patients with migraine, may result in the development of pleural pain, shortness of breath, fever and malaise after several months of continuous therapy (Graham, 1967). The pleural lesion is usually described as fibrosis, although substantial improvement may occur after therapy when the drug is stopped. Kok-Jensen & Lindeneg (1970) found persisting severe disability in only two out of 12 cases in which treatment with methysergide had been stopped because of pleural fibrosis. Methysergide may also cause mediastinal fibrosis.

Practolol, the first selective beta-adrenergic beta-blocker to be introduced into clinical practice, was found, after many years of useful therapy, to produce kerato conjunctivitis and fibrosing peritonitis, and has now been withdrawn from the market as oral treatment. More recently, pleural fibrosis has been described in patients who had received practolol (see Brewis, 1977). The mechanism of this reaction is unknown but may be related to the production of an unusual, and highly reactive metabolite, in a small minority of patients.

Drugs may produce pulmonary damage indirectly by interfering with either the respiratory muscles or the central nervous control. Thus sedatives such as barbiturates and many benzodiazepines may produce respiratory depression which can be dangerous in patients with chronic bronchitis or asthma. Other drugs may produce paralysis of the respiratory muscles by affecting the neuromuscular junction. A number of antibiotics, particularly the aminoglycoside antibiotics (gentamicin, neomycin, kanamycin, streptomycin) may cause neuromuscular blockade, while colistin and polymyxin may also produce respiratory paralysis, particularly in patients with renal impairment.

Occupational and industrial causes

Pulmonary damage may be the result of short- or long-term exposure to a compound present in the environment of a particular work situation, usually in the air. A number of causes of allergic alveolitis are listed in Table 14.5, in which occupational exposure to an inhaled allergen is of prime

Table 14.5. Occupational lung diseases: allergic alveolitis.

Disease	Source of antigen	Nature of antigen
Farmer's Lung	Mouldy hay	Fungal spores *T. actinomycete*
Bird Fancier's Lung	Bird droppings	Avian protein
Vineyard Sprayer's Lung	Copper sulphated hydrated lime	? Antigen
Suberosis	Mouldy cork dust	Cork
Bagassosis	Mouldy bagasse	*T. sacchari*

importance. Some patients may show a type I hypersensitivity response and have symptoms, such as wheezing and shortness of breath, immediately after exposure to the antigen. In other cases, a type III hypersensitivity pattern is seen and symptoms will be noted some time (6-8 hours) after exposure. In these patients, symptoms may be indistinguishable from influenza, with cough, muscle aches and fever. In many cases the asthma is caused by precipitins in the blood, which react with the antigen, liberating histamine and other pharmacologically active mediators such as bradykinin

and slow-reacting substance A, which obstruct the airways through constriction of the smooth muscle in the bronchiolar wall. Byssinosis is a
similar condition in cotton or flax workers due to inhalation of dust, and
symptoms tend to worsen during the weekdays with continued exposure to
the dust, allowing some recovery at the weekend. This type of asthma is
probably caused by some direct histamine liberator present in the dust
(Douglas *et al.*, 1971).

A large variety of compounds may cause pulmonary oedema due to the
direct toxic effects of the compound on lung tissue following inhalation.
Figure 14.2 shows a radiograph of acute pulmonary oedema in a man who
had inhaled nitrogen dioxide (NO_2). Many of the oxides of nitrogen are
toxic in this way and are produced in a variety of industrial processes such
as in arc welding, shot blasting in mines and in forage tower silos. Other
compounds that produce similar toxic effects include phosgene, ozone,
cadmium oxide, vanadium and manganese fumes (see Parkes, 1974).

Air pollution is a common cause of pulmonary disease. Perhaps the
commonest pollution of the air we breathe comes from smoking. The list of
diseases now known to be associated with smoking is long; in particular,
carcinoma of the bronchus is twenty times more common in smokers than
in non-smokers. The incidence of lung cancer rises as the number of
cigarettes smoked per day increases. Chronic bronchitis is undoubtedly
caused in many cases by smoking. Pollutants of the air that are not under
individual control are either particulate, e.g. smoke and carbon particles, or
gaseous — notably sulphur dioxide. Excess mortality from chronic bronchitis is closely linked with the degree of air pollution and over the last 15
years the mean concentration of pollutants in urban air has fallen by a
factor of 3 (Lawther, 1973). Concern has also been expressed about pollution due to motor car exhaust fumes, containing in particular, carbon
monoxide and nitrogen dioxide, the latter producing a severe lachrymatory
haze in cities such as Los Angeles (see Lawther, 1973).

Pneumoconiosis

The most important industrial lung diseases induced by compounds in the
air are undoubtedly the pneumoconioses. These conditions arise from the
inhalation of dusts, usually over long periods during work. Simple pneumoconiosis may be recognized only by the appearance of small dense opacities
on the chest radiograph such as in tin workers (stannosis) and iron workers
(siderosis). In some pneumoconioses, however, fibrosis occurs and this is
particularly seen in silicosis, a typical radiograph of which is seen in Figure
14.4. Silicosis is popularly associated with coal miners, but may occur in the
mining of gold, graphite and copper as well as in sand blasters and iron
foundry workers amongst others. The patients often suffer from shortness
of breath, cyanosis and fever; the shortness of breath is due to both a
reduction in total lung capacity and secondary emphysema which causes
decreased airflow. It seems likely that immunological factors play a role in
the development of fibrosis in susceptible individuals (Soutar, Turner-
Warwick & Parkes, 1974).

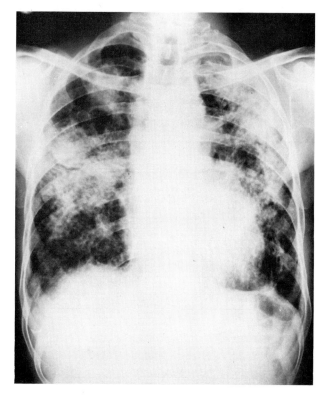

Fig. 14.4.   Chest radiograph of a 52-year-old man who had worked in the coal mines for 25 years. The features of massive pulmonary fibrosis due to silicosis are seen with fibrotic nodules in both lung fields.

Asbestos is responsible not only for pneumoconiosis (asbestosis) but also for pleural fibrosis and calcification as well as for a carcinogenic effect. Asbestos, a naturally fibrous mineral, is used in three main forms, crocidolite (blue), amosite (brown) and crysolite (white). Most diseases are associated with previous exposure to crocidolite, possibly because its particles are smaller and more readily reach the smaller bronchioles. Asbestosis usually presents with increasing shortness of breath due to impaired oxygen transfer across the fibrosed alveoli and later with cough, weakness and loss of weight. A typical chest radiograph is seen in Figure 14.5. Exposure to asbestos predisposes to carcinoma of the lung as well as to the rare tumour malignant mesothelioma of the pleura (Wagner, 1971).

Other materials

Paraquat

Some compounds are toxic to the lung but are neither drugs nor industrial hazards; paraquat is an example. Paraquat is a widely used herbicide

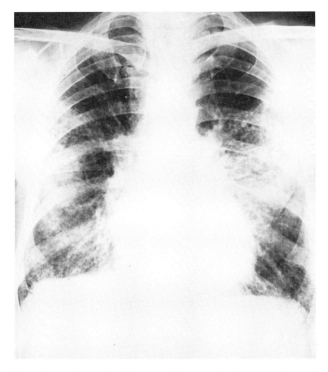

Fig. 14.5.   Chest radiograph of 48-year-old man with pulmonary fibrosis following
exposure to asbestos particles in the air over many years.

produced for general use as granules (Weedol) or for agricultural use as a
liquid concentrate (20-40% — Gramoxone, Ortho paraquat CL). It is a very
useful directly acting weed-killer and is inactivated on contact with the soil.
It is, however, toxic to man, producing many local irritant effects (e.g. to
skin and eye) from accidental splashes and may be fatal if ingested.
Paraquat is most often ingested by mistake after having been transferred
from its original container to a beer or orange squash bottle, but it is sometimes used in a deliberate attempt to kill. The fatal dose of paraquat is
probably 15-30 ml for an adult and, after small doses, death occurs only
after a prolonged and unpleasant illness. Paraquat is probably toxic
through the production of superoxide free radicals (O_2^-) which have a high
affinity for oxygen-rich tissues such as the lung and the kidney (Fisher,
Clements & Wright, 1973). Local soreness of the mouth, tongue and
oesophagus usually predominates at first, perhaps, in more severe cases,
with renal damage. After a temporary improvement, increasing shortness of breath with tachycardia and cyanosis develops, death being due
to steadily progressive asphyxia over the next one or two weeks. Examination of the chest radiograph reveals pulmonary oedema which progress
to pulmonary fibrosis. Eventually the alveolar area is occupied by so

much fibrous tissue that the lung is no longer functional.

Many different methods of treating paraquat poisoning have been tried, usually with little success. Paraquat is poorly absorbed from the gut and excreted unchanged in the urine. The most effective form of treatment appears to be the use of Fullers Earth or magnesium sulphate by mouth, as soon as possible after ingestion of paraquat, in order to prevent absorption. Haemodialysis may be of value if renal damage has occurred, which would limit the excretion of the compound from the body. Hypoxic atmospheres should be created to produce a PaO_2 of 40-45 mmHg (Fairshter *et al.*, 1976). Other forms of treatment which are more controversial involve the use of *D*-propranolol to displace paraquat from lung tissue, and superoxide dismutase to eliminate the superoxide radicals (Autor, 1974). Lung transplantation has been tried but was unsuccessful due to subsequent paraquat-induced damage to the transplanted lung.

Oxygen toxicity

High concentrations of oxygen are toxic to the alveoli and the pulmonary capillaries. Proliferative changes may develop in the walls of capillaries within a few hours of exposure to 100% oxygen at atmospheric pressure. The mechanism of this toxicity is uncertain but may, as with paraquat, involve the production of superoxide radicals. Normal subjects breathing pure oxygen will develop intolerable distress after 48-72 hours (Doleval, 1962), but all the changes seen are fully reversed after 48 hours breathing a normal oxygen tension. The lung tissue undergoes pathological changes similar to that seen with paraquat but usually without the development of fibrosis. Oxygen can be inhaled at concentrations below about 45% for long periods without harm, but in patients maintained on respirators without interruption, there is a risk of developing oxygen toxicity.

References

Autor, A. (1974). *Life Sci.*, 14, 130.
Boyles, P.W. (1969). *Clin. Med.*, 76, 11.
Brewis, R.A.L. (1977). In *Textbook of Adverse Drug Reactions*, Editor: Davies, D.M. Oxford Medical publications.
British Medical Journal (1972). 4, 378.
British Medical Journal (1973). iii, 490.
Brooks, S.M., Werk, E.E., Ackerman, S.J., Sullivan, I. and Thrasher, K. (1972). *New Engl. J. Med.*, 286, 1125.
Byrd, R.B. and Schanzer, B. (1969). *Chest*, 55, 170.
Conolly, M.E., Davies, D.S., Dollery, C.T. and George, C.F. (1971). *Br. J. Pharmac.*, 43, 389.
Davies, P. (1976). *Medicine*, 2nd Series, p. 1074.
Doleval, V. (1962). *Riv. Med. Aeronaut.*, 25, 219.
Doniach, I., Morrison, B. and Steiner, R.E. (1954). *Br. Heart J.*, 16, 101.
Douglas, J.S., Zuckerman, A., Ridgeway, P. and Bouhuys, A. (1971). In *International Conference on Respiratory Disease in Textile Workers*. Barcelona Spain, p. 133.
Evans, D.A.P. (1971). *Acta Pharmac. Tox.*, 29, (Suppl. 3), 156.
Fairshter, R.D., Rosen, S.M., Smith, W.R., Glauser, F.L., McRae, D.M. and Wilson, A.F. (1976). *Q. J. Med.*, 40, 551.
Fiegenberg, D.S., Weiss, H. and Krishman, H. (1967). *Arch. intern. Med.*, 120, 85.

Fisher, H.K., Clements, J.A. and Wright, R.R. (1973). *Am. Rev. resp. Dis.*, 107, 246.

Follath, F., Burkart, F. and Schweizer, W. (1971). *Br. med. J.*, i, 265.

Frand, U.I., Shim, C.S. and Williams, M.H. (1972). *Ann. intern. Med.*, 77, 29.

Garrod, L.P., Lambert, H.P. and O'Grady, F. (1973). *Antibiotic and Chemotherapy*, 4th edn., p. 62. Edinburgh: Churchill Livingstone.

Graham, J.R. (1967). *Am. J. med. Sci.*, 254, 1.

Hailey, F.J., Glascock, H.W.J. and Hewitt, W.F. (1969). *New Engl. J. Med.*, 281, 1087.

Harpey, J.P. (1973). *Adv. Drug Reaction Bull.*, p. 43.

Heard, B.E. (1962). *J. Path. Bact.*, 83, 159.

Heard, B.E. and Cooke, R.A. (1968). *Thorax*, 23, 187.

Hildeen, T., Krogsgaard, A.R. and Vimtrup, B.J. (1958). *Lancet*, ii, 830.

Horne, N.W. (1976). *Br. J. Hosp. Med.*, 15, 440.

Israel, H.I. and Diamond, P. (1962). *New Engl. J. Med.*, 266, 1024.

Israel, K.S., Brashear, R.E., Sharma, H.M., Yum, M.N. and Glover, J.L. (1973). *Am. Rev. resp Dis.*, 108, 353.

Jick, H. (1974). *New Engl. J. Med.*, 291, 824.

Jones, G.R. and Malone, D.N.S. (1972). *Thorax*, 27, 713.

Kay, J.M. (1974). *Thorax,* 29, 266.

Kok-Jensen, A. and Lindeneg, O. (1970). *Scand. J. resp. Dis.*, 51, 218.

Lawther, P. (1973). *Medicine*, 1st series, p. 840.

Levy, M., Nir, I., Birnbaum, D., Superstine, E. and Eliakim, M. (1973). *Israel J. Med. Sci.*, 9, 619.

Lippmann, M. (1977). *Med. Clin. N. Amer.*, 61, 1353.

Littler, W.A. and Ogilvie, C. (1970). *Br. med. J.*, iv, 530.

Parkes, W.R. (1974). *Occupational Lung Disorders.* London: Butterworth.

Passmore, R. and Robinson, J.S. (eds.) (1974). *A Companion to Medical Studies*, Vol. 3, part 1. Oxford and London: Blackwell Scientific Publication.

Paterson, J.W., Conolly, M.E., Davies, D.S. and Dollery, C.T. (1968). *Lancet*, ii, 426.

Perry, H.M. (1973). *Am. J. Med.*, 54, 58.

Royal College of General Practitioners (1974). *Oral Contraceptives and Health*, London.

Royal College of General Practitioners (1977). *Lancet*, 2, 727.

Samter, M. and Beers, R.F. (1967). *J. Allergy*, 40, 281.

Soutar, C.A., Turner-Warwick, M. and Parkes, W.R. (1974). *Br. med. J.*, 3, 145.

Speizer, F.E., Doll, R. and Heaf, P. (1968). *Br. med. J.*, i, 335.

Vessey, M.P. and Doll, R. (1969). *Br. med. J.*, ii, 651.

Wagner, J.C. (1971). *J. nat. Cancer Inst.*, 46, 1.

Whitcomb, M.E., Schwarz, M.I. and Tormey, D.C. (1972). *Thorax*, 27, 636.

15. Prospects for the therapeutic control of fibrosis

C. I. Levene

Introduction

This chapter is concerned with the effect of drugs on the connective tissues. Those diseases of the connective tissues which are generally referred to as the 'collagen diseases' include rheumatoid arthritis, disseminated lupus erythematosus, scleroderma and dermatomyositis; a second large group of connective tissue disease consists of the inherited diseases so well described by McKusick (1972). On the whole, the collagen diseases still lack specific therapeutic measures and so the prognosis, in general, is poor. The toxicity of drugs in relation to the connective tissues could be dealt with by discussing those drugs which are at present available for the treatment of the collagen diseases, such as aspirin, gold salts, steroids or anti-malarial compounds. These diseases, however, have three things in common — their aetiologies remain obscure, the prognosis, if not hopeless, remains poor, and the specificity of available drugs questionable. There are also diseases of the connective tissues whose aetiology is less obscure — these are diseases of collagen which have been experimentally induced by drugs, whose effect was clearly toxic. However, these toxic effects may be put to beneficial therapeutic use in the prevention of what is undoubtedly, the largest group of connective tissue diseases which truly involve collagen — *fibrosis*, or the formation of scar tissue.

While working on an experimentally induced connective tissue disease, we noted that the causative agent, β-aminopropionitrile (BAPN) produced bizarre, disastrous results in the test animals; this compound had a most unusual effect — it inhibited the cross-linking of collagen, a protein whose main physiological function of stability depends on intact cross-linking (Levene & Gross, 1959). Fibrosis, which essentially involves the deposition of collagen in a pathological situation, is both the result *and* the cause of a great deal of disease; it is also an inexorable process, since, once laid down, it generally remains, and yet BAPN did affect its deposition; further exploration appeared worthwhile.

Some 30 years ago, Klemperer coined the term 'collagen diseases' to include the diseases previously mentioned, on the basis that they all showed the presence histologically of fibrinoid necrosis and had a somewhat similar clinical picture (Klemperer, Pollack & Baehr, 1947), the patients tending to be treated in rheumatological clinics. The use of the term had the beneficial effect of allowing the clinicians to think about these diseases in a more orderly fashion; it was not meant to imply a collagenous aetiology, its use being strategic.

The Department of Medicine at the Massachussetts General Hospital was then headed by a very distinguished rheumatologist, Walter Bauer; his observations of patients suffering from the collagen diseases, and their poor prognosis, had led him to the belief that these diseases would need to be dealt with, in research terms, at both the clinical level and at the basic level, dealing with a particular protein or mucopolysaccharide component of the connective tissues, in the hope that useful leads would emerge. The vehicle he helped forge and which he used for advancing the basic studies was the Helen Hay Whitney Foundation. The question he posed its research fellows was: 'If I gave you a piece of the patient's tissues, what could you tell me about the disease?' Despite their seemingly disappointed responses, Bauer maintained his dual approach to attempt to understand these diseases.

Just before this episode, the connective tissues had not even been considered as an entity — in fact, Wasserman in his review on the 'Intracellular components of the connective tissues' (1956) depicts the uncertainty of histologists at that time about the actual existence of ground substance, by describing the oblique phenomenological experiments of Bensley (1934), Duran-Reynals (1942), McLean (1930) and Day (1948), as well as the discovery of the PAS reaction for glycoproteins (McManus, 1946; Hotchkiss, 1948) and of metachromasia for the acid mucopolysaccharides (Sylven, 1941). It had taken 20 years of indirect evidence for morphologists to accept the existence of a ground substance, and only then were the chemists to begin to come to grips with its nature.

In the field of the fibrous proteins of the connective tissues, however, a much rosier prospect was emerging. A number of findings slowly unravelled, culminating in such a clear understanding of the structure of collagen that it is now possibly the best documented of all proteins. The basis of what we know about collagen had been laid by industry — the leather industry in which Gustavson had been a pioneer (1956), the textile industry which had interested Astbury, a pioneer of X-ray diffraction studies on fibrous proteins (1950-51), the glue and gelatin industries representing also photography and food technology. Later, Schmitt and his group at M.I.T. became deeply involved — in particular, mention must be made of Gross. During the last 10-15 years, great advances have been made in elucidation of the pathway of collagen biosynthesis; at present, attempts are being made to understand its cellular biology. How did the explosion in the understanding of collagen structure and biosynthesis come about?

The structure of collagen

Three events contributed to the elucidation of collagen structure — wide angle X-ray diffraction studies first demonstrated its crystalline nature; electron microscopy revealed the 64 nm axial periodicity characteristic of the fibril, and finally the phenomena of the solubility of collagen in acid, alkali and neutral saline which eventually led to the purification of collagen by Gross and to its characterization chemically and physico-chemically by many others. Four other events played a key role in the subsequent characterization of the molecule; these included the discovery that BAPN increased the solubility of collagens such as bone collagen which had been hitherto unavailable for study without prior denaturation; secondly, the demonstration that the three chains comprising the molecule could be separated using a chromatographic column following thermal denaturation; thirdly, the use of cyanogen bromide to break up the chains of 1000 amino acids into small manageable peptides, and finally the use of sodium boro[³H]hydride to isolate the intra- and intermolecular reducible cross-links.

Properties of collagen

Collagen is no longer considered to be as inert a protein as it once was — turnover does occur and varies with location in the animal. It is the body's most abundant protein, comprising one third of its total protein. Its role is mostly tensile; it is a crystalline protein which exhibits a 64 nm axial periodicity in the electron microscope and which stains red histologically with the Van Gieson stain. The collagen molecule is called tropocollagen and consists of a triple helix with a molecular weight of 300 000 daltons, measuring 280 x 1.4 nm. At the ends of each chain, non-helical regions exist which are important in cross-linking and in the immunological specificity of collagen; these are called telopeptides.

The amino acid composition of the helical body of the chain is characteristic — every third residue consists of glycine; proline and hydroxyproline comprise 25%, and hydroxylysine 0.5%. Hydroxyproline and hydroxylysine are virtually specific to collagen for which they form chemical fingerprints. Glucose and galactose form part of the molecule. Analysis of the separated chains reveals that at least four different types of collagen exist, designated types I-IV.

The work of Prockop's group has shown that hydroxyproline, whose role was a mystery until recently, stabilizes the molecule — in its absence, as in scurvy, the molecule is probably rapidly degraded *in vivo*.

A solution of collagen will, under the correct ionic conditions, gel at 37°C to form fibrils, and form a sol at 5°C; this transformation is reversible. In order to give the 64 nm periodicity normally found in native collagen, the molecules align end-to-end, and side-to-side but staggered at approximately 1/4 of their 280 nm length; a space of 40 nm remains as a hole region which may play a role in mineralization. The cross-links which need to be formed intra- and intermolecularly are particularly important, since it is from them that collagen derives its tensile strength, the function it is basically required to fulfil.

Experimental diseases of collagen

Since the time when Wolbach first investigated scurvy in the guinea-pig

(1933), this disease has been considered as the model in which to study collagen biosynthesis. It was supplemented in 1959 by the demonstration of the molecular lesion in the experimental disease, osteolathyrism; the advantages of this condition that would easily yield whole, undenatured and uncross-linked collagen soon became evident.

Human neurolathyrism

Human lathyrism has been known for hundreds of years; it produces a complex of symptoms including spinal paralysis, following consumption of the seeds of the *lathyrus sativus*; this pulse is grown extensively in Central India because it is hardy and survives drought conditions. Since it is also cheap and constitutes the bulk of the diet of the poor under famine conditions, as much as 7% of the population may be afflicted with neuro-lathyrism in times of drought.

During the search for the neurotoxic agent, a factor was found in the seeds of another member of the lathyrus family — the sweet pea (*Lathyrus odoratus*). When fed to young rats, the 'lathyrus factor' present in the sweet pea seed produced a disease of the skeleton and connective tissues called osteolathyrism, but bearing no apparent relationship to the human condi-tion of neurolathyrism (Geiger, Steenbock & Parsons, 1933). Only the experimental condition, osteolathyrism, will be discussed in this chapter.

Osteolathyrism

Osteolathyrism was first produced in young growing rats by feeding them on a diet rich in the seed of the sweet pea, *Lathyrus odoratus* (for review, see Levene, 1973). This resulted in severe skeletal deformities, hernias, loosening and detachments of ligaments, slipping of epiphyses and aortic aneurysm, which often ruptured. The 'lathyrus factor' was first isolated in 1954 (McKay *et al.*, 1954; Dasler, 1954) and shown to be β-aminopropio-nitrile (BAPN), $NH_2CH_2CH_2CN$; it was first manufactured by Abbotts of North Chicago. Apart from BAPN, certain other aliphatic nitriles such as aminoacetonitrile and methylene aminoacetonitrile had been observed to be lathyrogenic in the rat. Studies with ^{14}C-labelled aminoacetonitrile or ^{14}C-BAPN proved disappointing; a major metabolite of BAPN turned out to be cyanoacetic acid, itself a non-lathyrogen. This suggested to Lalich (1958) that an amine oxidase might be involved in the detoxication of BAPN, since Blaschko had suggested that some toxic amines might be detoxicated by amine oxidases (Blaschko, 1952).

Chick embryo lathyrism

Treatment of chick embryos with BAPN at 14 days of incubation by injection onto the chorioallantoic membrane via the shell produced a striking fragility of the tissues 2 days later, so that when the survivors were picked up by the head, the body separated at the neck. Exhaustive histological and biochemical analyses failed to reveal significant connective tissue differences from the normal; however, extraction of skin, aorta or bone with cold saline showed that in contrast to the normal, most of the collagen was extractable from the lathyritic tissues (Levene & Gross, 1959). This collagen was thought to come in part from pre-existing fibrillar collagens, since electron microscopic examination of the skin showed that fibrils present before extraction were almost completely absent after extraction (Van den Hooff, Levene & Gross, 1959). By all the criteria then available — chemical and physico-chemical — lathyritic collagen was normal. The lesion was therefore considered to be a defect in intermolecular cross-linking; later it was shown that intra-molecular cross-linking too was affected.

Structural requirements for lathyrogenic agents

This study was prompted by the hope that the mode of action of lathyrogenic compounds would be deducible from their general chemical structure and properties, since the radioactivity work had failed to clarify these points. For this purpose an assay system was required, since the rat proved to be inadequate. A lathyrogenic compound was defined as any compound which induced an increase in the connective tissue fragility and in the collagen solubility in the 14-day-old chick embryo. The system used therefore, was the chick embryo at 14 days (Gross, Levene & Orloff, 1960); originally the effect of the injection of 0.05 mM of the test compound on the fragility of the neck after 2 days of further incubation, was measured, followed by measurement of the relative viscosity of saline extracts of the bones; the extracts were prepared by separating the supernatant by centrifugation and the relative viscosity of each extract measured at 5°C in an Ostwald viscometer, this reading giving a direct measure in this system of the amount of collagen present in solution (Gross, 1958). When it was subsequently observed that a direct relation existed between the fragility and the relative viscosity, the lathyrogenic activity of various compounds was measured by comparing the relative viscosity of the extracts but omitting the fragility indices. Because the relative viscosity from normal chick embryo bone never exceeded 3.0, any compound producing a high value was considered lathyrogenic. With the use of this assay system, a critical evaluation was then attempted of compounds known to be, or suspected of being, lathyrogenic (Levene, 1961).

Lathyrogens

Nitriles. The substitution in aminoacetonitrile or BAPN of either the nitrile group (Table 15.1) or the terminal amine group (Table 15.2) resulted in a complete loss of activity with the exception of methylene aminoacetonitrile and cyanoacetic acid hydrazide.

Semicarbazide. The effect of substituting the NH_2NH- ending was to destroy all activity (Table 15.3). However, substitution of the amide ending, leaving intact the NH_2NHCO- ending indicated (Table 15.4) that activity clearly resided in the hydrazide grouping NH_2NHCO-C as well as within

Table 15.1. Effect of modifying CN-ending on lathyrogenic activity of two nitriles.

Name of compound	Formula	η rel of extracts
Aminoacetonitrile	NH_2CH_2CN	41.2
Methyl glycine ester	$NH_2CH_2COOCH_3$	2.0
Glycine	NH_2CH_2COOH	1.7
Methylamine	NH_2CH_2H	2.0
Aminoacetaldehyde acetal	$NH_2CH_2CH(OC_2H_5)_2$	2.0
Glycine amide	$NH_2CH_2CONH_2$	2.1
β-Aminopropionitrile	$NH_2CH_2CH_2CN$	35.6
β-Alanine	$NH_2CH_2CH_2COOH$	1.7
Ethylene diamine	$NH_2CH_2CH_2NH_2$	1.7
β-Mercaptoethylamine	$NH_2CH_2CH_2SH$	1.7

From Levene (1961) with permission.

Table 15.2. Effect of modifying NH_2-ending on lathyrogenic activity of two nitriles.

Name of compound	Formula	η rel of extracts
Aminoacetonitrile	NH_2CH_2CN	41.2
Cyanoacetic acid	$COOHCH_2CN$	1.9
α-Cyanoacetonitrile	$CNCH_2CN$	2.3
Benzyl nitrile	$\langle\bigcirc\rangle-CH_2CN$	2.5
Acetonitrile	HCH_2CN	2.1
Propionitrile	CH_3CH_2CN	1.9
Methylene aminoacetonitrile	$CH_2=NCH_2CN$	44.2
Cyanoacetic acid hydrazide	$NH_2NHCOCH_2CN$	17.1
β-Aminopropionitrile	$NH_2CH_2CH_2CN$	35.6
β-Hydroxypropionitrile	$HOCH_2CH_2CN$	2.1
β-β'-Iminodipropionitrile	$NH(CH_2CH_2CN)_2$	2.5
Succinonitrile	$CNCH_2CH_2CN$	2.0
β-Dimethylaminopropionitrile	$\begin{matrix}CH_3\\ \searrow N-CH_2CH_2CN\\ CH_3\nearrow\end{matrix}$	1.9
Butyronitrile	$CH_3CH_2CH_2CN$	2.3

From Levene (1961) with permission.

the ureide grouping $NH_2NHCO-N$, but that in the case of the ureides, substitution of the hydrogens of the terminal amine resulted in loss of activity.

Hydrazine. The lathyrogenic activity of the hydrazides suggested testing hydrazine for activity; hydrazine was found to be active (Table 15.5) but substitution of any of the hydrogens diminished the amount of activity.

Comparison of the degree of lathyrogenic activity of the compounds tested, on an equimolar basis (0.05 mM/egg) indicated a spectrum, with nitriles as the most powerful, followed by ureides, hydrazides and lastly, hydrazine (Table 15.6).

Table 15.3.   Effect of modifying NH_2NH-ending on lathyrogenic activity of semicarbazide.

Name of compound	Formula	η rel of extracts
Semicarbazide	$NH_2NHCONH_2$	24.6
1-Phenyl semicarbazide	⟨phenyl⟩$-NHNHCONH_2$	1.8
Acetone semicarbazone	$(CH_3)_2C=N\cdot NHCONH_2$	21.7
Oxamide	$NH_2COCONH_2$	2.2
Acetamide	CH_3CONH_2	1.9
Iodoacetamide	ICH_2CONH_2	All died
Glycine amide	$NH_2CH_2CONH_2$	2.1
Nicotinamide	⟨pyridine⟩$-CONH_2$	1.8
6-Aminonicotinamide	NH_2-⟨pyridine⟩$-CONH_2$	2.2
Benzamide	⟨phenyl⟩$-CONH_2$	2.1
Acrylamide	$CH_2\cdot CHCONH_2$	1.9
Urea	NH_2CONH_2	2.2
Asparagine	CH_2-CONH_2 $\mid$ $CHCOOH$ $\mid$ NH_2	1.8
Glutamine	$COOHCH(NH_2)(CH_2)_2CONH_2$	1.5

From Levene (1961) with permission.

Interpretation of results of assay

Three of the foregoing four groups act as carbonyl-blocking agents, and the fourth, the nitriles, probably break down to produce cyanide which also acts as a carbonyl-blocking group. A hypothesis was therefore proposed that lathyrogenic compounds act by blocking carbonyl groups, theoretically postulated as essential for the normal polymerization of collagen. The minimal requirements for this hypothesis to be upheld would be, firstly, the demonstration of carbonyl groups on the collagen molecule, and secondly, blockage of such groups by lathyrogenic compounds. Studies with purified normal and lathyritic guinea-pig skin collagen *in vitro* (Levene, 1962) showed that normal collagen reacted with 2,4-dinitrophenylhydrazine, a carbonyl-blocking agent, whereas lathyritic collagen did not, suggesting that carbonyl groups had either been blocked or were absent. Since then it has become clear that carbonyl groups *do* exist in collagen and play a critical role in its cross-linking; lysyl oxidase, the cross-linking enzyme (Figure 15.1) is responsible for the oxidative deamination of specific lysine or hydroxylysine residues in the collagen molecule (Pinnell & Martin, 1968) to form aldehydes which then form Schiff base aldimine cross-links with

Table 15.4. Effect of modifying NH_2-ending on lathyrogenic activity of semicarbazide.

Name of compound	Formula	η rel of extracts
Semicarbazide	$NH_2NHCONH_2$	24.6
4,4-Diphenylsemicarbazide	NH_2NHCON (diphenyl)	2.3
Isonicotinic acid hydrazide	NH_2NHCO (pyridine)	15.1
Nicotinic acid hydrazide	NH_2NHCO (pyridine)	17.8
Benzhydrazide	NH_2NHCO (phenyl)	17.3
Cyanoacetic acid hydrazide	$NH_2NHCOCH_2CN$	14.1
γ-L-Glutamylhydrazide	$NH_2NHCOCH_2CH_2CH(NH_2)COOH$	10.9
Glycine hydrazide	$NH_2NHCOCH_2NH_2$	11.1
p-Nitrobenzhydrazide	NH_2NHCO (phenyl) NO_2	14.1

From Levene (1961) with permission.

Table 15.5. Effect of substitution of H's on lathyrogenic activity of hydrazine.

Name of compound	Formula	η rel of extracts
Hydrazine hydrate	$H_2N\cdot NH_2\cdot H_2O$	12.8
Unsym. dimethylhydrazine	$H_2N\cdot N \begin{smallmatrix} CH_3 \\ CH_3 \end{smallmatrix}$	5.3
Sym. dimethylhydrazine	$H_3C\cdot HN\cdot NH\cdot CH_3$	4.7.
Hydrazobenzene	(phenyl)$-HN\cdot NH-$(phenyl)	3.1
2,4-Dinitrophenylhydrazine	NO_2-(phenyl, NO_2)$-NH\cdot NH_2$	2.1
Phenylhydrazine	(phenyl)$-NH\cdot NH_2$	All died

From Levene (1961) with permission.

amino groups on neighbouring collagen chains or aldol condensation groups with neighbouring aldehydes. It is also clear that lysyl oxidase is inhibited by BAPN — exactly how is still obscure — it may block the

Table 15.6.   Classification of compounds found to be lathyrogenic in the chick embryo based on the salt-extractibility of collagen from their bones.

Lathyrogenic compound (0.054mmol/egg)	Relative viscosity of bone extracts
Normal control	2
I. *Organic nitriles*	
Methylene aminoacetonitrile	44
Aminoacetonitrile	41
β-Aminopropionitrile	36
II. *Ureides*	
Semicarbazide	25
Acetone semicarbazone	22
III. *Hydrazides*	
Nicotinic acid hydrazide	18
Benzhydrazide	18
Isonicotinic acid hydrazide	15
Cyanoacetic acid hydrazide	14
p-Nitrobenzhydrazide	14
Glycine hydrazide	11
γ-L-Glutamylhydrazide	11
IV. *Hydrazines*	
Hydrazine hydrate	13
Unsym. dimethylhydrazine	5
Sym. dimethylhydrazine	5

enzyme's active site or possibly chelate a cofactor, copper, but whichever the mechanism, the result is seen in the drastic connective tissue changes observed in the rat and the chick. If one studies the effects of lathyrogenic compounds on the cross-linking of collagen in cultured fibroblasts, it is possible to inhibit cross-linking without affecting either cell growth or protein synthesis; the action of lathyrogens at extremely low concentration suggests that they have a very specific effect on lysyl oxidase alone (Levene, Bates & Bailey, 1972).

Sequelae of lathyrism

Effect on tensile strength. The tensile strength of many tissues, particularly those which have a high collagen or elastin content, is diminished following treatment with lathyrogens, since the degree of cross-linkage of collagen and elastin is diminished. This only occurs in young growing animals, or where collagen and elastin synthesis is actively proceeding; lathyrogens will not affect tissues whose collagen and elastin have already undergone the cross-linking and the maturation process.

Effect on wound healing and on the repair of fractures. The strength of such wounds and fractures is diminished; however, withdrawal of treatment permits healing and recovery of wound strength to proceed normally.

Effect on tissue hydration. Treatment of chick embryos with lathyrogens produces great swelling of the cartilages (Levene, 1966); their water content increases by 20-30% (Table 15.7); since the proteoglycans appear

Cross - link formation in collagen

Enzyme : lysyl oxidase (Cu; pyridoxal)

Substrates : peptidyl lysine, hydroxylysine

Oxidative deamination :

$$R - CH_2 - NH_3^+ \longrightarrow R - CHO + NH_4^+$$

Schiff base formation :

$$R_1 - CHO + H_2N - CH_2 - R_2 \rightleftharpoons R_1 - CH = N - CH_2 - R_2 + H_2O$$

Aldol reaction :

$$R_1 - CH_2 - CHO + \underset{CHO}{CH_2 - R_2} \longrightarrow R_1 - CH_2 - \underset{OH}{CH} - \overset{CHO}{CH} - R_2$$

Fig. 15.1.   Scheme representing the formation of the aldehydic precursors of collagen cross-links by the enzyme, lysyl oxidase.

Table 15.7.   Effect of lathyrogenic compounds on the water content of the cartilage of 16-day-old chick embryos treated two days earlier.

Test compound (0.054 mmol/egg)	Class	Excess hydration %
β-Aminopropionitrile (BAPN)	Nitrile	21
Semicarbazide	Ureide	31
Isonicotinic acid hydrazide	Hydrazide	19
Hydrazine	Hydrazine	31

to be normal (Levene, Kranzler & Franco-Browder, 1966), this finding has been interpreted as a direct result of the inhibition of collagen cross-linking so that the proteoglycans can express their physico-chemical affinity for water, a property clearly seen physiologically in hyaluronic acid, as in the vitreous humour of the eye, or in Wharton's jelly in the umbilical cord.

Teratogenic effect. When lathyrogens were injected into chick embryos at the much earlier age of 4-6 days (Levene & Gross, 1959), they produced a typical malformation of the lower beak and a bowing of the leg bones (Figure 15.2). The probable explanation is that these represent the effect of unequal muscular tension upon a bone rudiment which has been weakened

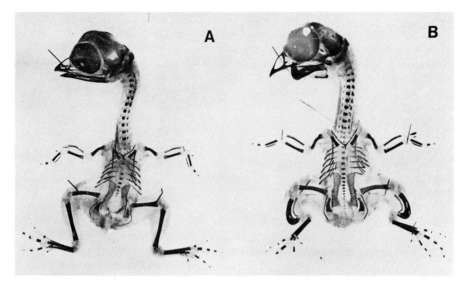

Fig. 15.2. The effect of BAPN on the skeleton of 16-day-old chicks when treated at 4 days: (*a*) normal alizarin-stained embryo (*b*) BAPN-treated alizarin-stained embryo.

early in its development by inadequate cross-linkage of the collagenous matrix. The effect of a single dose of a lathyrogen wears off with time, leaving the malformed limb, but it is a strong bone which shows no abnormal collagen solubility changes. The result has been called a pheno-copy of Marfan's Syndrome, a heritable human disorder of the connective tissues, and may perhaps one day illuminate the process producing this disease.

Penicillamine

In 1965 penicillamine treatment of rats was shown to increase the solubility of their collagen (Nimni & Bavetta, 1965); penicillamine did not affect collagen synthesis but did affect its cross-linking. Nimni has proposed that, in contrast to BAPN where the aldehydic cross-link precursor is not made, penicillamine does not prevent formation of the aldehydes but reacts with it once it is formed, possibly by forming a thiazolidine complex, and thus rendering it inaccessible for normal cross-link formation. The net result is therefore similar to the effect of BAPN, but the mechanism is different.

Penicillamine represents an important therapeutic weapon in the treat-ment of Wilson's disease in which it is believed to act by chelating copper and thus preventing excessive deposition in the brain (Walshe, 1977); it may not be widely known that a toxic side effect of penicillamine therapy is the spontaneous rupture of tendons. It is believed that penicillamine may break the Schiff-base type of cross-links; this could explain tendon rupture since collagen does turn over faster than was once believed to be the case; however, the mechanism is still incompletely understood.

Fibrosis

Three events may occur following acute inflammation — resolution, regeneration and repair; repair means the replacement of tissues which have been destroyed and which cannot regenerate, as can liver, epidermis and mesenchyme, by scar tissue formation. Scar tissue is clearly helpful in the healing of a surgical incision, a fractured bone or a myocardial infarct, but in general it is harmful — e.g. mitral stenosis, corneal scarring, silicosis, urethral stenosis etc. The three major ways in which it is deleterious are by damaging function, as in cirrhosis of the liver, by obliterating the lumen of a duct as in coronary atherosclerosis, gonococcal urethritis or in Crohn's disease, or by contraction, as may be seen following severe skin burns. Fibrosis has always tended to be thought of as an inexorable and immutable process about which nothing could be done and which is responsible for a considerable proportion of all disease. Following the lathyrism work, an attempt was made to see whether the toxic effects of lathyrism which have been described could be put to good use by trying to inhibit the harmful effects of fibrosis. The principle use was that since BAPN inhibited not synthesis but cross-linking of the tropocollagen molecules, BAPN should theoretically affect only newly synthesized collagen and thus prevent its effective deposition as fibrosis; it would not, by definition, affect collagen which had already been cross-linked.

Silicosis

As a model system for severe, progressive and eventually lethal fibrosis, pulmonary silicosis in the rat was selected and induced by the intratracheal administration of a fibrogenic quartz (Levene, Bye & Saffiotti, 1968). The type of lesion produced is a nodular fibrosis. The result of treating half of these animals with BAPN was that although the BAPN-treated silicotic rats had the same body weight as the untreated silicotic controls, the collagen content of their lungs was considerably diminished (Table 15.8); it was not,

Table 15.8.   Effect of BAPN treatment on the body weight gain and on the total collagen content of lungs of rats after silicosis of 8 weeks duration.

Treatment	Average weight gain ± s.e.m. (g)	Total collagen content ± s.e.m. (mg)	
		Right lungs	Left lungs
Normal controls	+ 129 ± 7.9	21.3 ± 1.4	12.0 ± 1.1
Silicotic controls	+ 21.8 ± 26.2	76.1 ± 18.1	21.9 ± 3.2
Silicotics treated with BAPN	+ 60.9 ± 12.5	34.7 ± 1.8	16.8 ± 1.6

therefore, a general non-specific inanition effect but was due to the treatment with BAPN. Since BAPN does not inhibit collagen synthesis, how then, did this inhibition of fibrosis occur? From experiments carried out with rats where it was not found possible to inhibit experimentally produced peritoneal adhesions by BAPN treatment (Levene, unpublished data), it was considered that the lung effects were probably due to the constant respiratory movement, resulting in degradation of any uncross-linked collagen. The fact remained that it was possible to stem a progressive fibrosis with a drug despite the constant presence of the fibrogenic quartz.

Collagen biosynthetic pathway — choice of system

The next step seemed clear; BAPN was not ideal — it had some toxic effects — and so it appeared desirable to investigate the biosynthetic pathway of collagen to see whether any other points existed, such as enzymes and their cofactors which might prove amenable to therapeutic assault. The first question was which system to use — animals presented problems; slices and granulomas such as those induced by carrageenan, or abscesses such as those induced by turpentine, or implanted Ivalon sponges or metal cylinders all had associated difficulties. Attempts were therefore made to evolve a test system containing the least number of variables and in which it might be possible to quantitate the amount of collagen synthesized at any one time per fibroblastic cell. This resulted in the use of the 3T6 mouse fibroblast line in culture (Levene & Bates, 1970); Todaro & Green (1963) had isolated 3T6 and shown that it was a good collagen-forming cell. The advantages of using a line versus a normal cell and of mouse species versus a human cell, were outweighed, on consideration, by the advantages of using a reproducible and quantifiable system. One would, no doubt, be obliged eventually to extrapolate from a line to the normal, and from a mouse to the human, but this problem is true for all model systems. It was therefore decided to use a model which worked rather than face the difficulties of using normal human cells with their finite numbers of divisions and the logistic problems of biopsies; the results, it is thought, justify the choice (Levene & Bates, 1973).

Fifteen years ago, the pathway for collagen biosynthesis was unknown; today, due to the efforts of a number of groups throughout the world, this pathway has been perhaps completely elucidated and the characteristic feature of collagen biosynthesis — the many post-translational modifications required — stand clearly documented (Grant & Prockop, 1972). Briefly, what happens in the fibroblast during collagen synthesis is as follows: after ribosomal synthesis of the precursor, which is larger than the product, due to the presence of N- and C- terminal extension peptides, and whose proline and lysine is completely unhydroxylated, hydroxylation of specific peptidyl proline and lysine residues occurs via the enzymes prolyl and lysyl hydroxylase (Figure 15.3). The cofactors of these enzymes are molecular oxygen, ferrous iron, ascorbic acid and α-ketoglutarate, the latter being a co-substrate since these enzymes are mixed-function oxidases. The next step is glycosylation of specific hydroxylysine residues by galactosyl or glucosyl transferase both of which are manganese-dependent. Following this, the three precursor chains assemble to form the precursor of the tropocollagen molecule; this is extruded by the cell and the N- and C-terminal extension peptides cleaved by the enzyme procollagen peptidase, which has

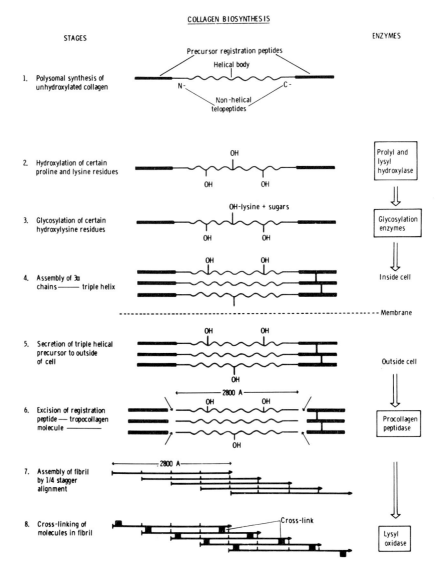

Fig. 15.3. Diagram illustrating the pathway for the biosynthesis of collagen.

no known cofactor. The tropocollagen molecules then align in end-to-end and side-to-side fashion but in a 1/4 stagger mode to give the classical fibril which shows a 64 nm axial periodicity. The final step consists of cross-link formation by the enzyme lysyl oxidase whose two cofactors are copper and pyridoxal phosphate (Murray & Levene, 1977); this gives the fibril the strength to perform its major tensile role.

A system has been evolved using 3T6 fibroblasts to study the role of ascorbic acid in collagen biosynthesis (Levene & Bates, 1975). Using added

[³H]proline, we isolated collagen and [³H]hydroxyproline in both the cell layer and the supernatant medium, and have shown, either directly or indirectly, that the system contains all of the enzymes essential for the synthesis of collagen fibrils, if the feed is supplemented with ascorbic acid. The system is a sturdy and reproducible one in which it is possible to study the effect of drugs on collagen synthesis and on the enzymes involved. Levene & Bates (1973) have been able to show, using this system, that ascorbate deficiency does not prevent the synthesis of collagen protein — the underhydroxylated precursor is synthesized in normal amounts but the subsequent hydroxylation of this precursor, particularly of proline, is dependent on the ascorbate concentration. It was also possible to demonstrate three new roles for ascorbate in this system: firstly, ascorbate is essential for the hydroxylation of critical hydroxylysine-dependent cross-link precursors; secondly, ascorbate was shown to activate the inactive precursor of prolyl hydroxylase in culture; thirdly, ascorbate was shown to be essential for the correct assembly of collagen fibrils in culture — in its absence no 64 nm banding was evident in the extracellular fibrils (Levene, Ockleford & Barber, 1977).

To summarize, little is understood of the causes of the so-called 'collagen diseases', but many chemicals are known to cause osteolathyrism. The structure and biosynthesis of collagen have recently become clear. The notion has been advanced that the major collagen disease is fibrosis, a major response of the body to disease processes and one which has been considered to be unpreventable. It is suggested that the toxic effects of lathyrogenic compounds could be used in the prevention of fibrosis. Finally, a tissue culture system has been described in which it is possible to test the effect of chemicals on the formation of collagen and so, hopefully, eventually provide drugs which may prove to be of use clinically in the prevention of the undesirable effects of fibrosis.

References

Astbury, W.T. (1950-1951). *The Harvey Lectures*, Series XI, VI. Springfield, Ill.: Charles C. Thomas, 3.
Bensley, H.S. (1934). *Anat. Res.*, 60, 93.
Blaschko, H. (1952). *Pharmac. Rev.*, 4, 415.
Dasler, W. (1954). *Science*, 120, 307.
Day, T.D. (1948). *J. Path. Bact.*, 60, 150.
Duran-Reynals, F. (1942). *Bacteriol. Rev.*, 6, 197.
Geiger, B.J., Steenbock, J. and Parsons, H.T. (1933). *J. Nutr.*, 6, 247.
Grant, M.E. and Prockop, D.J. (1972). *New Engl. J. Med.*, 286, 194, 242, 291.
Gross, J. (1958). *J. exp. Med.*, 107, 265.
Gross, J., Levene, C.I. and Orloff, S. (1960). *Proc. Soc. exp. Biol. Med.*, 105, 148.
Gustavson, K.H. (1956). *The Chemistry and Reactivity of Collagen*. New York: Academic Press.
Hooff, A. van den, Levene, C.I. and Gross, J. (1959). *J. exp. Med.*, 110, 1017.
Hotchkiss, R.D. (1948). *Arch. Biochem.*, 16, 131.
Klemperer, P., Pollack, A.D. and Baehr, G. (1942). *J. Am. med. Assoc.*, 119, 331.
Lalich, J.J. (1958). *Science*, 128, 206.
Levene, C.I. (1961). *J. exp. Med.*, 114, 295.
Levene, C.I. (1962). *J. exp. Med.*, 116, 119.
Levene, C.I. (1966). *Biochem. J.*, 101, 441.

Levene, C.I. (1973). In *Molecular Pathology of Connective Tissues*, Editors: Perez-Tamayo, R. and Rojkind, M., p. 175. New York: M. Dekker.

Levene, C.I. and Bates, C.J. (1970). *J. Cell Sci.*, 7, 671.

Levene, C.I. and Bates, C.J. (1973). In *Biology of the Fibroblast*. Editors: Kulonen, E. and Pikkarainen, J., p. 397. New York and London: Academic Press.

Levene, C.I. and Bates, C.J. (1975). *Ann. N.Y. Acad. Sci.*, 258, 288.

Levene, C.I., Bates, C.J. and Bailey, A.J. (1972). *Biochim. Biophys. Acta*, 263, 574.

Levene, C.I., Bye, I. and Saffiotti, U. (1968). *Br. J. exp. Path.*, 49, 152.

Levene, C.I. and Gross, J. (1959). *J. exp. Med.*, 110, 771.

Levene, C.I., Kranzler, J. and Franco-Browder, S. (1966). *Biochem. J.*, 101, 435.

Levene, C.I., Ockleford, C.D. and Barber, C.L. (1977). *Virchows. Arch. B. Cell Path.*, 23, 325.

McKay, G.F., Lalich, J.J., Schilling, E.D. and Strong, F.M. (1954). *Arch. Biochem. Biophys.*, 52, 313.

McKusick, V.A. (1972). *Heritable Disorders of Connective Tissue*, 4th Ed. St. Louis, Mo.: C.V. Mosby Co.

McLean, D. (1930). *J. Path. Bact.*, 33, 1045.

McManus, J.F.A. (1946). *Nature (Lond.)*, 158, 202.

Murray, J.C. and Levene, C.I. (1977). *Biochem. J.*, 167, 463.

Nimni, M.E. and Bavetta, L.A. (1965). *Science*, 150, 905.

Pinnell, S.R. and Martin, G.R. (1968). *Proc. Natl. Acad. Sci. (U.S.A.)*, 61, 708.

Sylven, B. (1941). *Acta chir. scand. (Stockholm)*, 86, 1.

Todaro, G.J. and Green, H. (1963). *J. cell Biol.*, 17, 299.

Walshe, J.M. (1977). *Proc. Roy. Soc. Med.*, 70, 1.

Wasserman, F. (1956). *Ergeb. Anat. Entwick.*, 35, 240.

Wolbach, S.B. (1933). *Am. J. Path.*, 9, 689.

16. Side effects associated with the use of radiopharmaceuticals

D. H. Keeling

The term radiopharmaceutical is used to cover a very wide spectrum of materials used in clinical medicine and research, whose only common point is the possession of a radioactive nuclide or nuclides in the preparation. There is an extensive amount of metabolic testing to be done on new drugs and compounds of biochemical interest. Radiotracers are now an indispensable part of this work, and although much of this work is done in animals, it is frequently necessary to carry out trials in normal and pathological states in patients. The study of these varieties of compound, which one might categorize as pharmacological and biochemical investigation, is by its nature a research procedure which, once done, need not be repeated. In these cases, the number of patients exposed to a given material is quite small and is governed by the usual controls on research investigations and clinical trials.

The second main grouping is of radioactive materials used for therapeutic purposes. We exclude from any consideration here the sealed sources of radionuclides used for external radiotherapy treatment, e.g. cobalt 60 teletherapy machines, and also small sealed sources of radionuclides placed internally in the body and used in the treatment of bladder tumours, ablation of the pituitary gland etc. These function simply as radiation sources and have none of the biochemical attributes of their constituents. However, there are an important, if small, group of radiochemicals which have been used for therapeutic purposes and which are allowed to distribute themselves within the body. These date back forty years or more to the very beginnings of nuclear medicine. At that time [^{131}I]iodide and [^{32}P]phosphate were first introduced into clinical medicine and used in the treatment of malignant disease. The rationale for this lies in the specialized metabolism of the thyroid and bone marrow such that these tissues concentrate the materials and thus receive localized high doses of radiation. Since that time, a few further examples have been added to this list including radiopharmaceuticals given for treatment of some types of malignancy disseminated in the peritoneum and pleura. More recently, radioisotopes have been used in the local treatment of some types of chronic synovitis and are given by intra-articular injection.

The third main group of radiopharmaceuticals is numerically by far the largest and includes all the materials given to patients in the routine investigation of disease. This work has come to make up the bulk of the clinical content of nuclear medicine and the last ten to fifteen years have seen an enormous increase, not just in the number of patients investigated, but in the number and complexity of the radiopharmaceuticals used. At the beginning of that time, most of the radiopharmaceuticals used were relatively simple inorganic chemicals and the isotope store of a nuclear medicine department would have contained perhaps a dozen different radionuclides, all decaying away more or less wastefully! By the very nature of human biochemistry, there are relatively few of the higher atomic weight elements which play an important part in human metabolism, though it is these which have been the more readily available from reactor sources. Nevertheless a number of useful chance findings were made and a considerable number of more or less obscure elements have been used in clinical practice. Such a trend has of course been relatively expensive in cost and effort in producing radioisotopes and relatively unrewarding in producing results of value to doctors. The last ten years have seen a very considerable swing in emphasis to the present state where a nuclear medicine department may carry a stock of only four or five radioisotopes, the great bulk of the work being done with just one or two. The introduction of generator produced radionuclides and in particular the production of technetium-99m — a most convenient radionuclide from its physical characteristics — has meant that there has been a great attraction in using just one or two radionuclides and varying the chemical and physical form as necessary to obtain the required distribution in the body. Virtually every major hospital in the country with radionuclide facilities now has a constant daily supply of this radioisotope — ^{99m}Tc — with its convenient six-hour physical half life, radiation suited to modern detecting instruments such as the gamma camera and the freedom to give relatively large quantities and obtain good statistically reliable data without a worrying radiation dose. At first the chemistry of technetium seemed a most unpromising one and indeed, as pertechnetate, TcO_4^-, the big brother of permanganate, MnO_4^-, from the Periodic Table, it has a limited application in human biochemical studies. However, in its reduced forms it can be attached to a great many molecules of pharmacological interest, and it is this widespread use which accounts for its considerable representation in the following 'Table of adverse reactions' (Table 16.1).

Like so many of the radionuclides used in medicine, ^{99m}Tc is present in only infinitesimal quantities in its radiopharmaceuticals — the relevant unit would be picograms — and cannot contribute chemically to any observable reaction *in vivo*.

The Medicines Act of 1968 makes no specific mention of radiopharmaceuticals but equally it is clear that they are to be regarded as medicinal products as defined in the Act since they are administered to human beings for the purpose of 'diagnosing disease or ascertaining the existence, degree or extent of a physiological condition'. The great majority of radiopharmaceuticals are produced in hospitals and labelled with short-lived radionuclides,

Table 16.1. Reported adverse reactions to radiopharmaceuticals.

		USA		UK	
		1972 (a)	1976 (b)	1974 (c)	1978 (d)
Particulates.	MAA	11	1	8	2
	Microspheres	–	20	–	3
	Iron hydroxide	16	–	45	–
Colloids	various	51	10	23	8
Albumin		19	1	–	–
T.3 and T.4 in 50% P.G.		–	–.	–	8
Rose Bengal–^{131}I		–	2	–	1
Iodo Me-norCholesterol		–	2	–	1
[^{203}Hg] Chlormerodrin		3	–	–	–
^{99m}Tc DMSA		–	2	–	1
o-[^{131}I] Iodohippurate		14	1	–	1
^{99m}Tc Glucoheptonate		–	1	–	–
^{99m}Tc DTPA		1	1	1	–
^{113m}In DTPA		1	2	1	–
Sodium [^{131}I] iodide		14	2	–	–
Sodium [^{99m}Tc] pertechnetate		4	1	–	4
[^{67}Ga] Gallium citrate		–	1	–	–
[^{85}Sr] Strontium nitrate		3	–	–	–
Chromic [^{32}P] phosphate		1	–	–	–
^{99m}Tc pyrophosphate		–	7	–	–
^{99m}Tc diphosphonate		–	2	–	–

Sources: (a) Atkins *et al.* (1972); (b) Ford *et al.* (1978); (c) Williams, E.S. (1974); (d) Keeling, D.H., unpublished.

involve quite large quantities of radioactivity, but very small individual batches. This has meant there are special handling problems and that much of the testing of any manufacturing procedure must be done in retrospect. In practice, dummy runs are done extensively to sort out the problems during the initial production of a new pharmaceutical and the procedure then adhered to closely in all future runs. Random tests are taken for retrospective quality-control checks where there are no suitable tests of immediate applicability. There are still several radiopharmaceuticals of acknowledged clinical value whose exact chemical formula is uncertain. They are known to be mixtures of several radiolabelled molecules, and opinions differ as to which confers the desirable properties.

The developments in modern radiopharmaceuticals have meant that preparations in use today are not only basically of a more complex organic or even biological nature, but that these preparations may have to contain additional bacteriostats, radiolysis inhibitors, physiological blocking agents and various classes of stabilizer. Virtually all these materials have been implicated at one time or another as causes of adverse reactions.

One other basic difference between virtually all radiopharmaceuticals and the other varieties of drug causing adverse reactions which have been considered in this volume is the difference in pattern of dosage and quantities used. Most drugs exhibiting adverse reactions do so after a considerable quantity has been taken in repeated daily doses. By their very nature, most radiopharmaceuticals are given only once (or a relatively few times) to any one patient, and the physical amount of materials being given is usually extremely small. Chronic toxicity is therefore never a problem. These factors have a considerable bearing on the pattern of adverse reactions which we find in nuclear medicine.

It is only in the last five or six years that any attempt has been made to collate data on adverse reactions and still much of the data is in the form of case reports in literature. In the early 1970s attempts were made to collect such data both in the USA and in the UK through the professional societies involved in nuclear medicine. The first reports appeared in 1972 (Atkins *et al.*) and 1974 (Williams) but there has been a discernable alteration in the varieties of adverse reaction seen in the last decade. The earlier radiopharmaceuticals were essentially relatively simple radiochemicals, often produced in the hospital or university scientific department with relatively little pharmacy skill or expertise. Indeed, in those days there were very few hospital pharmacists prepared to get involved in this work. Inevitably many were untrained for work with radioactivity and most of the starting materials for these radiochemicals were not to be found in any Pharmacopoeia. Today there can be very few departments of nuclear medicine where pharmacy help is not readily available both in the direction and advisory aspects of radiopharmaceutical preparation and frequently in their day-to-day working.

It is convenient to consider the general classification of radiopharmaceuticals under the separate headings of 'radio' and 'pharmaceutical'. This is obviously something of an artificial division, but it helps. By 'radio' is meant the unstable radionuclide that labels the material. This will define the physical half-life and the nature and energy of its radiations, and has a very considerable bearing upon the subsequent radiation dose administered to the tissues. It also affects the choice of suitable instrumentation for its detection and measurement. The term 'pharmaceutical' covers the physical and chemical nature of the molecule involved. This determines the mode and pathway of its metabolism in the body and its excretion etc., which, together with the physical half-life of the nuclide, determine the actual site and quantity of radiation delivered.

Radiopharmaceuticals in current use cover such diverse physical forms as gases, aerosols, true solutions, macromolecular and colloidal solutions, particulates and, on occasions, powdered forms.

In much the same way, it is helpful to consider the types of adverse reactions under the separate headings of 'radio' and 'pharmaceutical'. Under the first we must strictly speaking include over-irradiation as an adverse reaction, even though nothing tangible may occur at the time, and even in the long term, nothing more than the statistical risks associated with radiation may have arisen. Overdosage is usually due to error by the operator, very probably abetted by a faulty calibration meter. The older but still widely used ionization chambers with picoammeter readout are usually reliable; however, the subsequent calculation, comparing a standard source of radioactivity with the dose to be assayed, involves factors of the order of 10^{-11} and is an invitation for decimal point trouble. Checking by a second person is an obvious safeguard but it is remarkably easy to read quickly through someone else's calculation and miss a decimal point error. The result can be, and indeed has been, an over-dosage by a factor of 10. If the original dose intended was of a therapeutic quantity of radionuclide, then there is certainly not room for an error of this order of magnitude. Many modern radiopharmacy laboratories make the second check by a calibration meter that does its own calculation and gives a direct numerical result. All these electronic 'black boxes' go wrong from time to time, but they can be easily checked each day against a known standard and when they do go wrong, the answer is usually ridiculous and not a decimal point slip. Thus as a second check on a calculation, they are extremely valuable.

A further problem from over-irradiation can arise with radionuclidic impurities. These can occur in several ways. A common cyclotron production method for iodine-123, a valuable short-lived isotope of iodine, inevitably gives a small yield of the longer-lived and undesirable iodine-124. When first produced, the irradiation due to the small quantity of contaminating ^{124}I in a dose of ^{123}I will be acceptable. With the decay of the short-lived ^{123}I, the same dose of ^{123}I withdrawn two or three days later will likely contain an unacceptable quantity of ^{124}I. Here it is necessary to enforce a strict shelf-life of the material based on calculation of relative decay rates of the two radionuclides.

A common hazard in this context is present whenever a radionuclide generator is eluted to obtain the useful daughter isotope for clinical use. By far the commonest example today is the molybdenum-99 — technetium-99m generator system. In this and in most other similar generators, the longer-lived parent nuclide is absorbed on an ion-exchange chromatography column and the daughter isotope, which 'grows in' by decay of the parent isotope, is eluted when required. The elution agent for a generator is chosen as a convenient solvent which will give a safe separation of the nuclides and in particular not elute the parent nuclide. Errors can and have arisen when the wrong solution is used to elute the column. A useful safeguard here is to see that the reagents for use with a particular generator are physically segregated with it and further precautions such as colour-coding help. Generators can be checked for the break-through of the parent nuclide but this is usually done when they are first delivered. Subsequent daily elutions cannot always be so fully checked.

There are, of course, the usual opportunities in nuclear medicine, as in medicine generally, to misread or even not read the label on the container. There is perhaps one small extenuating circumstance in nuclear medicine in that the final glass container is an unshielded radiation source and will usually be kept in its outer lead travelling container, which is also labelled. Instances have occurred in which the wrong product was supplied by a commercial producer and the error not immediately noticed. In one instance, mercury-203 chlormerodrin was supplied, whereas the outer lead container was labelled mercury-197 chlormerodrin — the required radio-pharmaceutical. Although the inner label was glanced at, the minor difference in mass number — the only difference in the two labels — was not immediately noticed.

There is a further variety of untoward reaction of the over-irradiation type due to maldistribution of the radiopharmaceutical in the body. Examples have been the long delay in clearance of colloidal gold from intra-dermal injection sites which can occur in the investigation of some types of lymphoedema. This has, on a few occasions, resulted in a small area of radiation burn to the overlying skin. Another example was found with certain preparations of ytterbium-169 diethylene triamine pentaacetate (DTPA) chelate used for studying the flow of the cerebro-spinal fluid. Whereas the original work had been done on low specific activity ytterbium-169, and the molar ratio of 1:10 ytterbium: DTPA found to be safe, manufacture by a second supplier with high specific activity ytterbium — although the molar ratio of DTPA excess was maintained — resulted, once in the cerebro-spinal fluid, in competition from calcium with the gradual release of ytterbium in ionic form, which rapidly becomes fixed to the meninges. Its relatively long physical half-life, which had seemed a useful attribute in giving it a good shelf-life, then led to unnecessary irradiation of the brain and meninges, and highlighted the potential problem with any radiopharmaceutical in which biological pathways are relied on to keep the radiation dose within intended limits.

These examples highlight the necessity of having dose limits related to the worst probable tissue distribution and the resultant level of local irradiation. However, to put these in perspective, most diagnostic nuclear medicine tests involve a tissue radiation dose less than a comparable X-ray diagnostic study.

The varieties of adverse reaction which have been attributed to the 'pharmaceutical' part of the molecule are as diverse as the radiopharmaceuticals themselves. Nevertheless it seems more helpful to consider these under the general classifications of the radiopharmaceuticals.

One finds by looking at the collected experience on both sides of the Atlantic that the adverse reactions commonly attributed to three main groups of radiopharmaceuticals make up the bulk of the reports, though there is a generous assortment of 'others'. These main groups are the radiocolloids used in the investigation of the reticulo-endothelial system (and more particularly liver scanning), the particulate preparations which deliberately micro-embolize the capillary system to which they are fed, and the third group includes the particular problems associated with intra-thecal preparations. Taking them in reverse order, problems with intra-thecal radiopharmaceuticals have highlighted deficiencies in standard pharmacopoeial testing. In the mid 1960s, radio-iodinated human serum albumin was first introduced as a tracer for CSF flow and was very useful in the investigation of certain forms of hydrocephalus and in detecting CSF leaks. From the earliest days, sporadic cases of aseptic meningitis were reported (Detmer & Blacker, 1965; Nicol, 1967; Oldham & Staab, 1970) following its use, for which no adequate explanation could be found.

Preparations passed the standard pharmacopoeial rabbit test for pyrogens and of course were sterile. It was postulated that the reaction might have been to the overall quantity of albumin used, frequently in excess of 20 mg, or to chemical irritants acting directly on the brain. Because of dosage limitation due to ^{131}I irradiation, the radio-iodinated albumin images were frequently poor, and fresh radiopharmaceuticals were looked for. Subsequently, chelates of indium-111 and ytterbium-169 with DTPA were widely used. However, this did not lead to any fall in the incidence of aseptic meningitis (Alderson & Siegel, 1973) and it was not until the introduction of the Limulus test for pyrogens that the answer became clear. A classic investigation by Cooper & Harbert (1973, 1975) in the USA showed that the presence of bacterial endotoxin was the cause of these reactions. The standard USP pyrogen test in three rabbits had been quite normal. Cooper and Harbert investigated no less than 39 reactions associated with cisterno-graphic investigations and found that 20 of these cases related to ten commercial samples of radiopharmaceutical. In these ten they found a strongly positive Limulus test and their findings provided the clinical evidence for the observation made in animals, namely that endotoxin is at least 1000 times more toxic intra-thecally than intravenously. At the same time, it was noted that the source of endotoxin in the radio-iodinated albumin preparations was not the albumin itself, but came from an anion exchange resin used to remove unbound iodine. These columns can be extremely difficult to wash free of the large quantities of pyrogen present in them. In the DTPA preparations, it was again not the primary material itself but a phosphate buffer which contained the endotoxin. Their findings, corroborated by a number of workers since, underline the necessity for the strictest quality control of the starting materials for the production of intra-thecal radiopharmaceuticals and highlight a deficiency of the present Pharmacopoeia.

A number of important reactions with particulate radiopharmaceuticals have been reported and can be broadly classified under three headings. These materials are used by intravenous injection, for lung perfusion scanning (looking for pulmonary emboli, etc.) and by intra-arterial injection, for measurement of blood flow (all the particles will be removed in the first capillary bed they reach).

The use in lung perfusion scanning is extremely widespread and many thousands of such tests are performed each year in the UK. Three main types of adverse reaction have been reported with these. The first is a fairly obvious haemodynamic problem and is essentially a relative overdosage. Too many particles or particles of the wrong size can block a dangerous proportion of the pulmonary capillary bed — particularly in pathological states such as severe pulmonary hypertension when this may be grossly reduced and result in immediate cardiac problems (Dworkin, Smith & Bull, 1966; Vincent, Goldberg & Desilets, 1968; Williams, J. O., 1974). Measurements by Harding *et al.* (1973) have shed further light on the number and diameter of vessels in the pulmonary circulation. Their calculations show that from 1 mg of albumin, any of a range of sizes of albumin spheres from over 500 μm diameter down to 15 μm diameter would block a maximum of

0.31% of the normal pulmonary circulation. This small fraction is clearly not going to cause clinical trouble, but in pathological states the simple mechanical blockage of a proportion of the pulmonary circulation may be an important factor.

The second and somewhat surprising variety of reaction which has been reported in the last two to three years is of an anaphylactoid type of reaction to human albumin preparations (Ford *et al.*, 1978; Littenberg, 1975), though of course these are heat-denatured. These reactions have mostly occurred in patients with a past history of asthma; following injection there was a fairly quick skin flush followed by pallor, dyspnoea, hypotension, tightness in the chest and cyanosis which recovered without specific treatment. Other cases have received intravenous steroids and antihistamines. At least three deaths have been reported following the use of intravenous albumin macro-aggregates or microspheres for pulmonary perfusion scanning. In these the patient apparently dies of acute heart failure due to pulmonary hypertension. Another worrying variety of adverse reaction has been associated with iron hydroxide particles. These are a simple inorganic preparation and were first introduced as a co-precipitate with indium-113m for lung scanning. Two varieties of adverse reactions were reported. The commoner was the onset, within one to two minutes of intravenous injection of only 100-200 μg iron (ferric or occasionally ferrous) hydroxide of a flush reaction from the mid chest upwards. This was usually associated with a slight tachycardia, occasionally with tightness in the chest and sometimes a strange sensation passing down all the limbs, apprehension, nausea and even vomiting. Of particular interest here is that some departments using apparently identical methods saw a very low incidence of these reactions and others saw a relatively high percentage — as much as 10%. The reaction could be reproduced absolutely in standard form in this author and was, within limits, dose dependent. Between 50 and 100 μg of ferric hydroxide gave rise to a cutaneous 'blush' from the mid chest up and including the conjunctivae, starting 90 seconds after intravenous injection. At this dose level there were relatively few generalized signs and no ECG changes. The reaction passed off in 4-5 minutes. Attempts to show which drugs could inhibit this reaction showed no result whatsoever with large doses of various antihistamines, and the only drug which inhibited the reaction in the author was methysergide and for obvious reasons it was not to be used in patients as a routine preventative and the use of the iron hydroxide agent was subsequently dropped.

There had been a very small number of more serious reactions with the ferric hydroxide particles. One assumed from the previous observations that these reactions were due to or aggravated by serotonin release, either directly or indirectly instigated by the iron particles lodging in pulmonary capillaries. Such a release would be likely to cause constriction of other pulmonary vessels and a further rise in pulmonary artery pressure, in a patient in whom this was already a severe problem. This reaction probably accounts for the deaths reported, and usually occurs about 15-20 minutes after the injection. In a case observed in the author's department, a young woman with 'idiopathic' pulmonary hypertension, developed the signs and symptoms of acute pulmonary oedema during the scan which was abandoned and although emergency treatment was instigated, she finally suffered a cardiac arrest which could not be reversed. Five similar fatal cases occurred in this country and several were reported in the USA.

Problems have arisen, presumably on a simple haemodynamic basis, following the intra-arterial use of macroaggregates and microspheres of albumin in studies of blood flow measurement. The coronary artery injection of such material has resulted in immediate cardiac arrest which has proved irreversible. The total number of particles injected is obviously crucial.

Colloids have been implicated in a considerable number of reactions (Williams, E.S., 1974; Ford *et al.*, 1978). There are several varieties in clinical use, but by far the commonest are sulphur colloids with a ^{99m}Tc tracer adsorbed. Also popular is a colloid of antimony sulphide which can be labelled with ^{99m}Tc. This is a stable preparation and can be made in large batches before use; full quality control can, therefore, be exercised on each batch; even so occasional reactions still occur. Though not common, they are a drawback for a very frequently used form of radiopharmaceutical.

The more frequent type of adverse reaction with these colloids is a form of vasomotor upset, frequently with an initial flush followed by pallor, hypotension, tachycardia and occasionally with a burning sensation in the skin (not related to the injection site). Bronchospasm and dyspnoea have been described, and in at least one seriously ill patient, death occurred shortly afterwards. Similar reactions have been reported with ^{99m}Tc-labelled phytate 'colloids'. Although several of the reactions to colloids have occurred following a second or subsequent injection, the majority occur after the first use in a patient, and the underlying cause is uncertain.

Following the adverse affects related to these three main groups of radiopharmaceuticals, there are a significant number of reports relating to a heterogeneous group of radiopharmaceuticals. Perhaps the commonest, and this is likely to be just a reflection of the frequency of its use, is to pertechnetate ion in aqueous solution. As this is present in only picogram quantities, it seems inconceivable that it is the causative agent, and indeed it is unusual to have any clear cause-and-effect relationship. Oxidants and impurities in the generator eluant are present in much larger quantities that the technetium, and alumina from the column is occasionally detected (though its main effect seems to be to precipitate any colloids being made).

Most of the reactions attributed to simple pertechnetate solution have been of a more or less prompt vasomotor nature, and could well be psychogenic, but cases with urticaria appearing 24 or 48 hours later are known. Not all have a definite history of atopy, but in some, uncertainty arises about causation, such as prior anti-tetanus inoculation. In a personal case, oral potassium perchlorate (200 mg) had been given before the pertechnetate, and facial oedema and urticaria was noted at 48 hours, which responded to antihistamine treatment. A repeat pertechnetate scan on the same patient without perchlorate but with 15 mg chlorpheniramine maleate was uneventful.

In the past there have been several cases where Lugol's iodine was given to block thyroidal uptake of radio-iodine and has been the probable cause of untoward reaction in iodine sensitive patients (Bliek & Bachynski, 1971).

Colloid-stabilizing agents, such as gelatin, caused some pyrogen reaction earlier, but awareness of the problem and the need for pharmaceutical quality agents, and the hazards of storage, seem to have solved this difficulty. A colleague has recently reported eight cases of reactions associated with two batches of thyroxine and triiodothyronine in aqueous propylene glycol. Five out of seven patients receiving physiological doses of the thyroid hormones in 50% aqueous propylene glycol noted local discomfort in the arm on intravenous injection and subsequent malaise, headache, etc. for a day. Subsequently, three of seven patients receiving these hormones in 5% aqueous propylene glycol complained of 'extreme tightness of the skin' following intravenous injection. A careful investigation failed to indicate the cause — possibly contaminants in the hormone preparations or in the aqueous propylene glycol.

There remain a number of isolated cases where a report has been made though the reactions are almost invariably like those with colloids — of an immediate vasomotor nature. o-[^{131}I]Iodohippurate, ^{99m}Tc DMSA (dimercaptosuccinic acid) and several inorganic radiopharmaceuticals such as sodium [^{131}I]iodide and [^{67}Ga]gallium citrate have also been mentioned (Ford *et al.*, 1978). No coherent pattern emerges.

However, in an effort to coordinate the reporting of these untoward effects associated with radiopharmaceuticals, and to try to identify any patterns when individual experience is almost bound to be small, several professional bodies in the UK are now co-operating in a scheme backed by the D.H.S.S. Committee on Safety of Medicine. The British Institute of Radiology supplies the central secretariat, and the British Nuclear Medicine Society, the Hospital Physicists' Association, and the Hospital Pharmacists Group of the Pharmaceutical Society of Great Britain have all arranged to circularize their members with a short 'reporting questionnaire'. The information obtained is also banked in the data files of the main Committee on Safety of Medicine's Reporting Scheme computer as a valuable cross check in case relevant information should come in, based on (non-radioactive) medicinal products. May I, as the current Medical Assessor for this radiopharmaceutical reporting scheme, take this opportunity of asking for your help and support.

References

Alderson, P.O. and Siegel, B.A. (1973). *J. nucl. Med.*, 14, 609.
Atkins, H.L., Hauser, W., Richards, P. and Klopper, J. (1972). *J. nucl. Med.*, 13, 232.
Blieck, A.J. and Bachynski, J.E. (1971). *J. nucl. Med.*, 12, 90.
Cooper, J.F. and Harbert, J.C. (1973). Abstract in *J. nucl. Med.*, 14, 387.
Cooper, J.F. and Harbert, J.C. (1975). *J. nucl. Med.*, 16, 809.
Dworkin, H.J., Smith, J.R. and Bull, F.E. (1966). *Am. J. Roentgen.*, 98, 427.
Detmer, D.E. and Blacker, H.M. (1965). *Neurology*, 15, 642.
Ford, L., Shroff, A., Bensen, W., Atkins, H. and Rhodes, B.A. (1978). *J. nucl. Med.*, 19, 116.
Harding, L.K., Horsfield, K., Singhal, S.S. and Cumming, G. (1973). *J. nucl. Med.*, 14, 579.

Littenberg, R.L. (1975). *J. nucl. Med.*, 16, 236.
Nicol, C.F. (1967). *Neurology*, 17, 199.
Oldham, R.K. and Staab, E.V. (1970). *Radiology*, 97, 317.
Vincent, W.R., Goldberg, S.J. and Desilets, D. (1968). *Radiology*, 91, 1181.
Williams, E.S. (1974). *Br. J. Radiol.*, 47, 54.
Williams, J.O. (1974). *Br. J. Radiol.*, 47, 61.

Author index

Subject index